LECTURES ON TUNG'S ACUPUNCTURE Therapeutic System

By Dr. Wei-Chieh Young

American Chinese Medical Culture Center

Lectures on Tung's Acupuncture: Therapeutic System

By Young, Wei Chieh
Translated by Tao, Jin Wen
Illustrations by Alice Young
Published by American Chinese Medical Culture Center

LOC Cataloging-in-Publication Data
ISBN: 978-0-9779026-5-1
First Edition: July 2008
Second Print: January 2010
Third Print: February 2012
Fourth Print: November 2013
Fifth Print: April 2017

Printed in Taiwan

For More Information Contact:

Chinese Medical Center
19161 Colima Road,
Rowland Heights, CA 91748 U.S.A.
Telephone: 626-581-1755
Fax: 626-581-1688
Website: www.drweichiehyoung.com
e-mail: cmcyoung18@yahoo.com

Contents

Preface to the Second Edition

Ever since the *Lectures on Tung's Acupuncture – Therapeutic System* was firstly published in July 2008; it has been popular among the readers around the world. The first edition was quickly sold out. We received many feedback letters from the readers. Some were to give praises; and some were to offer suggestions. The praises encouraged us to work harder and inspired us to progress further. The suggestions helped us discover the errors and make corrections. We would like to thank particularly the Turkish doctor Dr. Erk Ozkaya for making some finer revisions of medical terms often lost in translation from Chinese to English. We do our best to revise and correct the errors and omissions. Our endeavors were to make sure the readers harvest the most from reading the book.

At the moment of the second edition publication, we would like to take this opportunity to thank our readers for their love and support. We also hope our readers continue to send us their comments and suggestions.

Wei Chieh Young

January 2010

Directions to the English Edition

1. The translation of this book is based upon volume II (Lectures on Tung's Acupuncture: Therapeutics System) of Collected Works of Young, Wei Chieh (*Yang Weijie Quan Ji*). The main contents are the lectures of Dr. Young, Wei Chieh for Qinxi University in Seoul, Korea in 2003 and completed by the lectures in Korean Shiming University. There are Chinese and Korean editions before this publication.

2. The book takes therapeutics of Tung's acupuncture as the main content. In addition to the selection of Tung's acupuncture points for treatment of each disease introduced, the reason for selection of the points and mechanism are also presented. Besides, based upon Dr. Young's personal experience, the effective points of the fourteen meridians are also introduced as well together with the ancient and contemporary needling techniques. Comparison of Tung's acupuncture points and the points of the fourteen meridians is clear and practical, and the readers will know how to select either of the two or both in application. Therefore the book is not only the therapeutics of Tung's acupuncture points but also the therapeutics of the points of the fourteen meridians.

3. During the lectures, the audience often put forward various kinds of questions, some of which are not very much related with the focus of the lectures. Answers were thrust between chapters in the form of "Question" and "Answer" to make it different from the main text. Requested by the audience, Dr. Young also introduced certain herbal formulas and herbs for some diseases. Though it is not very complete, it is very practical and can be taken as reference in the clinic.

4. "The extraordinary connections of the *zangfu* organs," "Acupuncture based upon correspondence between different parts of the body," "Acupuncture based upon *Taiji* holographic correspondence," and "Method of Selecting Five-*shu* Points of the Same Five-element Category" are important theoretical basis of Tung's acupuncture. In addition to selection of points and explanation with examples, more detailed explanation and systemic application are give after introduction to treatment of diseases of one category (one chapter) so that the readers may learn the method of drawing inferences about other cases from one instance and applying Tung's acupuncture points and the points of the fourteen meridians in a creative way.

5. Appendix 1 "Application of Bloodletting Therapy" and Appendix 2 "A Collection of Application of Tung's Extraordinary Points" are originally the contents of the book Tung's Acupuncture. They also attached to the Chinese edition. They may serve as the reference to the

Therapeutics and are therefore collected in this book with some revision.

6. Since many books such as Strategy of Acupuncture (*Zhen Jiu Jing Wei*), Meridians and Points of Acupuncture (*Zhen Jiu Jing Xue Xue*), Application of Five-*shu* Points in Acupuncture (*Zhen Jiu Wu Shu Xue Ying Yong*) and Annotation of Yellow Emperor's Inner Classic (*Huang Di Nei Jing Yi Jie*) are very popular and taken as textbooks in Korea and Taiwan, the biggest publishing house of Chinese medicine in Korea Daxing Press of Medicine intends to publish all these works as Collected Works of Young, Wei Chieh with revision. Being appreciated to his teacher Master Tung, Dr. Young takes the most popular lectures on Tung's Acupuncture in Korea as Volume 1 and Volume 2, "Points of Tung's Acupuncture" and "Therapeutics of Tung's Acupuncture," of the Collected Works.

7. The Korean edition of the book was translated and compiled by the outstanding doctor Dr. Chu, Xianyu in Korea, and Dr. Wenji Piao, Dr. Yumin Zhou, and Mandy Young made great effort in the translation of the Chinese edition. I would like to take this opportunity to thank them all.

I want to express my appreciation to those who helped with the preparation of this edition. First, I want to thank the professor of Nanjing University of TCM, Tao Jin Wen, who translated the text. I want to also thank the President of the Academy of Oriental Medicine at Austin, William Morris, and Dr. Michael Chung, Dr. Anita Marshall, Dr. Chiung Hui Tseng and Dr. Christine Chang, who gave some comments and revision. Thanks for all of them.

Mandy M. Young

July 2008

Preface to the Chinese Edition

Tung's Points in the World and Taiwan

It is great that the book "Lectures on Tung's Acupuncture: Therapeutics System" is published. This book mainly covers the lectures given by Dr. Young Wei Chieh in Qinxi University and Shiming University in Korea during the period from 2000 to 2003 that were recorded, sorted out and published by Korean Daxing Press of Medicine. The original text was published in Korean, and the Chinese edition has given it revision and supplementation, making it more complete and practical.

Since Tung's acupuncture spread to Korea by Young Wei Chieh, the offspring of Tung's acupuncture, it has been popular in the country for 20 years and well-known by everyone in the medical field. When Dr. Young gave lectures in Korea during the period from 2000 to 2003, almost all the audience brought the book Therapeutics of Tung's Acupuncture to the lectures. In many bookstores in Korea, there are a lot of books with focus on study of Tung's acupuncture or clinical case studies. In recent years, there has established National Research Association of Tung's Acupuncture. From this, it can be seen that the standard of the research of and importance attached to Tung's acupuncture is very high.

Tung's acupuncture has been greatly developed in the United States of America in the last 20 years. Successively, Dr. Young has given lectures on Tung's acupuncture for doctoral programs in Samra University of Chinese Medicine in Los Angeles and San Francisco University of Chinese Medicine in 1984, and for American Acupuncture Association for 6 months in 1987. After that, some of the students such as Mariam Lee, Susan Johnson and Esther Su have been teaching Tung's acupuncture in many places in the United States and Europe. In recent years, there is always a special report on Tung's acupuncture in every national academic conference of acupuncture in America and hundreds of participants listened to the lectures every time. In 2003, the American Acupuncture Licensure listed Tung's acupuncture as one of the subjects in continuous education of acupuncture, showing that Tung's acupuncture has been highly emphasized and greatly developed in the United States of America.

Tung's acupuncture has been rapidly developed in the mainland of China in recent years. Five editions of the book Tung's Acupuncture (Dong Shi Qi Xue Zhen Jiu Xue) has been published in simplified Chinese. Successively, Dr. Young has given lectures for Shanghai Acupuncture Association, Shanghai University of Traditional Chinese Medicine, and in the cities such as Wuhan, Guangzhou and Nanjing. Beijing Higher School of Chinese Medicine has run many training courses on Tung's acupuncture for the students of the whole country, and it was the student of Dr. Yang, Zuo Changpo that gave the lectures for the courses. In 2003, China Association of Acupuncture listed Tung's acupuncture as a credit subject in continuous education for acupuncturists of the whole country. In recent years, the national periodicals of acupuncture also often published articles with focus on discussion of Tung's acupuncture. Tung's acupuncture has been affirmed and greatly developed in the mainland of China.

"Tung's Acupuncture" (English first edition) written by Dr. Young was published in September of 2005. Not long after, there came many orders of the book from different places of the United States and Europe, Turkey and Israel. It shows the Tung's acupuncture has become well-known and drawn more attractions in Europe, America and middle Asia. The admiration and respect to Tung's acupuncture in the world is the pride of Taiwan, where the therapy originated. However, the situation of Tung's acupuncture in Taiwan makes me feel sad. This is because, when Tung's acupuncture is getting more and more popular in the world, it is still being persecuted in Taiwan.

Early in 1972, Master Tung applied to the Ministry of Home Affairs of Taiwan for copyright of Tung's acupuncture and the answer was that "the therapy is absurd, departed from the classics and rebel against orthodoxy, and the application is therefore rejected." Because of this, Tung's acupuncture was plagiarized and the copyright was illegally taken by a doctor named Zhuang with nowhere to accuse. For this reason, Master Tung finally passed away depressively. When this lost learning was taken as a treasure abroad, the authority of Taiwan still throw it away like a pair of broken shoes. Only by 1990 when international book number system started to be practiced, the book Tung's Acupuncture was registered and obtained the copyright.

In early 1999 when the first conference of whole Taiwan on Tung's acupuncture was held, some people who considered themselves as authority of acupuncture made carding comments on newspaper and smeared Tung's acupuncture. I wander what kind of intention drove them to tread on such scholastic attainment. My understanding is they have neither learning nor skill. Having a general view to the professionals who have gained achievements in the studies on Tung's acupuncture in the world, they all have a solid foundation of the theory of the fourteen meridians. Dr. Young Wei Chieh is an example. The book Strategy of Acupuncture (Zhen Jiu Jing Wei) he wrote made a record in publications (20 editions) in Taiwan, and is honored as the best acupuncture book of 20th century in Korea. His treatise on the fourteen meridians "Meridians and Points of Acupuncture (Zhen Jiu Jing Xue Xue)" obtained academic prize issued by Ministry of Education in Taiwan. This book was also published 20 editions and considered as the best book of meridians and points as well in Korea. We may say that, without solid foundation of the fourteen meridians, it is impossible to understand the deep implications of Tung's acupuncture.

Tung's acupuncture therapy was not affirmed by Taiwan authorities of medicine yet even in 2005. The medical insurance doesn't cover the treatment with Tung's acupuncture therapy. How sad it is! It is even worse that the acupuncturists who use Tung's acupuncture are persecuted. There was a doctor who had such a patient unfortunately. The patient smoke cigarettes two packs or more per day and he is also addicted to alcohol, and finally affected by heart disease and died. Because the patient received acupuncture treatment few days ago with needling the points on the legs, the appraisal group of the ministry of health put the blame on the acupuncture treatment, though anatomical examination confirmed the death was natural. They not only denied the conclusion made by the anatomical examination but also made some false materials to prove their behavior. They dared not and avoided debate in the court. The administration of medicine is so rude and unreasonable in Taiwan and the public procurator is so low-leveled that they denied the conclusion of anatomical examination and determined the cause of death with conjecture. It is the biggest joke in the world! I would like to ask: what is the responsibility of medical legal expert?

The Taiwan authorities keep on saying that they want to join the World Heath Organization (WHO). Just imagine, if the technique of anatomy is so backward and determination of cause of death needs to be judged by conjecture, the medical appraise system is acting with utter disregard for human life, the level of administration of justice is so low, and the learning and practice of this acupuncture therapy which is affirmed and accepted by the whole world is so badly persecuted, is Taiwan qualified for joining WHO?

This book contains the experience of 40 years in application of the points of the fourteen meridians and the Tung's extraordinary points with profound theoretical explanation. The publication of the book in Korea aroused great echo. Hope the publication of the Chinese edition may change the point view of those who dispel Tung's acupuncture, and more people will get benefit from it, and in this way to carry forward Tung's acupuncture and let the learning of acupuncture in Taiwan shines in the world.

Editor

March, 2006

Preface to the Korean Edition

As stated by Dr. Young Wei Chieh, this is a guiding book that formally describes and explains the Tung's acupuncture and corrects the mistakes in misconception.

Luckily, we have been in touch with Tung's acupuncture quite early in the medical field in Korea. Because the points have excellent and rapid therapeutic effect, this therapy has been loved by many clinicians. The profound academic thought of Master Tung and Dr. Young Wei Chieh who has inherited, developed and completed this thought has been mostly left out and misunderstood, the importance has been therefore attached to its clinical application only and the basic theory has been neglected. Many Korean doctors that the translator has met misunderstood that "Tung's acupuncture only pays attention to the clinical practice without guiding theory," or "it is enough to remember the indication," or "the points are effective for pain syndrome only," or "there are too many points and the needling technique is difficult," etc.

With the appreciation to Dr. Young Wei Chieh for his instruction in the medical field of Korea, I have translated this book to show our thanks to him.

When I saw Dr. Young during his lecturing visit in Seoul, I was impressed by his great enthusiasm and opening mind. He is an example of great master of medicine in this century with his academic knowledge, clinical ability and moral character. His books include Strategy of Acupuncture and Moxibustion (Zhen Jiu Jing Wei) that was appraised to be one of the most complete and best acupuncture books of the 20th century and many other medical and philosophical books, which could be finished by twenty generations. Even with such talent, he started to follow Master Tung Jinchang and many other masters in his study when he was yang. He is a great master with both natural endowments and knowledge obtained through studies.

It is difficult to understand the realm of his great learning with imaginative power of an ordinary person. Excessive introduction will possibly decrease the great image of the master and hope the readers will get the proof from Collected Works of Young Wei Chieh which is to be published continuously in future.

Zhu Xianyu

August, 2003

Seoul

The Author

Young, Wei Chieh, born in Qingdao, Shandong Province and brought up in Taiwan, now lives in the United States. He is doctoral student of Beijing University, doctoral student of Beijing University of Traditional Chinese Medicine, doctoral student of Chinese and Western Medicine University, and visiting scholar of Zhongshan University. He has made extensive studies in literature, history and philosophy and has great attainments especially in medicine and study of *Yi Jing*. He passed the special examination for Chinese medicine doctors and in his pursuit of the knowledge of Chinese medicine has followed several famous doctors: as the only disciple of the prestigious acupuncturist Tung Jingchang (Master Tung), and the doctoral student of the Chinese medicine master Liu Duzhou and the renowned *Yi Jing* scholar Zhu Bokun. He took the initiative among doctors of Chinese medicine in Taiwan to give lectures in the mainland, as well as in Taiwan, Japan, Korea, Singapore and the United States. He wrote articles for three major newspapers in Taiwan. He was once director of the Union for Chinese Medicine Doctors in Taipei, executive director of China Medicine Research Institute in Taipei, academic leader of the Acupuncture Society in the United States, and chairman of the China Society of Chinese Medicine Academic Theories. He has thirty-five years of clinical experience in Chinese medicine, and has won the first *Huatuo* Prize for doctors of Chinese medicine and acupuncturists in Taiwan in 1990 and the Prize for Most Outstanding Figure at the World Chinese Medicine Conference in 2000. He has written over 35 books, including *Zhong Yi Xue Gai Lun* (An Outline of Chinese Medicine), *Zhen Jiu Jing Wei* (The Longitude and Latitude of Acupuncture and Moxibustion), *Zhen Jiu Jing Xue Xue* (Channels and Acupuncture Points), *Tung Shi Qi Xue Zhen Jiu Xue* (Tung's Extraordinary Points), *Zhen Jiu Wu Shu Xue Ying Yong* (Application of Five Shu Points in Acupuncture), *Zhong Yi Nei Ke Zheng Zhi* (Differential Diagnosis and Treatment of Internal Diseases with Chinese Medicine), *Tong Zheng Bai Jie* (One Hundred Solutions to Painful Syndromes), *Yang Sheng Shi Liao Bao Dian* (A Valuable Book on Health Preservation and Dietetic Therapy), etc., many of which have been translated into Korean, English and simplified Chinese. He has also published several hundred research papers and ranks among famous doctors and scholars in the world.

Introduction

Essentials of Tung's Acupuncture Therapy

Tung's acupuncture therapy has now been popularized in many countries and regions such ad Korea, United States, China and Taiwan, and the Tung's extraordinary acupuncture points are now listed together with the points of the fourteen channels and could even have better therapeutic results. A good command of Tung's extraordinary acupuncture points may even help deepen the understanding to the acupuncture points of the fourteen channels.

Then, what is the difference between Tung's extraordinary acupuncture points and the points of the fourteen channels? It is common knowledge in the profession that the points of the fourteen channels operate through the channels and collaterals:

1. Select the points along the diseased channel.
2. Select the points from the externally-internally related channel.
3. Select the points from the same-named channel of hand or foot.

In fact, in the use of the points of the fourteen channels, distal points are also often selected. As stated chapter "Ode to Elucidate Mysteries" (Biao You Fu) of the book "*Compendium of Acupuncture and Moxibustion*" (*Zhen Jiu Da Cheng*): "To dredge the channels with distal points, needle the points on the foot to treat diseases of the head." "Using contra lateral insertion, needle the right points for left diseases." It means when a disease is located on the left side, we needle the points on the right side, and when a disease is located on the head, we needle the points on the leg and foot, and vice versa. The contra lateral selection of acupuncture points functions to balance the two sides of the body, while selection of the lower points to treat the upper disease functions to dredge the channels. The method of selecting the right lower points for left and upper disease and vice versa is known as *Ju Ci* (opposite needling). This method is often used in selection of the points of the fourteen channels as well as Tung's acupuncture.

The core of the connotation of Tung's acupuncture is the extraordinary connection between the *Zang-Fu* organs. For instance, the Liver is connected with the Large Intestine. The Large Intestine channel runs on the hand and arm, and the Liver channel runs on the foot and leg. One pertains to *Yin* and the other pertains to *Yang*. One is a *Fu* organ and the other is a *Zang* organ. With such connection between the upper and lower, and the left and right, a balance is maintained. Therefore, the therapeutic effect of Tung's acupuncture is even better than just selecting the points of the diseased channel. Take *Quchi* (LI 11) as an example.

Since it is a point of the Large Intestine channel, it has very good therapeutic effect for diarrhea. However, it can also successfully treat vertigo, headache, Ménière's syndrome, and lower blood pressure. This is because the Large Intestine channel is connected with the Liver channel.

Here is another example, using *Quchi* (LI 11) for the treatment of tennis elbow. This point is not very close to the bone; however, if we needle this point closer to the bone, the therapeutic effect will be faster and better. This method is the based upon the second important theory of Tung's acupuncture – Local Treatment – which includes "needling the bone to treat bone diseases." This method suggests that bone diseases must be treated by needling close to the border of the bone or into the bone. Chapter 7 of the *Lingshu* (*Miraculous Pivot*) explains the basis for this acupuncture method. *Chize* (LU 5) is located by the side of *Quchi* (LI 11) and close to the big piece of tendon. If we needle this point with its location close to the tendon, it can treat periarthritis of the shoulder with special effect. This is because dysfunction of the shoulder in raising arm is a disease of tendon and "needling tendon can treat tendon diseases." In Tung's acupuncture, the therapeutic effect of "needling the bone for bone diseases," "needling the tendon for tendon diseases," "needling the vessel for vessel diseases," "needling the muscle for muscle diseases" and "needling the skin for skin diseases" gives remarkable results, and is a distinct feature of his work.

A detailed introduction to the extraordinary connections between *Zang-Fu* organs will be given later in the book. The theory derives from the *Neijing* (*Yellow Emperor's Inner Classic*). A deeper study will reveal originations of these theories in the *Yi-Jing* (*The Book of Changes*). Without the *Yi-Jing*, there would be no channels and collaterals theory. *Yi-Jing* is the origin of the theory of channels and collaterals. More studies on the theory of symmetry and balance in *Yi-Jing* will help you become a master of acupuncture.

While the extraordinary points are the focus of Tung's acupuncture, the theory of five elements is still used. Studies on the five-*Shu* points may assist in the practical use of Tung's extra points.

Holography is another important principle in Tung's system. Master Tung considered that each part of the body has correspondence to the Triple Energizers (*Sanjiao*), the upper, middle and lower. Take the forearm as an example. Its anterior part corresponds to the Upper Energizer (*Shangjiao*) and can therefore treat diseases of head and face; its middle part corresponds to the Middle Energizer (*Zhongjiao*)and can therefore treat diseases of the Middle Energizer, and points *Ganmen* (33.11) and *Changmen* (33.10) are located in this part; its posterior part corresponds to the lower energizer and point *Xinmen* (33.12) is located in this part and can be selected to treat coccygeal pain and knee joint pain. Point *Yunbai* (44.11) and *Libai* (44.12) are located on the posterior part of the upper arm and can be selected to treat women's diseases. The second metacarpal bone is also divided into three parts corresponding to the Triple Energizers. Point *Sanjian* (LI 3) corresponds to the Upper Energizer and is good at treating diseases of the head and face; *Hegu* (LI 4) corresponds to the Middle Energizer and is good at treating gastrointestinal diseases (the medical classics also state that it is useful for treating diseases of the head and face). *Linggu* (22.05) corresponds to the Lower Energizer and is good at treating diseases of the Lower Energizer such as lower back pain, sciatica and heel pain.

The head is also divided into three parts corresponding to the Triple Energizer. Point *Yintang* (Extra) and *Zhenjing* (1010.08) are in the Upper Energizer and can therefore calm the mind; *Renzhong* (DU 26) and *Majinshui* (1010.13) are located at the junction of the Middle and Lower energizers and are therefore good at treating lower back pain; Point *Chengjiang* (Ren 24) is located in the Lower Energizer and can be used to treat amenorrhea. (Point *Chengjiang* is the crossing point of hand and foot *Yangming* channels and the *Ren* channel. It is connected with perineum and can regulate *qi* and blood and thus the therapeutic effect.) On the thigh, three points corresponding to the Triple Energizer are often selected together to treat the Upper, Middle and Lower Energizers simultaneously such as the Upper, Middle and Lower point *Sima* (88.17, 18, 19), and *Tianhuang* (88.13), *Minghuang* (88.12) and *Qihuang* (88.14). Point *Shenguan* (77.18) on the leg corresponds to the Upper Energizer and is good at treating headache and periarthritis of the shoulder; Point *Renhuang* (77.21) is located in the Lower Energizer and *Dihuang* (77.19) in the Middle Energizer. The combination of the three points in application can treat diseases of all the three Energizers simultaneously. Point *Dadun* (Liv1) and *Yinbai* (Sp1) are all located at the distal end of the foot and they are therefore good at treating diseases of the lower part of the body. For instance, *Dadun* (Liv1) is good for hernia and impotence, and selection of both treats uterine bleeding (Hematuria).

Further Introduction to the Difference Between Tung's Extraordinary Points and the Points of the Fourteen Channels

More than once I have emphasized that it is important to understand the title of Master Tung's first book "Tung's Extra Acupuncture Points and the Points of the Regular Channels." The "regular channels" here refer to the fourteen channels. It implies the connections between Tung's Extra Acupuncture Points and the points of the 14 channels. Tung's extra points are different from other extraordinary points, which don't have their own system and mechanism.

Like the points of the 14 channels, Tung's extra points are also often selected from the diseased channel, the same-named channel or externally-internally related channel. The principle in selection follows that in application of the fourteen channels. It is most important to attach importance to the connections between *Zang-Fu* organs. To go deep in the study on such connections will give great help to the application of the theory of Treatise on Attack by Cold (*Shang Han Lun*) and Warm Diseases (*Wen Bing*), and treatment of difficult problems.

Chinese medicine takes the human body as integrity. The fundamental theory of acupuncture and that of *Shang Han Lun* (Attack by Cold) are the same. Only when you have a good command of internal medicine, can you raise your acupuncture treatment to a higher level.

Another characteristic of Tung's extra points is that they affect not the points needled but cover a large area and thus the therapeutic effect is faster and better than that of the points of the 14 channels. Take neck sprain as an example, which is clinically characterized by pain of the head, shoulder and upper back at the same time and difficulty of the neck in rotation. How do we treat neck sprain with selection of the points of the fourteen channels? It is stated in Chapter 26 (Miscellaneous Diseases) of book *Lingshu* (*Spiritual Pivot*): "In case of difficulty of the neck in flexion and extension, needle the UB channel of foot-*taiyang*; in case of difficulty of the neck in rotation, needle the SI channel of hand-*taiyang*." Dr. Zhang Jingyue of Ming dynasty considered the point of the hand-*taiyang* channel for neck sprain should be *Houxi* (SI 3) and that of the foot-*taiyang* channel should be *Kunlun* (BL 60). Selection of *Houxi* (SI 3) is correct, while *Kunlun* (BL60) is incorrect and its therapeutic effect is poor. Why? It is stated in Chapter 68 of book *Nanjing* (*The Classic of Difficulties*): "*Shu*-stream points are indicated in heaviness of the body and pain of the joints." The *Shu*-stream point of the *Yin* channel pertains to earth and is related to the Spleen and its functions of: transformation and transportation, in this case, of water and damp. The *Shu*-stream point of the *Yang* channel pertains to wood and is related to the Liver; it maintains free flow of *qi* and dispels wind. Heaviness of the body and joint pain often result from wind and damp. The *Shu*-stream point of *Yang* channel pertains to wood and is more closely related to the tendons. Difficulty in rotation of the neck must be related to the tendons, and therefore point *Shugu* (BL65) should be needled which pertains to wood and is *Shu*-stream point, not *Kunlun* (BL60) which is a *Yuan*-source point and pertains to fire.

Neck sprain may also present discomfort at point *Jianjing* (GB21), in which *Shaoyang* channel is involved. Some doctors often select point *Xuanzhong* (GB39) to treat neck sprain but cannot cure the problem in one treatment. Neck sprain is a small problem and covers multiple channels. However, in Tung's acupuncture, with selection of *Chongzi* (22.01) and *Chongxian* (22.02), a single treatment may resolve the problem quickly. If point *Chengjiang* (Ren24) is added, the therapeutic result will be even better. In the most of the classical medical odes, the selection of *Chengjiang* (Ren24) for rigidity of the neck is mentioned. Selection of this point for neck sprain is actually based upon the theory of correspondence between the anterior and posterior. Use the anterior point *Chengjiang* to treat posterior neck rigidity. Master Tung also often selected the posterior point *Zongshu* (1010.07) which is between *Fengfu* (DU16) and *Yamen* (DU 15) to treat hoarse voice, nausea and vomiting and dysphagia in the front. It is one of the important needling techniques of Master Tung.

The method of selecting one point for multiple channels and areas is often seen in Tung's acupuncture. Take sciatica which is commonly seen as another example. Generally *Huantiao* (GB30), *Chengfu* (BL36), *Zhibian* (BL54) and *Fengshi* (GB31) are selected with some additional points along the affected channels such as *Weizhong* (BL40), *Chengshan* (BL57) and *Kunlun* (BL60) when *Taiyang* channel is involved and *Yanglingquan* (GB34), *Xuanzhong* (GB39) and *Qiuxu* (GB40) when *Shaoyang* channel is involved. This method uses more points with less effect. If both *Taiyang* and *Shaoyang* channels are involved, points of both channels have to be selected, altogether more than ten needles are used and the results may not be satisfactory. In some cases of sciatica, there is pain radiating to the groin and medial aspect of the thigh where *Yin* channels are distributed. In this case even more needles are used. When multiple channels are affected in pathological conditions, selection of Tung's extra points is an improvement because it uses lesser needles and the results are typically better. For these forms of sciatica, select the two points, *Linggu* and *Dabai* on the opposite hand in order to obtain immediate analgesic effect for all channels of the *Taiyang*, *Shaoyang* and *Jueyin* channel. Additionally, these points are distal, and therefore safe and convenient. Though the method is simple, the connotation is deep. From these two case examples we can see the difference between Tung's extraordinary points and the points of the fourteen channels.

1. Question: What is the *Qian Yin* (Guiding) needling method? How is it applied?

Answer: It is a needling method that is used to attract the *qi* flowing to the desired area. It is based on the theory of "attracting effect." If we needle two points at the same time and then withdraw one needle, the *qi* of the other point will be attracted and flows towards and finally arrives at the area of the withdrawn needle. If you give a short stimulation to one of the two points, the *qi* will flow towards the retained needle. This is the basic mechanism of the attracting needling technique. If you want to go deeper into this method, you could read my book *Zhen Jiu Jing Wei* (The Strategy of Acupuncture). In the chapter "Tung's Extra Acupuncture points," there is an introduction to "Tung's Commonly Used Three Needling Methods."

Following are few case examples often seen in the clinic and they might help you better understand this method.

Take knee joint pain as an example. Needle the therapeutic point on the healthy side first. In this case, the needle is inserted into *Neiguan* (PC 6) or *Xinmen* (33.12) which are on the healthy side, then needle a distal point on the diseased side as the attracting point. If the pain is on the stomach channel, needle the *Shu*-stream point of the stomach channel which is *Xiangu* (ST43); if the pain is medial, along the path of the liver channel, needle *Taichong* (LR 3), the *shu*-stream point of the liver. In this way, *Neiguan* (PC 6) and *Taichong* (LR3) (or *Xiangu* ST 43) form an attracting group. The *qi* of *Neiguan* and that of *Taichong* attract each other and the flow of *qi* must pass through the painful area. This method is very effective in the treatment of knee joint pain. During treatment, if the patient can make some local exercise, then the therapeutic effects will be improved. If no exercise is made by the patient, treatment is still effective and better than local massage.

The *Shu*-stream points of various channels are typically used for the attracting points. As stated in Chapter 68 of the book *Nanjing* (A Classic of Difficulties): "*Shu*-stream points are indicated in heaviness of the body and pain of the joints." The *Neijing* (The Yellow Emperor's Inner Classic) also states, "When pain in a disease aggravates and alleviates alternatively, *Shu*-stream point should be needled." An example of this is the pain caused by cancer which tends to fluctuate. *Shu*-stream points in the *Yang* channels correlate with wood while on the *Yin* channels, it is earth. Wood dominates tendons and earth dominates muscles, therefore these points give good results in the treatment of muscles and tendons, heaviness of the body and joint pain in particular.

For shoulder joint pain, needling *Shenguan* (77.18) can be very effective. Once the needle is inserted into the point, the pain is typically alleviated immediately. In addition, the corresponding *Shu*-stream point should be selected for better result according to diseased channels. That is to select the *Shu*-stream point *Sanjian* (LI 3) for *Yangming* channel, *Zhongzhu* (SJ 3) for triple energizer channel and *Houxi* (SI 3) for *Taiyang* channel.

For sciatic pain, we often use *Linggu* (22.05), *Dabai* (22.04) on the healthy side to treat multiple channel involvement. To these, add the *Shu*-stream points as attracting points: *Sanjian* (LI 3), *Zhongzhu* (SJ 3) and *Houxi* (SI 3) on the diseased side. Even if the patient cannot exercise due to pain, the treatment is still effective because the attracted *qi* flows through the diseased area. Massage is not indicated for the attracting method since it may lead to local tissue fatigue and aggravate the pathology.

The *Qian Yin* (Guiding) technique has another advantage: the use of *Juci* (contra lateral needling). In such treatment, points are selected from both the upper and lower, and the left and right to dredge the upper and lower and balance the left and right. The *Qian Yin* (guiding) needling method is that I derived from Tung's *Dong Qi* (active *qi*) needling method. In general, the selection of one point from the diseased channel is sufficient.

Selecting a point from diseased channel can be very effective. The ancient physicians often selected *Shu*-stream point to treat pain which can serve as the main point or the attracting point. Typically, *Zusanli* (ST36), *Yanglingquan* (GB34), *Liangqiu* (ST34), or similar points are selected for knee joint pain. However, *Taichong* (LR3) is mostly selected for knee joint pain in ancient classics. Now we select this point plus *Neiguan* (PC3), one upper and one lower, to obtain both therapeutic and attracting effect, which is incomparable.

Another example is tennis elbow. Puncture point *Quchi* (LI11) and *Shousanli* (LI10) on the healthy side first as therapeutic points, and then needle *Linggu* (22.05) as the attracting point. Then ask the patient to exercise the disease elbow in order to obtain very good therapeutic effects. *Linggu* is taken as attracting point in this instance; it also serves as a therapeutic point.

Depth of insertion and retention of needles

Needling a point with correct location might not have the desired effect: this is because of incorrect insertion depth. There is an ancient saying in Chinese medicine, do not divulge the secret: for herbal medicine, it is the dosage and for acupuncture it is the depth of insertion. Therefore, great importance should be attached to the depth of insertion.

Point *Zusanli* (ST36) can treat many diseases of the body. However, there is not much information regarding therapeutics related to the depth of insertion. Generally speaking, needling this point with the depth of 0.5 to 1 *cun* (heaven) treats pain or other diseases of the leg; needling this point with the depth of about 1.5 *cun* (man) can treat diseases of the Spleen and Stomach and other middle energizer diseases, and needling this point with deep insertion (about 2 *cun*) with long needle retention is very effective for heart disease and asthmatic breathing. This point is also very effective for facial paralysis, however, the depth of insertion should be at least 2 *cun* with the needle directing obliquely upward.

In chapter "Channels and Points" of the book *Dong Shi Qi Xue* (*Tung's Extraordinary Acupuncture Points*), the description of the first point *dajian* (11.01) says: "Needling the point with the depth of 0.1 to 0.2 *cun* treats pathological changes of the heart; needling the point with the depth of 0.2 to 0.3 *cun* treats diseases of the small intestine, hernia and knee joint pain. The point is needled unilaterally on the healthy side." At the very beginning, Master Tung attached the importance to the depth of insertion and put forward the principle of contra lateral needling. In the description of the second point *Xiaojian* (11.02), he also says: "Needling the point with the depth of 0.1 to 0.2 *cun* when a half *cun* needle is used treats diseases of heart and lung; needling the point with the depth of 0.2 to 0.25 *cun* treats hernia and knee joint pain." In the description of point *Dizong* (44.09), he says: "Needling this point with insertion of 1 *cun* treats mild diseases and 2 *cun* treats severe diseases." In the description of *dishi* (33.14), he says: "Needling the point with insertion of 1 *cun* treats asthmatic breathing and 1.5 *cun* treats heart disease." The above mentioned are just few examples and the other Tung's extra points are also needled following the same principle.

Master Tung's theory of insertion depth has various theoretical bases and the most important is that "Shallow insertion is indicated in local or adjacent diseases and deep insertion is indicated in distal diseases." It means shallow needling treats near and new diseases and deep needling treats distal and old diseases. This principle can also be applied in acupuncture points of the fourteen channels. Take *Houxi* (SI 3) as an example. Needling this point with the depth to the heaven can treat the upper diseases such as facial spasm, trigeminal neuralgia and rigidity of the neck; needling this point with the depth to the man can treat lower back pain; and needling this point with the depth to the earth can treat sciatica and pain of the lower limbs. In general, the main cause of the therapeutic effect of either the acupuncture points of the fourteen channels or Tung's extra points is the depth of insertion.

Once the depth of insertion is well controlled, a single point may act as several points, saving the number of the points to be selected and the time of treatment. During last thirty years of practice, I have treated tens of patients daily in average and sometimes over one hundred patients per day. This would be impossible if I hadn't selected fewer points and used few needles for each treatment. On average, I use four needles per patient (not more than eight needles and minimally one needle). The points should be selected as minimally as possible and flexibly.

I attended the national acupuncture conference of America in Washington D.C., and gave a lecture on "The Twelve Commonly Used Points of the 14 Channels." The introduction to the twelve commonly used points of the fourteen channels is based upon the summary of the experience of ancient physicians and ancient classics as well as that of my own. The introduction to the twelve frequently used Tung's extra points is based upon the summary of master Tung's experience and that of my own obtained during my clinical practice over last thirty years. These points are essential in clinical practice. A good command of the twenty-four points may help treat pathological changes of the whole body. These points will be introduced in the related chapters.

Lastly, I would like to talk about needle retention. Master Tung typically retained the needles for 45 minutes. This is based upon the *Lingsu* (Spiritual Pivot) which states that one whole circulation of *qi* and blood in the body takes twenty-eight minutes and forty-eight seconds. To make it more convenient in calculation, we take it as 29 minutes, and 30 minutes even better. The Shanghai Journal of Traditional Chinese Medicine published one article in 1980 mentioning that the highest pain threshold was achieved with needle retention for between 40 and 50 minutes at point *Hegu* (LI 4). It can be seen that the author of that articles and Master Tung coincidentally had the same idea. I often retain needles in points for forty-five minutes. In case there are not enough beds or the patient is in a hurry, the needles should be retained for at least 30 minutes. The duration of needle retention should be prolonged for chronic conditions, severe diseases, cold syndromes and acute abdomens. I will retain needles for 60 minutes in cases of facial paralysis; 90 minutes could be even better. Thirty years ago, I saw a senior TCM doctor retaining needles in points for two hours in treatment of heart disease and chronic asthmatic breathing. In the industrial and commercial times, people are busy and it is difficult to retain needles for 60 minutes and such long needle retention is rarely seen.

Tung's system is remarkable. Following is the application of Tung's extraordinary point in treatment of various kinds of diseases.

Chapter One

Head, Face, Neck and Nape

1. Head

1) Headache

a. *Dabai* (22.04) is very effective. The combination of *dabai* and *zhongbai* (22.06) or *chasan* (A.04) may have a better result.
b. Needle *Cesanli* (77.22), *Cexiasanli* (77.23) and *Shenguan* (77.18). Retain the needles for 45 minutes. Mild cases may be cured in 2-3 treatments. A severe case may be cured within 4-5 treatments without recurrence. These points may have good results for chronic and stubborn headaches.
c. *Linggu* (22.05) may immediately alleviate headaches.
d. Blood-letting *Wuling* (DT.04) in order to immediately stop headache.
e. Blood-letting point *Taiyang* (Extra) has a special effect for chronic headaches. For mild attacks, give 1-2 treatments; for severe attacks give 3-4 treatments for cure.

I like to supplement points of the fourteen channels with Tung's major points. Generally speaking, *Dabai* (22.04) and *Sanchasan* (A.04) may immediately stop pain. In addition, *Sanchasan* (A.04) is one of the frequently used 10 important Tung's extraordinary points; it is also a very good point for the common cold. It is located on the course of Triple Energizer channel of hand-*shaoyang* and improves immunity. It is very close to *Yemen* (SJ2), which is the *Ying*-spring point of the Triple Energizer (*San Jiao*) channel. It is stated in the book *Neijing* (Yellow Emperor's Inner Classic): "*Ying*-spring and *Shu*-stream points are indicated in disorders of external channels." It is therefore a commonly used point for exogenous diseases. For headache due to common cold, this point plus *Dabai* (22.04) is sufficient. *Dabai* is located on the same level of *Sanjian* (LI3). Needling this point along the border of the bone may stop headache quickly. Further, *dabai* is located on the course of the large intestine channel and the large intestine is externally-internally related to the lung has therefore good therapeutic effect for diseases of the lung. Thus, it has remarkable effect in treatment of headache due to cold. According to the theory of holography, *Dabai* (22.04) is located on the area of head and face. It is close to *Sanjian* (LI3) which pertains to wood. *Dabai* (22.04) has the same property and it is therefore effective for liver (wood) and wind diseases.

According to the theory of connections between *zangfu* organs, the liver is connected with the large intestine. Therefore the points are also effective for headache due to liver disorders. In conclusion, *Sanchasan*

(A.04) plus *Dabai* (22.04) has special effect in treatment of headache due to cold, and is also effective for general headache. *Sanchasan* (A.04) combined with *Tushui* (22.11), they work together to treat sore throat very effectively. *Sanchasan* (A.04) is also a special point for relieving fatigue. Another point for fatigue is *Biyi* (1010.22). If somebody is sleepy or tired, the two points may be needled. The same treatment can be used for driving long-distances since it heightens the spirit.

I have another story about point *Sanchasan* (A.04). There was a *gongfu* competition in Taiwan in 1975 and I was one of the judges, taking a rest at the site. One of the athletes came to me because he was suffering from shoulder pain. I needled *Sanchasan* (A.04) for him. After needle retention for 30 minutes, the pain was relieved. Right after that he went to the competition and he didn't feel tired when he finished the first round. By the second round, he was more and more competent and finally won the game and became the champion. *Sanchasan* (A.04) is a very effective point for fatigue relief. It is also an important point for disorders of the five sense organs. It can be selected for all the disorders of the five sense organs, based upon the theory of holography.

I once gave lectures in San Francisco and one audience who was a female doctor at present was suffering from an attack of allergic rhinitis. I needled *Sanchsan* (A.04) for her and the running nose immediately stopped. This point is a very good point for disorders of the five sense organs. For shoulder pain, it is advisable to needle this point on the diseased side, and in case of pain of the thigh, it is advisable to needle the point on the healthy side. It also has very good therapeutic effect for nausea, vomit, neck sprain, hypochondriac pain, lower back pain, palpitation and itching of the skin due to various kinds of allergy.

I would like to return to headaches. I want to emphasize that the first points to select for headaches are *Dabai* (22.04) and *Sanchasan* (A.04). The combination of these two points is extremely effective. The second points are *Cesanli* (77.22) and *Cexiasanli* (77.23) plus *Shenguan* (77.18). They are also very good, since the first two points are located between *Yangming* and *shaoyang* channels and they are therefore able to treat disorders of the two channels such as *yangming* and *shaoyang* headache. *Shenguan* (77.18) governs on the kidney, which is externally-internally related to the urinary bladder and it is therefore effective for *Taiyang* headache. It is also good for various kinds of chronic diseases because prolonged illness will finally affect the kidney. If, on the basis of this, *Linggu* (22.05) is added, the analgesic effect will be even heightened. Besides, Master Tung has another special method to treat headache. That is to bleed point *Taiyang* (Extra). Even if the headache is prolonged and chronic, one treatment may obtain remarkable effect. The maximum duration for cure will not go beyond 2-3 treatments.

2) **Migraine**

a. Needle *Cesanli* (77.22) and *Cexiasanli* (77.23). They have good therapeutic effect.
b. Needle *Zhongjiuli* (88.25) (point *Fengshi* GB31). The result is also good.
c. Pricking *Sanchong* (77.07) and *Sihuawai* (77.14) to cause bleeding may immediately stop pain.
d. If the pain is at *Taiyang* (Extra), needling *Menjin* (66.05) is very effective.
e. Blood-letting *Taiyang* (Extra) has special effect for chronic migraine, one treatment in mild case and 2-3 treatments in severe case may cure the condition.
f. Needle *Shuiqu* (66.09).

3) **Occipital Headache**

a. Blood-letting *Chongxiao* (DT.17) may immediately stop pain.
b. Needling *Zhengjin* (77.01) and *Zhengzong* (77.02) may also have good effect.
c. Blood-letting *Weizhong* (BL40) is very effective for chronic posterior headache.

Now let's discuss migraine. *Cesanli* (77.22) and *Cexiasanli* (77.23) are effective for the disorders of *Yangming* channel. They also have therapeutic effect for migraine. Since *Cesanli* (77.22) and *Cexiasanli* (77.23) are located between *Yangming* and *Shaoyang* channels, they are able to treat pain of the two channels. If the pain is located on the *Yangming* channel or at *Taiyang* (Extra), needling point *Menjin* (66.05) would be enough, which is located behind point *Xiangu* (ST43). It is needled along the border of the bone. If *Menjin* (66.05) is not found, *Xiangu* (ST43) can also be selected because it is the *shu*-stream point of the *yangming* channel, which is indicated in heaviness and pain of the body and joints.

In cases of chronic headache, the point should be needled along the border of the bone and combined with point *Menjin* (66.05) would be the best. There is a saying in TCM that a prolonged illness will finally affect the kidney. It means if an illness lasts for long, it will weaken the function of the kidney, leading to deficiency of either kidney *Yin* of kidney *Yang*. This is why the point should be needled along the border of the bone or with the tip of the needle hitting the bone for chronic diseases. It is the principle in TCM so called "treating the bone for bone diseases" and "treating the bone for kidney diseases." For migraine, *Zhongjiuli* (88.25) which is actually point *Fengshi* (GB31) is also a good point. It is one of the most frequently selected points of Master Tung. It works for all kinds of pain, the pain of *shaoyang* channel in particular.

If you don't know what to start with in treatment of a difficult miscellaneous disease, you may select point *Zhongjiuli* (88.25) first to at least alleviate pain, and then seek the cause of the disease and needle other points accordingly. The method can help heighten the therapeutic effect.

Here I'd like to detail the explanation about *Zhongjiuli* (88.25) and *Fengshi* (GB31). In ancient time *fengshi* was taken as an extraordinary point. It was not introduced in *Zhen Jiu Jia Yi Jing* (The Systematic Classic of Acupuncture and Moxibustion), *Qian Jin Yao Fang* (Thousand Ducat Formulas), *Wai Tai Mi Yao* (Secrets of a Frontier Official) or *Tong Ren Zhen Jiu Shu Xue Tu Jing* (Illustrated Classic of Acupuncture Points on the Bronze Man). It was first introduced in *Zhen Jiu Da Cheng* (The Great Compendium of Acupuncture and Moxibustion) and *Zhen Jiu Zi Sheng Jing* (The Classic of Supplementing Life with Acupuncture and Moxibustion). Chinese medicine considers that pain syndrome and wind syndrome are often related to wind. "*Feng* (wind) *shi*" means the place where pain due to wind comes and goes. When Master Tung treated patients with pain of one or two places, he selected corresponding extraordinary points. If the patient has pain all over the body, he needled *Fengshi* (GB31) plus *Zhongdu* (GB32) with *Dao Ma* (Coupling) technique. The combination of the two points effectively alleviates pain of the whole body. The point *Zhongdu* (GB32) is very much related to pathogenic damp because "*du*" means water passage. Wind and damp often cause pain together and the two points are therefore selected. Moreover, following the principle of "treating muscle for muscle disorders" and "treating muscle for disorder caused by damp," the two points are selected. The muscles at *Fengshi* (GB31) is thick, it is good at treating damp diseases. Besides, *Fengshi* (GB31) is located on the gallbladder channel, which is externally-internally related with the liver, it can treat diseases of both the liver and gallbladder. Both the liver and gallbladder dominate tendons. If the point is needled with the needle tip touching the bone, the therapeutic effect will go to the kidney, treating kidney diseases. In this way, it treats all the disorders of the tendons, bones and muscles. According to the theory of the five elements, it treats all the disorders due to wind, cold and damp. The theory of *zangfu* considers that the liver dominates tendons and kidney dominates bones. However, this does not conform to the book *Lingshu* (Spiritual Pivot). It is stated in Chapter 10 of *Lingshu* (Spiritual Pivot) that *shaoyang* dominates bones and *taiyang* dominates tendons. That's why I often select *Fengshi* (GB31) to treat bone spur.

Further, Chapter 9 of the *Suwen* (Essential Questions) states: "All the other eleven *zangfu* organs rely on the gallbladder." From this statement, we can understand why *Fengshi* (GB31) is selected to treat so many diseases. My teacher, Prof. Liu Duzhou is very famous in mainland, China. He is an academic authority of *Shang Han Lun* (Treatise on Fabrile

Diseases), and is expert with the formula *Xiao Chai Hu Tang* (Minor Decoction of Bupleurum). He was my supervisor when I was doing my doctoral degree of *Shang Han Lun* in Beijing University of Traditional Chinese Medicine. I began teaching *Shang Han Lun* in 1976. In 1980, I was invited by Tongji Hospital of Singapore to teach *Shang Han Lun*. In the last tens of year of clinical practice, I have often used *Xiao Chai Hu Tang* with modification which affects the *shaoyang* channels and successfully treated many diseases. Based upon the same theory, point *Fengshi* (GB31) of *shaoyang* channel has good effect for all kinds of pain. It has good therapeutic effect for all kinds of headache, migraine in particular. For chronic headache, blood-letting point *Taiyang* (Extra) is the best because prolonged illness gives rise to blood stasis. In the points for treating headache, the point with special effect is *Zhengjin* (77.01). The therapeutic effect is even better when it is combined with *Zhengzong* (77.02) with *Dao Ma* (Coupling) technique. *Zhengjin* (77.01) is located between *Taixi* (K3) and *Kunlun* (BL60), right on the Calcaneal (Achilles) tendon. We could say it is located on the urinary bladder channel. Therefore it is extremely good for posterior headache located on the urinary bladder channel. Since the point is located right on the Calcaneal tendon, many doctors dare not needle this point, but actually it is very safe. If you don't like to select this point, you could select point *Shugu* (BL65) instead for the same effect. *Shugu* (BL65) is the *shu*-stream point of the urinary bladder channel, which is effective for all kinds of pain of the urinary bladder channel. Some use the *xi*-cleft point which is effective for acute pain. For chronic pain, the *shu*-stream point is often used. Besides, blood-letting method is used to *He*-sea point for prolonged pain, and *Weizhong* (BL40) for posterior headache.

4) Frontal Headache (supraorbital headache, pain of nasal bone, *yangming* headache)

a. Point *Tianhuang* (77.17) or *Shenguan* (77.18) is very effective.
b. Needling point *Huoju* (66.11) may immediately stop pain.
c. Pricking point *Sihuazhong* (77.09) may also obtain good therapeutic effect. *Wuhu* 1 (11.27) and *Wuhu*2 (11.27) are also effective.

Now let's consider frontal headaches. To treat frontal headache, the first choice is point *Tianhuang* (77.17), which is actually *Yinlingquan* (SP9). It is a Tung's extraordinary point that overlaps the point of the fourteen channels. *Shenguan* (77.18) is also a good point for frontal headache as well as one of Master Tung's ten most commonly used extraordinary points. Point *Huoju* (66.11) is also very effective for frontal headache. It is located behind point *Gongsun* (SP4) and is needled along the border of the bone. "*Ju*" means chrysanthemum flower, which is a Chinese medicinal herb with the function to clear heat and benefit the head and eyes. Point *Huoju* (66.11) has therefore the same therapeutic function and is indicated in hypertension, vertigo, headache and soreness of the eyes.

The three points of *Wuhu* (11.27) are indicated in shoulder and arm pain as well as headache. Besides, it is indicated in frontal headache. There is another very effective point for frontal headache. I often used this point 30 years ago but I am almost not using it anymore now. The point is *Zhongwan* (REN12). All these points introduced above are effective for front headache. *Yinlingquan* (SP9) is the *He*-sea point of the spleen channel. "*He*-sea points are indicated in diseases of *Fu* organ." Based upon the theory of holography, the upper end of the leg corresponds to the head; Point *Huoju* (66.11) is close to *Gongsun* (SP4), which is *Luo*-connecting point of the spleen channel. The spleen channel is externally-internally related to the stomach and therefore the *Luo*-connecting point of the spleen can treat *yangming* headache. *Gongsun* (SP4) also has very good therapeutic effect for gastric spasm and gastritis, as well as pain of the shoulder and arm; *Zhongwan* (REN12) is the Front-*mu* point of the stomach and is indicated in frontal headache, the *yangming* headache. If you understand all these, it is easy to select correct points that are therapeutically effective. Though they are extraordinary points, they have close relations with the fourteen channels.

5) **Vertigo**

a. Point *Linggu* (22.05) is very effective for vertigo.
b. In case of hypertensive vertigo, blood-let point *Wuling* (DT. 04) on the back first and then needle *huoyin* (66.03), the blood pressure will be lowered and vertigo stopped immediately. This method is also effective for vertigo due to hypotension.
c. In case of vertigo due to cerebral anemia, needle *Tongguan* (88.01), *Tongshan* (88.02) and *Tongtian* (88.03).

To treat vertigo, point *Linggu* (22.05) is the best one. It has the function to supplement *qi* and tonify the kidney. Since it is located on the course the of large intestine channel, which is connected with the liver, it is very effective for vertigo. Among the points of the fourteen channels, the best point for vertigo is *Quchi* (LI11). If *Linggu* (22.05) is selected together with *Quchi* (LI11), the therapeutic effect is improved, no matter whether the vertigo is resulted from hypertension, hypotension or anemia. The large intestine channel is the one with ample *qi* and blood and is effective for treating disharmony of *qi* and blood.

As an aside, I would like to speak here about fainting due to needles at this point. *Jiexue* (88.28) is useful for fainting. *Jiexue* (88.28) is effective for incorrect needling, derangement of *qi* and blood or acute pain. Further, contusion injures *qi* and blood giving rise to pain due to stagnation. In some patients, the pain is wandering without fixed location, and in this case, *Jie* (88.28) may play the same role of *Liangqiu* (ST34) – the *Xi*-cleft point of the stomach channel – which is also the channel with ample *qi* and blood. Moreover, *Xi*-cleft points are the place where *qi* and blood gather and therefore they have strong therapeutic effect to regulate *qi* and blood. *Jiexue* (88.28) is very close to *Liangqiu* (ST34) and nearer to the knee and has more *qi* and blood gathering there, thus a good point. In case of derangement of *qi* and blood due to disharmony, *Jie* (88.28) is useful. To relieve fainting due to needling, *Renzhong* (RU26) of the fourteen channels may be selected. Further, this point is the point of the *Du* channel which travels towards the head and clears the mind, warms the *yang* and rescues collapse; it is therefore a good point for fainting due to needling. In Tung's extraordinary points, *Jiexue* (88.28) is often used to relieve fainting caused by needling. The goal of this method is also to regulate *qi* and blood. In brief, needling cannot be separated from *qi* and blood, and *yin* and *yang*. If you know more fundamental TCM theory, you will find good points and improve your therapeutic results.

In addition, needling *Tongguan* (88.01) and *Tongshan* (88.02) is also very effective for vertigo due to anemia. In case of vertigo in Meniere's syndrome which is usually accompanied by nausea and vomiting, I often select *linggu* (22.05) in combination with *Neiguan* (PC6) for good result. If *Quchi* (LI11) is added, the result may be faster and better. In many cases of Meniere's disease, the patient came into the clinic with the help of others by hand and independently immediately following treatment. If the vertigo is due to pathological changes of the cerebral nerves, *Xiasanhuang* (77.18, 19, 21) is better. This point supplements the kidney, which dominates brain. In severe cases, bleed point *Sanchong* (77.07). Point *Linggu* (22.05) also improves cerebro-vascular circulation. It is indicated in tens of diseases, hemiplegia in particular. Dr. Jiao Shunfa, the inventor of Chinese scalp-acupuncture, can rotate the scalp needle with the speed as fast as 200 times per minute and most practitioners cannot do it. However, *Linggu* (22.05) could be used instead of needle rotation to improve outcomes. This point improves cerebral blood circulation heightening the therapeutic effects for hemiplegia. If *Xiasanhuang* (77.18, 19, 21) is added, the effect may be improved.

6) Cloudiness Thinking and Fatigue (neurasthenia)

a. Needle point *Zhenghui* (1010.01) and *Zhenjing* (1010.08) and then bleed *Sanchong* (77.07).
b. Needling *Xiasanhuang* (77.18, 19, 21) may also obtain good therapeutic effect.

7) Meningitis

a. Needle *Sanchong* (77.07) with *Dao Ma* needling technique.
b. Prick *Sihuawai* (77.14) first and then needle *Zhengjin* (77.01).

8) Brain Tumor

a. Needle *Zhoukun* (1010.3), *Zhoulun* (1010.4) first, and then needle *Sanchong* (77.07) with *Dao Ma* needling technique.
b. If point *Shangliu* (55.06) is selected in combination with the above points, the effect could be even better.
c. Needle point *Zhengjin* (77.01).

9) Enlargement of Cranial Bone

a. Needling *Zhengjin* (77.01) may have good therapeutic effect, and if *Shangliu* (55.06) is added, the result will be even better.

10) Hydrocephalus

a. Needling *Zhengjin* (77.01) and *Shangliu* (55.06) may have favorable effect.
*Better results may be obtained if blood-letting is given to point *Sanchong* (77.07) in treatment of the last four diseases. (7-10).

Three cerebral diseases have been introduced: Meningitis, brain tumor and hydrocephalus. For all the three diseases, bleeding point *Sanchong* (77.07) is to improve effectiveness. *Sihuawai* (77.14) may also be bled. *Sihuawai* (77.14) is one of the most commonly used points of Master Tung. He also often bled *Chizi* (PC3) or *Weizhong* (BL40) for these brain conditions. Here I'd like to give a brief introduction to point *sihuawai*. It is located one *cun* lateral to *Tiaokou* (ST38). Bleed this point superiorly, inferiorly, medially and laterally to *fenglong* (ST40). As everybody knows, *Fenglong* (ST40) is the influential point of phlegm. It is because this is the *Luo*-connecting point of the stomach, which is internally-externally related to the spleen and is therefore able to treat disease of the spleen. Spleen is considered as the origin in production of phlegm and the lung the container of the phlegm. *Fenglong* (ST40) is a very effective point for phlegm. In terms of west medicine, hyperlipedemia or high cholesterol in the blood is considered to relate to phlegm greatly. Chinese medicine considers prolonged, strange, miscellaneous and difficult diseases to be related to blood stasis. But there is another consideration, and that is that they are all related to phlegm. Therefore, bleeding *Fenglong* (ST40) treats not only chronic, strange, miscellaneous and difficult diseases but also eliminates blood stasis. In the beginning of treatment for difficult and complex diseases and not knowing what to start with, we can bleed the four points superiorly, inferiorly, medially and laterally to *Fenglong* (ST40). If the condition easily leads to formation of nodules with phlegm, it is advisable to use bleeding methods. In case of brain tumor or hydrocephalus, needle *Shangliu* (55.06) on the foot. All these diseases may be treated by needling *Sihuawai* (77.14) or *Weizhong* (BL40).

2. Eye Diseases

1) Blurred Vision

a. In case of blurred vision due to hypertension, bleed point *Wuling* (DT04) first and then needle *Xiasanhuang* (77.18, 19, 21).
b. *Shenguan* (77.18) and *Guangming* (77.28) are also effective points.
c. Bleeding point *Erbei* (99.07) may have even better result.

2) Stye

a. Needle *Linggu* (22.05) with contralateral method. One or two treatments can cure the disease.
b. Bleeding ear apex for few drops of blood is also effective.
c. Bleeding point *Taiyang* (Extra) is extremely effective.

3) Redness of Eyes (Conjunctivitis)

a. Bleeding ear apex is very effective.

For some eye diseases such as blurred vision, *Shenguan* (77.18) and *Fuliu* (KI7) may be needled. Both acute excess and chronic eye diseases may be treated by bleeding *Taiyang* (Extra). For blurred vision needle *Shenguan* (77.18) and *Fuliu* (KI7) first. In case of stye, bleed ear apex or the vein on the ear back first. Then needle *Linggu* (22.05). For conjunctivitis, also bleed the ear apex.

The ear apex is one of most commonly used points for bleeding. This is a brief introduction to the ear apex. It is effective for all eye diseases. It also has good therapeutic effects for the common cold. For facial paralysis with no possibility of bleeding the buccal mucosa, the ear apex may be selected. Bleeding the ear apex may also treat insomnia and various kinds of skin diseases. Why does ear apex have therapeutic effect for so many diseases? Chinese medicine holds that *shaoyang* channel dominates wind and the *taiyang* channel dominates the exterior. The *taiyang* urinary bladder channel starts from the head, and then travels passing the temporal side of the head and reaches the ear; the *shaoyang* channel also winds around the ear. Exterior syndromes correlate with the *taiyang* channel, and skin diseases are related to both wind and the exterior. Thus, the ear apex is indicated for both wind and exterior syndromes. The *shaoyang* channels travel on both medial and lateral sides of the eye and bleeding given here may treat eye diseases, as *shaoyang* channels dominate wind. Moreover, the gallbladder is connected with the heart according to the theory of *Zang Fu Bie Tong* (the extraordinary connection of *zangfu*), the points of gallbladder channel are also indicated in insomnia. The kidney opens into the ear, however, *Su Wen* (Essential Questions) Chapter 4 states, "The heart opens into the ear." Base upon this theory, bleeding the ear apex may treat palpitations and hidrosis since the heart dominates perspiration.

We already mentioned that *Fengshi* (GB31) is important and is one of my ten most commonly used points. It is also one of the best points for insomnia. Insomnia has many etiological factors. The most common one is overthinking after that, disharmony of the stomach, deficiency of *yin* of the liver and kidney, and disharmony between the heart and kidney. Insomnia caused by overthinking is characterized by difficulty falling asleep which is related to fire of the heart and liver. In this case, opening the four gates (*Hegu* (LI4) and *Taichong* (LR3)) may obtain good therapeutic effects. For better results are necessary, needle *Sanjian* (LI3) and *Xingjian* (LR2). In other words, needle the four gates (*Hegu* and *Taichong*) with their locations placed distally. However, the best point for insomnia is *Jiangu* (Extra) located between *Sanjian* (LI3) and *Hegu* (LI4). According to the theory of holography, *Sanjian* (LR3) corresponds to the upper energizer and is more used for diseases of the head; *Hegu* (LI4) corresponds to the middle energizer and is more indicated in diseases of that region. For insomnia accompanied with the symptoms between the upper and middle energizers such as mental restlessness and stuffy chest, *Jangu* (Extra) has the best effect. Therefore, in treatment of insomnia, I often select *Fengshi* (GB31) and *Jiangu* (Extra). In case of chronic stubborn insomnia, I have also used *Xue Fu Zhu Yu Tang* (Decoction for Removing Blood Stasis from the Chest) and received good therapeutic effect, because this formula disperses blood stasis. For the same reasons, blood-letting may also help remove blood stasis, and bleeding ear apex is therefore used for insomnia. Since both the heart and kidney open into the ear, needle ear apex can harmonize the heart and kidney, and regulate water and fire, thus good results for insomnia.

For keratitis, bleeding the ear apex can be very effective. It can work faster than ophthalmic drugs in west medicine. For congestion around the eye due to trauma, filiform needling doesn't work as fast as bleeding *Taiyang* (Extra) on the diseased side. In case of chronic congestion, *Sima* (88.17, 18, 19) can be needled.

4) Dryness in the Eyes

a. Point *Mu* (11.17) has very good effect.
b. Needling *Minghuang* (88.12) is effective.
c. If *Fuliu* (KI7) or *Guangming* (77.28) is added, the effect will be even better.

5) Difficult Opening of the Eyes

a. Needling *Sanchasan* (A.04) and *Huoju* (66.11) may obtain immediate effect.
b. Needling *Gguanming* (77.28) and *Renhuang* (77.21).
c. Needling *Menjin* (66.05) has special effect.

6) Trachoma

a. Pricking the red spot on the inner wall of eyelid to cause bleeding has good effect.

7) Blurred Vision (Four fingers appearing like five fingers in front of the eyes)

a. Needling *Guangming* (77.28) with rotation of needle during needle retention. If *Fuliu* (KI7) is added, the therapeutic effect will be improved.

8) Astigmia

a. Needling *Zhongbai* (22.06) is effective.
b. *Shenguan* (77.18) and *Guangming* (77.28) are effective.

9) Deviation of Eyeballs

a. Needling *Xiasanhuang* (77.18, 19, 21) is effective.
b. Pricking *Taiyang* (Extra) to cause bleeding has extremely good results.

Point *Mu* (11.17) is the best point for dryness in the eyes. It is located on the medial aspect of the palmar side of the proximal segment of the index finger 0.2 *cun* toward the midline from the center of the phalanx. It has two points and the lower one has better effect. Point *Mu* (11.17) has special therapeutic effect for skin diseases of the hand such as eczema of house wife and tinea. It is also good for running nose, no matter the nasal discharge is white due to wind cold or yellow due to wind heat, or heat in the gallbladder channel. According to the meaning of the name, point *Mu* (11.17) dispels wind. It is indicated in diseases of the liver and gallbladder. When there is heat in the gallbladder, it dispels heat from the gallbladder. Master Tung often used this point to treat acute rhinitis and common cold. (Personally I treat common cold with point *Sanchasan* A.04). This point is also effective for dryness in the eyes and lacrimation due to wind. Further, point *Mu* (11.17) is located on the large intestine channel which is connected with the liver and is therefore effective for eye diseases. The large intestine channel is externally-internally related to the lung and this point is therefore effective for diseases of the lung. In Tung's acupuncture, the theory of the extraordinary connections among *zangfu* organs is often used.

Minghuang (88.12) and *Fuliu* (KI7) are also often selected for dryness in the eyes. For ptosis of the eyes due to myasthenia; *Sanchasan* (A.05) and *Huoju* (66.11) are effective. *Menjin* (66.05) is also applicable. Usually the points are needled with the depth of 1 *cun* or deeper. For difficulty in opening eyes, *Sima* (88.17, 18, 19) are also useful. The selection of these points is based on the theory of "treating the muscle for muscular diseases" and "treating the muscle for spleen diseases." These points are selected where the muscles are rich and thick since myasthenia is a condition of the muscles. *Sima* (88.17, 88.18 and 88.19) correspond to the spleen and therefore supplements *qi*. For these reasons, myasthenia due to deficiency of *qi* can be treated with this point. Further, *Hegu* (LI4) is also located at the thick muscle, supplementing the spleen and the *qi* it is therefore also useful for myasthenia. In general, the theories on which Tung's extraordinary acupuncture is based include the theory of the "extraordinary connections of the *zangfu* organs," "holography of human body" and "the method of correspondence."

Double vision due to strabismus can be treated with point *Minghuang* (88.12) and *Fuliu* (K7). For pediatric strabismus, *Shenguan* (77.18) and *Fuliu* (KI7) are better. In adults, strabismus can be caused by paralysis of ocular muscles. Normal functional activities of an eyeball are maintained by the six muscles around it, which must function in coordination on both sides. If a muscle sector is paralyzed, the eyeball will not function normally, causing double vision. Biomedicine allows six months for a cure or remission to occur, if the disease is not cured in six months, then the patient is referred to surgery. However, if the disease is treated with Chinese herbal medicine, it usually takes only three months for a cure. If we add blood-letting therapy, the duration of treatment may be even shorter. After taking Chinese herbal medicine, many patients improve about thirty percent. After bleeding *Taiyang* (Extra), the patient immediately improved another thirty percent. If bleeding is given again in one or two weeks, the patient improves another thirty percent. In general, three treatments of blood-letting may cure the case, while it could take at least three months to cure the problem if the patient take herbs only and western medicine takes at least six months. Another form of double vision due to diabetes is common in the senior population. For such condition, we can also bleed *Taiyang* (Extra). If there appears astigmia or visual confusion, needling *Zhongbai* (22.06) may have good therapeutic effect.

10) Cataract

a. Needling *Xiasanhuang* (77.18, 19, 21) for long time may have very good effect.
b. Needling *Shenguan* (77.18) and *guangming* (77.28).

11) Night Blindness

a. Needling point *Yemang* (A.07) has special therapeutic effect.

12) Lacrimation in Wind

a. Needling point *Mu* (11.17) has special good effect.
b. Needling *Xiasanhung* (77.18, 19, 21) is also very effective.
c. In prolonged cases, *Sanchong* (77.07) can be needled first.

13) Twitching of Ocular Muscle

a. Needle *Wanshunyi* (22.09) and *Wanshun'er* (22.08).
b. Needle *Cesanli* (77.22), *Cexiasanli* (77.23) and *Shenguan* (77.18).
c. Needle *Fengshi* (GB31) and *Fuliu* (KI7).
d. Needle *Shangquan* (88.22), *Zhongquan* (88.21) and *Xiaquan* (88.20).

Many people have lacrimation when exposed to wind and point *Mu* (11.17) has a special effect for the problem. Point *Xiasanhuang* (77.18, 19, 21) is also very effective. For chronic cases, bleed point *Sanchong* (77.07). If there is ocular muscle or facial twitching, *Wanshuyi* (22.09) and *Wanshun'er* (22.08) can be selected. Sometimes we can select *Houxi* (SI3), this is because *Houxi* (SI3) is connected with the Governing Vessel (DU) which goes upward and meets the liver channel at the vertex. Thus *Houxi* (SI3) dispels wind. Moreover, the small intestine channel goes upward and reaches the inner and outer canthus, then goes back to the zygoma, being closely related to the ocular muscle and trigeminal nerve. Point *Houxi* (SI3) is the *Shu*-stream point of the small intestine; it pertains to wood and corresponds to wind. Therefore the point is also indicated for trigeminal neuralgia and neuropathy of the face.

I would like to say something further about facial spasm and facial paralysis. Though facial spasm and facial paralysis are not difficult to treat, too much manipulation or electric stimulation may cause twitch of ocular muscle as a sequela. The facial nerves are close to the surface and shallow insertion is advisable. Manipulation of the needles is not advised in order to avoid over-stimulation. Improper treatment, long and strong stimulation in particular may cause sequela, which is difficult to cure, giving rise to twitching of the eye or muscles around the eye, or even myasthenia characterized by difficulty opening the eye. However, I usually select distal points for facial paralysis. Chinese herbal treatment for twitching of the eyelids works well with *Shao Yao Gan Cao Tang* (Decoction of Peony Root and Liquorice Root). If *Qian Zheng San* (Powder for Facial Paralysis) is added, the therapeutic effect is improved. *Zhimu* (Rhizoma Anemarrhenae) is then added to strengthen sedative function. If the pathological condition is severe, *Gouteng* (Ramulus Uncariae cum Uncis) should be added. The essential feature is the dosage of *Shaoyao* (Radix Paeoniae). It is usually 25-30 grams. As we know, each formula must have a principal ingredient and *Shaoyao* (Radix Paeoniae) is the principal herb of this formula since it mediates *yin*. Those people who stay up all night may be affected by facial spasm, because staying up all night may consume *yin* and *yin* deficiency produces wind.

14) Glaucoma

a. *Huoyin* (66.03) and *Huozhu* (66.04) are very effective.
b. Needling *Xiasanhuang* (77.18, 19, 21) and *Guangming* (77.28) may have excellent result.

15) Myiodesopsia

a. Needle *Shenguan* (77.18) and *Guangming* (77.28).

16) Optic Atrophy

a. Prick *Taiyang* (Extra) to cause bleeding.
b. *Shenguan* (77.18) and *Guangming* (77.28).

Among the fourteen channels, point *Xingjian* (LR2) is the best point for treating glaucoma. If *Xiasanhuan* (77.18, 19, 21) and *Guangming* (77.28) are added, the therapeutic effect can be improved. It is also advisable to bleed ear apex and ear back to lower intraocular pressure. In severe cases blood-letting *Taiyang* (Extra) may also be used. Not long ago I treated a patient who suffered from chronic glaucoma and often used pharmaceutical treatment. However, the drugs often caused oral ulceration, for which the patient came to my clinic. There is an autoimmune disorder that involves the mouth, eyes and genitals called Behcet's disease, causing ulceration of the oral cavity and genitals and poor vision. I first used several doses of *Gan Cao Xie Xin Tang* (Licorice Decoction for Purging the Stomach Fire) to treat oral ulceration. Together with the improvement of oral ulceration, his eyes also got better. Further, if the target treatment is for glaucoma, we need to use other agents. The best single drug for glaucoma is a large dose of *Cheqianzi* (Semen Plantaginis). It can be added to *Long Dan Xie Gan Tang* (Decoction of Gentiana for Purging the Liver Fire) since acute attacks of glaucoma are usually caused by liver fire. The dosage of *Cheqianzi* (Semen Plantaginis) is often up to 30 grams. In many cases of glaucoma, *taiyang* (Extra) bled in order to lower the intraocular pressure quickly. If there is myodesopsia known as vitreous opacity, the Tung's extraordinary point *Shenguan* (77.18) and point *Guangming* (77.28) are better. To treat most cases of optic atrophy, which is a very severe disease, point *Taiyang* (Extra) can be selected for blood-letting once every two weeks. It can be combined with needling *Shenguan* (77.18) and *Guangming* (77.28).

**2. Question: How long are needles retained in the points?
How are the needles manipulated?**

Answer: Master Tung often retained the needles in points for 45 minutes and manipulation was given once every 15 minutes. During the needle retention, ask the patient to have some exercise or give some massage. If the duration of needle retention is 30 minutes, manipulation should be given once every 10 minutes. The patient should also exercise through the range of motion while the needles are manipulated. Without manipulation, the results will be poor. However, excessive exercise will have opposite effect. The exercise every 10 minutes is the best and it can help move the flow of *qi*. Regarding the length of needle retention, there are two basic considerations. 1. In Chapter 15 of the *Lingshu* (Spiritual Pivot), it says: "The *qi* and blood circulate in the body day and night. One whole circulation of *qi* and blood in the body needs 28 minutes and 48 seconds." 2. In Chapter 18 of *Lingshu* (Spiritual Pivot), it says: "The *ying qi* (nutrient *qi*) circulates inside the vessels and *wei qi* (defensive qi) circulates outside the vessels. *Ying qi* circulates all over the body 50 times per day." Based upon this statement, one whole circulation takes 28 minutes and 48 seconds. For convenience, we take it as 30 minutes. It is generally considered that the duration of needle retention is 30 minutes. During the needle retention, manipulation is given once every 10 minutes.

3. Diseases of the Nose

Consider that all the nasal diseases can be treated with point *Sima* (88.17, 18, 19). All diseases respond better if two groups of points are used in alternation. However, in the treatment of nasal diseases, point *Sima* (88.17, 18, 19) is the best and most frequently used. Master Tung used to have his business card on which it was written: "Guaranteed to cure all nasal diseases," including allergic rhinitis, atrophic rhinitis, nasal pus retention (sinusitis) and hypertrophic rhinitis. With the selection of point *Sima* (88.17, 18, 19), a mild case can be cured in a few treatments and severe cases require more treatments with longer duration.

Master Tung didn't use Chinese herbal medicine very often and he gave acupuncture treatment about three times a week. 20-30 years ago, a single income could support the whole family and the life was slow. This made it possible for the patient to come for treatment 3 times a week or even more. There is much more stress in the life now and even both husband and wife working cannot support one child. So patients can only come to receive treatment once a week. In this case, blood-letting should be added to the treatment to strengthen and prolong the therapeutic effect. Of course, simultaneous application of Chinese herbs may improve the therapeutic effects. Here, I'd like to make it clear that, application of herbal medicine doesn't mean we are not confident in acupuncture and application of acupuncture doesn't mean the therapeutic function of herbs is weak. Either acupuncture or Chinese herbs should be effective, and the combination of both may have better results.

1) Dryness of the Nose

a. Needle point *Sima* (88.17, 18, 19).
b. Needle point *Mu* (11.17).

Many patients suffer from dryness and itching in the nose. For such patients, needling *Sima* (88.17, 18, 19) and *Yingxiang* (LI20) is very effective. Point *Yingxiang* (LI20) is the crossing point of *yangming* channels of hand and foot. Since the *yangming* channels of hand and foot have ample *qi* and blood and all travel to the nose, it has good function for regulating *qi* and blood and treating nasal diseases. Point *Mu* (11.17) is located on the large intestine channel, which travels by the side of the nose. The lung opens into the nose and is externally-internally related to the large intestine that is connected with the liver. The liver channel travels deep in the nasopharynx area. Based upon the above reasons, point *Mu* (11.17) can be selected to treat dryness in the nose.

2) Nasal Obstruction

a. In case of common cold with nasal obstruction, needling *Jianzhong* (44.06) has a very good effect.
b. Needling *Cesanli* (77.22) with needle retention is also effective.
c. Needling *Menjin* (66.05) is also effective.
d. Point *Mu* (11.17) is effective.
e. Point *Huofuhai* (33.07) is also effective.

There are many good points for nasal obstruction. The most commonly used one is *Yingxiang* (LI20), which has the fastest effect. In Tung's extraordinary points, point *Mu* (11.17) has best result. Point *Jianzhong* (44.06) or *Cesanli* (77.22) are also good for nasal obstruction. *Menjin* (66.05) is also effective. *Shousanli* (LI10) is also good for symptomatic treatment of nasal obstruction. *Sima* is also a good point. Though many points are indicated in nasal obstruction, *sima* is good enough for nasal obstruction due to chronic rhinitis. It is stated in *Nei Jing* (Yellow Emperor's Inner Classic): "The diseases of the heart and lung may affect the nose." Therefore, in the treatment of nasal disease, the use of additional points such as *Neiguan* (PC6) or *Tongguan* (88.01) and *Tongshan* (88.02) may improve the therapeutic effect. *Yingxiang* (LI20) can be added to any points selected for nasal diseases. It is both double treatment and attracting needling.

3) Nasal Allergy

a. Needle *Sima* (88.17, 18, 19), *Tongtian* (88.03) and *Tongguan* (88.01).
b. Needle point *Mu* (11.17).
c. Needle *Taibai* (SP3) and *Huozhu* (66.04).

Nasal allergies involve allergic and chronic rhinitis. Let's discuss allergic rhinitis first. In many cases, allergic rhinitis is caused by cold food. If drinking too much ice water in summer time, the person would be more liable to be affected by this disease in winter. Preference of cold food may lead to liability of sneezing and running nose in cold storage. This is so called "invasion of exogenous pathogenic cold or cold food or drink injures the lung." For the pathological condition, *Xiao Qing Long Tang* (Minor Decoction of Blue Dragon) is the best. The use of several doses would have therapeutic effect. Then use *Bu Zhong Yi Qi Tang* (Decoction for Strengthening the Spleen and Supplementing *Qi*) to strengthen the underlying condition and prevent recurrence. Allergic rhinitis is quite common in Taiwan, Los Angeles, and Korea. In Los Angeles, the rainy season starts from November and ends in March. It rains occasionally in April. There is no rain during the period after then till next November. Therefore, in April and May the air is full of pollen everywhere because Los Angeles doesn't have many high buildings, which gives rise to high morbidity of allergy caused by pollen. There are a lot of high buildings and rain in Taiwan. Though there are many allergy patients, not many of them are caused by pollen. To treat allergic rhinitis and pollen allergy, Tung's extraordinary point *Sima* (88.17, 18, 19) should be needled first. In herbal medicine, *Gui Zhi Tang* (Decoction of Ramulus Cinnamomi) combined with *Yu Ping Feng San* (Powder of Jade Screen) with modification can be taken. It raises the immunity and alleviates allergy to pollen.

To treat nasal diseases, ancient physicians often open (needle) the four gates (LI4 and LR3). The Tung's extraordinary point Ssima (88.17, 18, 19) is often used in combination with the four gates *Hegu* (LI4) and *Taichong* (LR3), with good therapeutic effect. Why select the four gates? *Hegu* (LI4) is the point of the large intestine channel. The trajectory travels around the nose and it is therefore indicated in the diseases of the nose. *Taichong* (LR3) is the point of the liver channel; it passes through deep layers of the throat and nose reaching the vertex, and is therefore closely related to the nose and throat. In other words, the large intestine channel is responsible for external nose and the liver channel is responsible for internal nose. Further, when heat in the gallbladder is transmitted to the brain, it can give rise to sinusitis. That's why application of *Xiao Chai Hu Tang* (Minor Decoction of Radix Bupleuri) plus *Ge Gen Tang* (Decoction of Radix Puerariae) has good therapeutic effect for pus retention (sinutitis). Nasal diseases are treated by taking the liver into consideration. In many cases, nasal problems are related to liver *qi* stagnation. Many doctors therefore like to treat the problems by either dispersing the liver *qi* stagnation or clearing liver heat. *Xiao Yao San* (Ease Powder) is often appropriate. Selection of *Hegu* (LI4) and *taichong* (LR3) follows the same principle. *Taichong* (LR3) has good effect for dispersing liver *qi* stagnation. This is a rationale for selecting the point in the treatment of nasal disorders.

Another frequently used and effective group of points are *Hegu* (LI4), *Quchi* (LI11) and *Zusanli* (ST36). The *yangming* channel and the liver channel are always considered in the treatment of nasal diseases. The three points above are from the *yangming* channels. *Taichong* (LR3) is the *Shu*-stream point and *Yuan*-source point of the liver. Point *Huozhu* (66.04) is just behind *Taichong* (LR3) and is needled along the border of the bone. Actually, the location of *Taichong* (LR3) in the ancient classics is close to the bone and overlaps Master Tung's extraordinary point *Huozhu* (66.04), which is also very effective for sore throat because the liver channel passes the throat and reaches the vertex. *Taichong* (LR3) is effective for chronic disorders of the throat and nose, as is point *Huozhu* (66.04). Since chronic diseases often affect the kidney, the point is therefore needled along the border of the bone, treating the kidney at the same time. Further, point *Mu* (11.17) is also good for treating nasal diseases. It is located on the large intestine channel, which is connected with the liver and is therefore effective for the nasal diseases. Moreover, the large intestine channel is externally-internally related with the lung that opens into the nose, and point *Mu* (11.17) is effective also because of this kind of relation.

4) Brandy Nose

a. Use three-edged needle or seven-star needle to blood-let point *Zhengben* (1010.12).
b. Blood-letting *Pishu* (BL20) and *Weishu* (BL21) is also very effective.

Brandy nose is characterized by redness of the nose tip. Many people who drink a lot of alcohol have this disease that is often resulted from damp heat in the spleen and stomach. Pricking point *Zhengben* (1010.12) with either three-edged needle or plum-blossom needle to cause bleeding is effective. Bleeding either *Pishu* (BL20) or *Weishu* (BL21) is also effective. This is because the nose is located in the center of the face, corresponding to the spleen and stomach according to the theory of holography.

5) Nasal Bleeding

a. Needling *Jianzhong* (44.06) may immediately stop bleeding.
b. Needling *Huozhu* (66.04) is effective.
c. Needling *Liuwan* (66.08) is effective.

For nasal bleeding, needling *Jianzhong* (44.06) is very effective. Needling *Liuwan* (66.08) is also effective. *Taichong* (LR3) or *Huozhu* (66.04) may also be selected. Since the liver has the function of storing blood, needling the point of liver has good effect. Further, needling *Hegu* (LI4) is also effective because the large intestine channel travels towards the nose. Since the liver is connected with the large intestine, nasal bleeding due to heat in the *yangming* channel can be treated with *Zhi Zi Bai Pi Tang* (Decoction of Fructus Gardeniae and Cortex Phellodendri) with modifications. If the ingredients of the formula *Zhizi* (Fructus Gardeniae), *Huangbai* (Cortex Phellodendri) and *Gancao* (Radix Glycyrrhizae) are combined with *xianhecao* (Herba Agrimoniae) and *Oujietan* (Nodus Nelumbinis Rhizomatis carbonized), the therapeutic effective is even better. *Zhi Zi Bai Pi Tang* can clear heat from the liver. This formula is listed in the "Jaundice" chapter of "*Yangming* Disorders." of *Shang Han Lun*. It is a formula for *yangming* channel and it is therefore effective for nasal bleeding. Generally, 3 to 5 doses of the herbal decoction would work effectively. This formula can also be used for infantile nasal bleeding. However, it doesn't work for nasal bleeding due to nasopharyngeal cancer.

6) Pus Retention in the Nose

Point *Mu* (11.17) is a very effective point for pus retention in the nose, so is *sima* (88.17, 18, 19). Pus retention in the nose often results from heat in the liver and gallbladder. This point is very effective because of the extraordinary connection between the large intestine and the liver. Selection of *Hegu* (LI4) and *Taichong* (LR3) is also very effective. If *Quchi* (LI11) is used in combination, the result is even better. *Taichong* (LR3) is a point of the liver channel, which goes up to the vertex via nose. *Hegu* (LI4) and *Quchi* (LI11) are all the points of the large intestine channel. Both are good for treating diseases of the head. The large intestine channel passes through the nose and is connected with the liver. It clears heat from the liver and gallbladder, and is therefore effective for pus retention. If point *Dabai* (22.04) is used instead of *Hegu* (LI4), the result is even better, because *Dabai* (22.04) is also located of the large intestine channel and has very good effect on regulating *qi*. From point of view of holography, it corresponds to the head and face. As we mentioned already, point *Sima* (88.17, 18, 19) is indicated in nasal pus retention. First, it is located on the stomach channel of foot-*yangming*, which passes by the side of the nose; second, it is located at the place where the muscles are rich and thick. Selection of this point follows the principle of "needling the muscle to treat diseases of the spleen." Needling this point has very good effect of regulating and supplementing *qi*. As mentioned before, application of modified *Xiao Chai Hu Tang* (Minor Decoction of Radix Bupleuri) is very effective, so is *Dan Zhi Xiao Yao San* (Ease Powder Modified with Cortex Moutan Radicis and Fructus Gardeniae).

4. Ear Diseases

1) Otitis Media

a. Prick *Cesanli* (77.22) and *Cexiasanli* (77.23) to cause bleeding.
b. Prick point *zhiwu* (11.26) to cause bleeding.

In the treatment of otitis media, Master Tung often gave blood-letting to the lateral side of lateral malleolus, and sometimes point *Diwuhui* (GB42) too. Personally I like to bleed point *Zhiwu* (11.26) to treat otitis media, which can help astringe the suppurating wound. A teacher from one of the universities in Beijing has a daughter who injured her sole. For three years, the wound was not healed by treatments of many doctors. However, one treatment by bleeding point *Zhiwu* (11.26) improved the condition and two treatments cured the case. Point *Zhiwu* (11.26) is located on the thumb and bleeding this point has good therapeutic result. Before bleeding, ask the patient to hold a tight fist so that the point becomes congested with blood. If wounds due to trauma or operation fail to heal, this point is always good. Further, this point assists recovery of herpes zosters. It is a good point for otitis media, the chronic case with pus flow in particular. Point *Zhiwu* (11.26) is close to the *Jing*-well point of the lung, which dominates the skin and *qi*. In Chinese medicine, the lung is often considered in treatment of skin diseases. In case of prolonged skin suppuration without cure, Chinese medicine often uses big dose of *Huangqi* (Radix Astragali seu Hedysari) to supplement *qi*. Therefore, it is reasonable to needle points of the lung in treatment of prolonged skin suppuration caused by various kinds of skin infection such as furuncles and carbuncles. Otitis media is situated on the course of foot-*shaoyang* channel, which runs around the ear, and thus bleeding therapy is used at the external malleolus.

2) Earache

a. Pricking *Cesanli* (77.22) and *Cexiasanli* (77.23) to cause bleeding.
b. Bleed *Sanchong* (77.07) and *Sihuawai* (77.14) simultaneously.
c. Needle *Sanchasan* (A.04).
d. Needle *Sima* (88.17, 18, 19).

The commonly used points for earache are *Cesanlii* (77.22) and *Cexiasanli* (77.23). Some other points such as *Sanchasan* (A.04) are also good. *Sanchasan* (A.04) treats diseases of the five sense organs, including the eye, ear, mouth, nose and skin. Point Sima (88.17, 18, 19) is also indicated in earache. If the earache is prolonged, bleeding therapy could be used to either *Sanchong* (77.07) or *Sihuawai* (77.14). Generally, when needling is not good enough, use blood-letting method.

3) Distention in the Ear

a. Needle *Quling* (33.16) and *Zhongbai* (22.06).
b. Needle *Sanchasan* (A.04).

4) Tinnitus

a. Needle *Sima* (88.17, 18, 19) with reducing method and *Shenguan* (77.18) with reinforcing method.
b. Needle *Quling* (33.16) with reducing method and *Minghuang* (88.12) with reinforcing method.
c. Needle *Sima* (88.17, 18, 19) and bleed the *Ashi* points around the external malleolus.
d. Needle *Wanshunyi* (22.09) and *Wanshun'er* (22.08).
e. Needle *Zhongjiuli* (88.25).
f. Needle *Linggu* (22.05).
g. Needle *Sanchasan* (A.04).

Both *Sanchasan* (A.04) and *Linggu* (22.05) are effective for distention in the ear. *Zhongbai* (22.06) is also a frequently used point. If it is combined with *sanchasan* (A.04), the effect is even better. In the treatment of tinnitus, Master Tung often selected *Sima* (88.17, 18, 19) and sometimes combined them with *Linggu* (22.05). I have often used *Sanchasan* (A.04) combined with *Fengshi* (GB31) with very good results. *Fengshi* (GB31) has sedative function and dispels wind. It is an important point of the foot-*shaoyang* channel, which passes and winds around the ear. Sometimes I also use *Sima* (88.17, 18, 19) or *Linggu* (22.05) in alternation. To treat tinnitus, it is mainly to supplement *qi* and strengthen the kidney. In my treatment for tinnitus, I use *Er Long Zuo Ci Wan* (Pills of Magnetitum for Deafness) for deficiency of kidney, which is composed of *Liu Wei Di Huang Wan* (Pills of Six Drugs Including Rehmanniae) plus *Wuweizi* (Fructus Schisandrae) and *Cishi* (Magnetitum). Additionally, I add *Shichangpu* (Rhizoma Acori Gaminei) and *Chaihu* (Radix Buleuri) for better results. *Shichangpu* (Rhizoma Acori Gaminei) helps open the orifices and *Chaihu* (Radix Bulerri) serves as the guiding drug to take the actions of the drugs to the *shaoyang* channel and ear. Moreover, there are many cases of tinnitus due to depressed *yang*, more in young people. It is advisable in this case to apply *Yi Qi Cong Ming Tang* (Decoction for supplementing *Qi* and Promoting Hearing) to supplement *qi* and lifting *yang*. In the prescription, *Gegen* (Radix Puerariae) is an important drug for treating tinnitus. The decoction has the function to tonify lung and supplement *qi*. The mechanism in application of herbs here is the same as that in application of point *Sima* (88.17, 18, 19) by Master Tung for tinnitus. In treatment of tinnitus, it is advisable to supplement *qi* first, and in chronic cases, take the kidney into consideration by needling *Shenguan* (77.18) and using *Er Long Zuo Ci Wan* (Pills of Magnetitum for Deafness) plus *Wuweizi* (Fructus Schisandrae), *Cishi* (Magnetitum), *Shichangpu* (Rhizoma Acori Gaminei) and *Chaihu* (Radix Buleuri). Selection of *Wanshunyi* (22.09) and *Wanshun'er* (22.08) is also related to the kidney. In the ancient acupuncture point songs for tinnitus, *Tnghui* (GB2) is almost always listed. In the application of the above Tung's extraordinary points, *tinghui* is therefore often used as the guiding point for good therapeutic effect.

5) Deaf-mutism

a. Bleed point *Sanchong* (77.07) first, then, needle Sima (88.17, 18, 19) with six needles.
b. Prick point *Zongshu* (1010.07) to cause bleeding.
c. Needle point *Shiyin* (88.32).

Deaf-mutism refers to deafness or double hearing plus aphasia. It is curable if it is mild and incurable if it is severe. It is often treated with *Tinggong* (SI19) and *Tinghui* (GB2) according to the medical classics. Master Tung often used *Sima* (88.17, 18, 19) in the treatment. For aphasia, he often used point *Shiyin* (88.32), and in severe case, bled *Sanchong* (77.07). Personally I needle *Tinggong* (SI19), *Tinghui* (GB2) and *Ermen* (SJ21) selectively for double hearing or poor hearing function, and *Sima* (88.17, 18, 19) or *Xiasanhuang* (77.18, 19, 21) in alternation additionally. For aphasia, pricking *Shiyin* (88.32) or *Zongshu* (1010.07) to cause bleeding is both safe and effective. In herbal medicine, *Mai Men Dong Tang* (Decoction of Radix Ophiopogonis) Modified with *Jiegeng* (Radix Platycodi) and *Fenghuangyi* (Membrana Follicularis Ovi) is often used.

5. Diseases of the Mouth and Teeth

1) Pain of the Mandible (difficulty in opening mouth)

a. Needle *Huoyin* (66.03). The therapeutic effect would be even better if *Jiexi* (ST41) is added.
b. Prick the ear back to cause bleeding.
c. Blood-letting *Taiyang* (Extra) is especially effective.

Huoyin (66.03) is effective for mandibular pain with difficulty in opening mouth as is *Huozhu* (66.04). Furthermore, *Waiguan* (SJ5) and *Yanglingquan* (GB34) of the fourteen channels are also effective. In 1989, I treated one case of oral cancer. The patient used to have the hobby of chewing areca, which contains lime that may make the oral membrane pale and cause cancer. Small amounts of pepper gave rise to pain in the oral cavity and the patient had difficulty opening the mouth to let even one finger in. This was due to fibrosing on both sides. When the patient came to my clinic, I bled *Taiyang* (Extra). Few days after bleeding, the patient could put two fingers into the mouth. The bleeding treatment was given once every two weeks and after three treatments the patient could put three fingers into the mouth. The patient then received few more treatments. The membrane in the oral cavity gradually became pink. At the same time, he drank the tea of *Danzhuye* (Herba Lophatheri). After three months of treatment, all the symptoms subsided and he is still alive after over 10 years. This patient didn't take medication, bleeding *Taiyang* (Extra) and occasionally *Chize* (Lu5) was the primary treatment. I treated another case of oral cancer which could not open the mouth after operation. I gave him bleeding treatment few times and he finally could open his mouth. These two cases were severe. In mild cases, *Huoyin* (66.03) and *Waiguan* (SJ5) is sufficient. Point *Menjin* (66.05) is also helpful since it is the wood point of the *yangming* channel and is needled along the border of the bone, treating both tendons and bones. Moreover, the *yangming* channel passes through the mandible, which is why *Menjin* (66.05) has special effect.

2) Deviation of the Mouth and Eye (facial paralysis)

a. Bleed *Sihuawai* (77.14) first and then needle *Cesanli* (77.22) and *Cexiasanli* (77.23).
b. Bleed *Sanchong* (77.07) first and then needle *Sima* (88.17, 18, 19) and *Tongshen* (88.09).
c. Bleeding the oral membrane on the diseased side has special therapeutic effect.
d. Bleeding the ear apex of the diseased side is also effective.

This facial paralysis does not involve apoplexy, but rather Bell's paralysis and facial neuritis. It is usually caused by cold or exposure in cold wind during sleep with windows open. After getting up the next morning, the patient had salivation while brushing the teeth and a deviated face. When I served as the member of the council of Taiwan Association of Traditional Chinese Medicine in 1980, the director of the board was suffering from facial paralysis at a meeting. I urged him to have timely treatment. Three weeks later he gave me a call and asked me for help. I asked him why he didn't receive any treatment for three weeks. He told me he was the director of the board and many doctors gave him treatment on their own initiative but received no effect. He also prescribed some herbal medicine for himself that didn't work either. I gave him blood-letting treatment on the oral membrane of the affected side twice and he was completely cured. This case report was published in The Annuals of Traditional Chinese Medicine, 1981. There are more such case examples. Among all the cases of facial paralysis, the youngest was a few month old newborn baby. For the treatment, I also used blood-letting therapy. The second treatment was given 3-4 days later. In general, 2-3 treatments may cure the patient.

There is one thing I'd like to make it clear: the pathological condition may get worse after the first treatment. This is because the first five to seven days after the attack are progressive stages of the disease. However, with continued treatment, the condition will not get worse but will become gradually alleviated. This statement should be given to the patient during the first week of treatment.

I once suffered from facial paralysis. In the winter of 1994, I was invited by the board director of Taiwan Association of Acupuncture to accompany the delegates of Hongkong Association of Chinese Medicine to dinner. Eight people drank 3 bottles of western liquor. I usually didn't drink alcohol, but I drank a lot that night. I had been busy writing articles for a special newspaper column for a few nights. I also had many patients in my clinic during the day and was tired. During the dinner, I was sitting close to the air conditioner. Suddenly, I was feeling abnormality like numbness and stiffness on my face. Some person sitting beside told me that my face was deviated. Immediately, I went home and asked one of my students to needle *Shangjuxu* (ST37), *Zusanli* (ST36) and do blood-letting. The next morning, the condition was even worse. I kept on working in clinic during the day with a plaster on my face. That evening I needled the points myself with no change. After treatment on the third day, the condition started to improve. I then asked my student to perform more bleeding. By the fourth day, most of the deviation was corrected. I received treatment with acupuncture twice a day and blood-letting once every other day. In addition, I took *Gui Zhi Jia Ge Gen Tang* (Decoction of Ramulus Cinnamomi and Radix Puerariae) plus *Qian Zheng San* (Powder for Treating Facial Paralysis). By the fourth day of treatment, the disease was almost cured and the fifth day it was completely cured when the herbal decoction was finished. Many people didn't believe I was cured in four days. However, I received treatment twice a day, for four days; this treatment is equal to regular treatment of eight days, and thus the effect. A correspondent reported my case in the newspaper and tens of patients with facial paralysis came to visit me in one week. I saw that there are many patients suffering from this disease.

If the duration of the disease goes beyond 3 weeks, the patient needs to take decoction of *Bu Yang Huan Wu Tang* (Decoction Invigorating Yang for Recuperation) plus *Qian Zheng San* (Powder for Treating Facial Paralysis). If the duration of the disease is more than one month, it is more difficult to treat. In general, the therapeutic effect of local points such as *Dicang* (ST4) and *Jiache* (ST6) are not good. For chronic cases, needle *Shangjuxu* (ST37) and *Zusanli* (ST36) bilaterally, or select *Cesanli* (77.22) and *Cexiasanli* (77.23) contralaterally. Retention of needles should be long. The two groups of points are often selected alternatively. If the duration is over two months, the patient should also take the herbal decoction, *Shun Feng Yun Qi San* (Powder for Dispelling Wind and Harmonizing Qi) for good therapeutic effect. In addition, needle *Shangjuxu* (ST37) and *Zusanli* (ST36) or *Cesanli* (77.22) and *Cexiasanli* (77.23). Moreover, blood-letting in the oral cavity may improve the results. When needling *Shangjuxu* (ST37) and *Zusanli* (ST36); insert the needles at a 45° angle obliquely upward. The depth of insertion should be 2 *cun* and the duration of needle retention should be at least 60 minutes. Blood-letting should be given once every other week. Generally speaking, a two-week treatment may cure an acute case completely. This requires that acupuncture be given 3 times a week. If receiving treatment twice a day like I did, the therapeutic effect can be faster. Attention should be given to the angle of needle insertion. It is the best to insert the needle along the stomach channel with the angle of 45 degrees upward. The stomach channel runs from the upper to the lower. Treatment is therefore given against the flow of *qi* in the channel. Such oblique insertion has better effect than perpendicular insertion. These two points are used because *Shangjuxu* (ST37) is the lower *He*-sea point of the large intestine and *Zusanli* (ST36) is the *He*-sea point of the stomach. Both of the two channels go up to the face and wind around the lips, and thus the two points are indicated in diseases of face and mouth. The therapeutic effect is also related to reinforcing or reducing method based on the needling direction along or against the channel. According to my experience, oblique insertion is more effective than perpendicular insertion. Long needle retention, at least 60 minutes may obtain better results.

3) Rigidity of the Tongue (aphasia due to apoplexy)

a. Needle *Jianzhong* (44.06). If point *Shangqiu* (SP5) is added, the effect is even better.
b. Needle *Zongshu* (1010.07) shallowly or prick the point to cause bleeding.
c. Select *Shuijin* (1010.20) and *Shuitong* (1010.19).

Rigidity of the tongue here refers to aphasia due to apoplexy, for which it is quite good to prick the points around *Fengfu* (DU16) and *Yamen* (DU15) to cause slight bleeding. Such treatment is usually given once every 3-4 days. Apoplectic aphasia is a form of stroke sequela and its principle of treatment is the same as that of apoplexy. This will be detailed later in discussion regarding to the selection of points and management of the acute condition. I have been invited to the hospitals to give emergency management to tens of apoplectic patients. Many of them had no hope of survival. However, after acupuncture treatment with blood-letting therapy and use of herbal medicine, they resuscitated and survived. My clinical practice has proven to me that acupuncture for the treatment of hemiplegia due to stroke has the best therapeutic result.

For aphasia due to apoplexy, *Shuijin* (1010.20) has good therapeutic effect. After needling *Shuijin* (1010.20), bleed *Fengfu* (DU16) and *Yamen* (DU15). *Fengfu* (DU16) and *Yamen* (DU15) are indicated for aphasia and vomiting. This is based upon the correspondence between the anterior and posterior. Bleeding the two points are very effective for nausea and vomiting which is a disease of the anterior while *Fengfu* (DU16) and *Yamen* (DU15) are the points of the posterior. In acupuncture, this method of treatment is known as correspondence between the anterior and posterior. It is also known as "treating *yin* diseases with *yang* points and treating *yang* diseases with *yin* points." The method of correspondence and treatment will be detailed later for diseases of the four limbs. Understanding the correspondence and symmetry of the four limbs is essential to treatment of their diseases. Such correspondence and symmetry exist between arm and arm, arm and leg, arm and trunk, arm and thigh, leg and leg, leg and trunk, left and right, upper and lower, and anterior and posterior. Some doctors don't study much about the theory of channels and collaterals but know the correspondence and symmetry, but they can still treat many diseases. If we have a good command of the knowledge of both, we will be able to treat diseases better. The more we know such knowledge, the better and more flexible we will be in treating diseases, especially knowing how to start the treatment for a patient. As a doctor of Chinese medicine, we need to have confidence for good therapeutic effect. If we doctors don't have confidence, there would be no therapeutic effect. It is therefore important to have confidence, which comes from a good command of such knowledge.

Point *Shangqiu* (SP5) is very effective for aphasia because the spleen channel reaches the bottom of the tongue. *Shangqiu* (SP5) is the metal and *Jing*-river point of the spleen channel. It has good therapeutic effect for pathological changes of phonation. Selection of this point is based upon the theory of the five elements. It is stated in the *Lingshu* (Spiritual Pivot), "When the disease is located in *zangfu* organs, select a *Jing*-well point." If *zangfu* organs are attacked in wind stroke, the patient will have unconsciousness and *Jing*-well point should be bled, "when the disease gives rise to the change of color, select *Ying*-spring point." For instance, if the patient faints due to needling and has a pale face, strengthen the heart by needling the *Ying*-spring of the heart *Shaofu* (HT8). In case of red face due to heat in the lung, select the *Ying*-spring point of the lung *Yuji* (LU8). If there is redness, swelling and itching of the skin, select the *Ying*-spring point of the heart *Shaofu* (HT8), the *Ying*-spring point of the triple energizer (*San Jiao*) channel *Yemen* (SJ3) and *Sanchasan* (A.04), which is located behind *Yemen* (SJ3). If the pathological condition is going up and down, select *Shu*-stream point. "When there is pathological change in phonation, select *Jing*-river point." It means when any pathological change happens to phonation, we may select *Jing*-river point in treatment. For instance, we may select point of pericardium channel to treat nausea and vomiting. This is because the stomach channel and pericardium channel are inter-connected. *Laogong* (PC8), *Daling* (PC7) and *Neiguan* (PC6) are all indicated in nausea and vomiting. However, point *Jianshi* (PC5) is the best. This is because *Jianshi* (PC5) is the *Jing*-river point and is indicated in abnormal voice that occurs with vomiting. In case of sudden aphonia caused by fright, which is considered to be an abnormal change of phonation related to heart and mind, we should select *Lingdao* (HT4), the point of the heart that dominates mind and the therapeutic effect is good. In general, any pathological changes of the phonation can be treated by *Jing*-river points. This consideration is originated from *Nei Jing* (The Yellow Emperor's Inner Classic).

Now let's see what is said in the book *Nei Jing* (The Yellow Emperor Inner Classic): "*Jing*-well point is indicated in fullness of epigastrium; *Ying*-spring point is indicated in hotness sensation of the body; *Shu*-stream point is indicated in heaviness and pain of the body and joints; *Jing*-river point is indicated in asthmatic breathing, cough, chills and fever; *He*-sea point is indicated in dysentery due to adverse flow of *qi*." Corresponding to the five elements, the *Jing*-river point pertains to metal; the *Shu*-stream point pertains to earth; the *Ying*-spring points pertain to fire; the *Jing*-river point pertains to wood. In the five elements, metal makes the loudest sound. When the metal is broken, its sound becomes lower. A broken bell doesn't make sound. On the contrary, a stuffed bell doesn't make sound either. Take the common cold as an example. It is often caused by an invasion of pathogenic cold, which causes *qi* stagnation in the lung, giving rise to hoarse voice. Both cough and asthmatic breathing are diseases related to change of voice, and the *Jing*-river point of the lung or other related channels can be selected in the treatment since the lung pertains to metal according to the theory of the five elements. The *Jing*-river point is also indicated for cold and heat syndromes of the common cold because *Jing*-river point, like the lung, pertains to metal. For aphasia due to wind stroke, the best choice is the *Jing*-river point of the spleen. This is because, for wind stroke, earth points (the points of the spleen and stomach) should be selected to promote metal. Further, the *Jing*-river points are empirical for treating aphasia. Moreover, the spleen channel goes to the root of the tongue. Therefore, the *Jing*-river point of the spleen channel *Shangqiu* (SP5) is very good for aphasia due to wind stroke. The herbal formula for such aphasia is *Di Huang Yin Zi* (Rehmannia Decoction), which is very good for stroke patients with hemiplegia and aphasia. This condition is also known as "*Fengfei*" and "*Yinfei*), for which the combination of both herbal medicine and acupuncture in the treatment is much better. Another problem caused by stroke is disphagia, which could be treated by bleeding

Fengfu (DU16), *Yamen* (DU15) or *Zongshu* (1010.07) plus *Di Huang Yin Zi* (Rehmannia Decoction).

4) Sublingual Swelling

a. Needling *Cesanli* (77.22) and *Cexiasanli* (77.23) is effective. Bleeding *jinjin* and *Yuye* (Extra) may have even better result.
b. Give blood-letting to the ear apex.

Sublingual swelling here refers to swelling of the tongue body, which can be treated by many points. In Tung's extraordinary points, *Cesanli* (77.22) and *Cexiasanli* (77.23) are often needled. Since the spleen channel is connected with the root of the tongue exteriorly and the heart interiorly (the heart opening into the tongue), the points of the heart and spleen should be selected if we use the points of the fourteen channels. In brief, bleeding *jinjin* and *Yuye* (Extra) has very good therapeutic effect. Since the heart opens into the tongue, we can also bleed ear apex.

5) Oral Ulceration

a. Prick point *Sihuazhong* (77.09) to cause bleeding and needle *Sihuashang* (77.08).
b. Prick point *Shangchun* (77.15) and *Xiachun* (77.16) to cause bleeding.
c. Give blood-letting to *Taiyang* (Extra).
d. Prick ear apex to cause bleeding.

Oral ulceration is a disease related to the heart and spleen. In treatment, we can bleed local points around the ulcer, or *Sihuazhong* (77.09), or *Shangchun* (77.15) and *Xiachun* (77.16). If the ulceration is multiple, bleeding *taiyang* (Extra) is the best. To make the treatment simple, bleeding *Ttaiyang* (Extra) is very effective.

6) Toothache

a. Needle *Linggu* (22.05) bilaterally, and *Cesanli* (77.22) and *Cexiasanli* (77.23) contralaterally.
b. Needling *Sihuawai* (77.14) is also effective.
c. Prick the dorsum of the foot.

Master Tung used to select many points to treat toothache. His most frequent strategy was bleeding the points located between *Xiangu* (ST43) and *Jiexi* (ST41), or the points on the dorsum of the foot along the gallbladder channel when there was inflammation. He usually punctured the points on the healthy side with filiform needles and bled the points on the diseased side, with good therapeutic effect. After that, *Linggu* (22.05) and *Cesanli* (77.22) were needled to consolidate the treatment. When using the fourteen channels, select *Neiting* (ST44) and *Zusanli* (ST36) for pain of the upper teeth, and *Hegu* (LI4) or *Sanjian* (LI3) for pain of the lower teeth. The pain of the tooth root is related to the kidney, and can therefore be treated with *Taixi* (KI3) and *Kunlun* (BL60).

There are effective herbal methods for toothache. Soak 30 grams of *Shigao* (Gypsum Fibrosum) and *Xixin* (Herba Asari) in boiling water. This is known as *Er Xin Tang* (Decoction of Two Pungent Drugs) because both ingredients are pungent. The decoction is used to rinse the mouth for an anesthetic effect. *Shigao* (Gypsum Fibrosum) is pungent and cold and has the function to clear heat from the stomach; *xixin* (Herba Asari) is pungent and warm affecting the kidney, and tonifies the kidney. 80-90% of such cases have fire in the stomach or kidney, therefore *Er Xin Tang* (Decoction of Two Pungent Drugs) is used for toothache. There is another formula used for toothache called *Yu Nu Jian* (The Jade Lady Decoction) that also clears fire from the stomach and kidney. In case of decayed teeth, treatment can include modified *Qing Wei San* (Powder for Clearing Heat from the Stomach). As previously mentioned, *Sanchasan* (A.04) is a good point for all the diseases of the five sense organs, including toothache.

6. DISEASES OF THE FACE

1) Facial Spasm (spasm and tremor)

a. Needle *Cesanli* (77.22) and *Cexiasanli* (77.23) and *Zhongjiuli* (88.25) which is actually point *Fengshi* (GB31).
b. For facial spasm, needle point *Sima* (88.17, 18, 19).
c. Needle *Wanshunyi* (22.09) and *Wanshun'er* (22.08).

2) Numbness of the Face

a. Bleed point *Sanchong* (77.07) and needle *Cesanli* (77.22) and *Cexiasanli* (77.23).
b. Unilateral facial paralysis: *Fengshi* (GB31) and *Cesanli* (77.22).

In the introduction to the facial diseases, we discussed facial spasm first, which has a larger affected area with higher frequency than twitching of the eyelid. However, both have the same treatment principle. As mentioned previously, *Wanshunyi* (22.09) and *Wanshun'er* (22.08) are very effective for these types of facial disease. Other useful points include *Cesanli* (77.22), *Cexiasanli* (77.23) and *Fengshi* (GB31) and point *Sima* (88.17, 18, 19). The indicated herbal formula is *Shao Yao Gan Cao Tang* (Decoction of Radix Paeoniae and Radix Glycyrrhizae) plus *Qian Zhen San* (Powder for Facial Paralysis) with modifications.

The facial paralysis mentioned here doesn't refer to deviation of mouth and eye. It is a kind of abnormality in sensibility of the face, a kind of dull sensation of the face. Such patients should pay attention to the prevention of apoplexy. In mild case, we needle *Cesanli* (77.22) and

Cexiasanli (77.23). For all diseases of the face, we can needle the two points contralaterally, these include: dull sensation of the face, facial spasm, zygomatic pain and trigeminal neuralgia. In severe cases, bleed *Sanchong* (77.07) because it is located between the stomach and gallbladder channels and is therefore very effective for the diseases of *yangming* and *shaoyang* channels. It is also helpful to bleed the ear apex.

3) Zygomatic Pain

a. Prick point *Sanchong* (77.07) to cause bleeding.
b. Needle *Cesanli* (77.22) and *Cexiasanli* (77.23).

In case of zygomatic pain, it is also advisable to needle *Cesanli* (77.22) and *Cexiasanli* (77.23). In severe case, bleed *Sanchong* (77.07). *Wanshunyi* (22.09) is also a good point. *Yanglingquan* (GB34) and *Houxi* (SI3) are also effective.

4) Trigeminal Neuralgia

a. Needle *Cesanli* (77.22) and *Cexiasanli* (77.23) (corresponding to *Dubi*, ST35).
b. Needle *Mudou* (66.07) and *Muliu* (66.06).
c. Needle *Dabai* (22.04).
d. Needle *Wanshunyi* (22.09) and *Wanshun'er* (22.08).
e. In chronic case, bleed *Taiyang* (Extra).

To treat trigeminal neuralgia needle *Cesanli* (77.22) and *Cexiasanli* (77.23) first. In severe cases, add *Waixiyan* (ST35). *Mudou* (66.07) and *Muliu* (66.06) are also very good, as are *Wanshunyi* (22.09), *Wanshun'er* (22.08) and especially *Dabai* (22.04). Select *Dabai* (22.04) on the healthy side as the therapeutic point and *Houxi* (SI3) on the diseased side as the guiding point, or vice versa. Both of these methods are effective. While the above groups of points have very good therapeutic effect for trigeminal neuralgia one can add *Cesanli* (77.22), *Cexiasanli* (77.23), and *Zhongjiuli* (88.25) on the leg. For very severe cases of trigeminal neuralgia, acupuncture treatment may stop the pain immediately. Bleed *Taiyang* (Extra) for severe conditions. Bleeding must be given to the diseased side while filiform needling the healthy side.

7. Diseases of the Throat

1) Fish bone in the Throat

a. Needling point *Zuqianjin* (77.24) has special effect.

Needling *Zuqianjin* (77.24) has very good therapeutic effect for fish bone in the throat. This point is considered to related to the external and internal relation between the lung and large intestine, and hence the name *Jin* (metal). Point *Jianshi* (PC5) of the pericardium channel is an important point for fish bone in the throat. It also pertains to metal according to the theory of the five elements. From this, it can be seen that Master Tung paid a lot of attention to the theory of the five elements in the use of Tung's extraordinary points.

2) Sore Throat

a. Bleed the vein on the ear back.
b. .Bleed point *Sanchong* (77.07).
c. Bleed *Zuqianjin* (77.24).
d. *Tushui'er* (22.11) and *Sanchasan* (A.04) are very effective for acute sore throat.
e. Point *Huoyin* (66.03) is very effective.

There are many points indicated for sore throat. *Sanchasan* (A.04) and *Tushui'er* (22.11) are extremely good for acute sore throat. The two points can cure a mild case in one treatment, and even a severe case may have the symptoms alleviated by 70-80%. *Sanchasan* (A.04) is an important point for exogenous diseases which are the primary cause of acute sore throat. The midpoint of *Tushui* (22.11) overlaps point *Yuji* (LU10), the *Ying*-spring point of the lung channel. *Ying*-spring and *Shu*-stream points dominate the exterior. They are therefore effective for sore throat. The combination of the two points mentioned above is very effective for the sore throat. However, in case of chronic sore throat, the best point is *Huozhu* (66.04), because the liver channel travels deeply in the throat. Sometimes sore throat is related to the kidney and *huozhu* (66.04) should be needled along the border of the bone. It is very effective for chronic sore throat related to the liver and kidney. Bleeding ear apex or ear back is also good for sore throat. It is also good for acute exogenous sore throat and can immediately stop pain.

8. Diseases of the Neck and Nape

1) Scrofula

a. Needling *Sanchong* (77.07) and *Liuwan* (66.08) on the diseased side is very effective.
b. Bleed *Sanchong* (77.07) and then needle *Chengfu* (BL36) and *Zhibian* (BL54). The effect is extremely good.

2) Enlargement of Thyroid Gland

a. Needle point *Sima* (88.17, 18, 19).
b. Needle *Zuqianjin* (77.24) and *Zuwujin* (77.25).
c. Bleed point *Sanchong* (77.07).

Scrofula is rarely seen during modern times. Master Tung used *Zhibian* (BL54) and *Chengfu* (BL36) to treat it with good results. I treated many such cases 30 years ago and few cases few years ago. Bleed

Sanchong (77.07) after needling and the therapeutic effect is improved. The ancient medical song said the point *Tianjing* (SJ10) of the triple energizer channel has the best therapeutic effect for scrofula. This consideration is also recorded in such books as *Yi Zong Jin Jian* (The Gold Mirror of Medicine), *Yu Long Ge* (The Song of Jade Dragon), *Yu Long Fu* (The Poem of Jade Dragon) and *Sheng Yu Ge* (Song More Precious than Jade). My clinical experience confirms the efficacy of *Zhibian* (BL54) and *Chengfu* (BL36).

3) Hyperthyroid Exophthalmus

a. Needle *Sima* (88.17, 18, 19).
b. Needle *Zuqianjin* (77.24) and *Zuwujin* (77.25).
c. Bleed *Sanchong* (77.07).

In the treatment of enlargement of thyroid gland, Master Tung used point *Sima* (88.17, 18, 19) the most. There is no better point. After *sima*, he selected *zuqianjin* (77.24) and *Zuwujin* (77.25). These two points are indicated in all the diseases around the neck. For neck disorders, bleeding *Sanchong* (77.07) is also very good. Needle *Sima* (88.17, 18, 19) for recent onset hyperthyroid exophthalmus. This treatment can help the eyeballs return to normal. The ancient physicians considered that "the neck and nape are the area where liver diseases happen." Needling *Sima* (88.17, 18, 19) strengthens the lung, supplements *qi* and soothes the liver.

4) Skin Diseases Around the Neck

a. Needling *Jianzhong* (44.06) is effective.
b. Needle *Sima* (88.17, 18, 19).
c. Bleed ear apex.

Point *Jianzhong* (44.06) is effective for skin diseases around the neck. *Sima* (88.17, 18, 19) are effective for all kinds of skin diseases. However, needling this point set requires special technique, which will be introduced in discussion on sternocostal diseases. Needling *Jianzhong* (44.06) or *Sima* (88.17, 18, 19) plus ear apex bleeding may have better results.

5) Stiffness of the Neck

a. Needling *Zhengjin* (77.01) and *Zhengzong* (77.02) may immediately help rotate the neck freely.
b. Needle point *Huaguyi* (55.02).
c. Needle *Shangbai* (22.03) and *Zhongbai* (22.06).

The best points for stiffness of the neck are *Zhengjin* (77.01) and *Zhengzong* (77.02). In severe case, bleeding *Weizhong* (BL40) is better. Point *Huaguyi* (55.02) is also applicable. Since it is located on the sole and needling this point is painful, *Zhengjin* (77.01) and *Zzhengzong* (77.02) may be chosen. We have introduced three groups of points here. However, that doesn't mean all points from the three groups must be selected in a single treatment. We just need to use one of the three groups. They are all effective. Usually, we introduce the most effective one first. In the points of the fourteen channels, the most effective point is *Chengjiang* (REN24). Selection of this point is based on the principle of correspondence between the anterior and posterior, using a *yin* channel point to treat disease of the *yang* channel (using Ren channel to treat Du channel). The point *Houxi* (SI3) and *Shugu* (BL65) of the hand and foot *taiyang* channels are also very good for stiffness of the neck. Both of the two points are *Shu*-stream points. *Shu*-stream points are indicated in heaviness and pain of the body and joints. They also pertain to wood in terms of the five elements. Therefore they are very effective in treatment of tendon disease. However, they are different in clinical application. As stated in Chapter 26 of *Lingshu* (Spiritual Pivot): "In case of difficult rotation of the neck, select *Houxi* (SI3); In case of difficult flexion and extension, select *Shugu* (BL65)." *Zhengjin* (77.01) and *Zhengzong* (77.02) should be selected first. However, for convenience, *Houxi* (SI3) and *Shugu* (BL65) may be selected instead. *Chengjiang* (REN24) could serve as the guiding point for either of the above two groups. Three points are therefore enough for one treatment. Both *Zhengjin* (77.01) and *Zhengzong* (77.02) are located on the ankle, corresponding to the neck in terms of holography. Moreover, the two points are on the Achilles tendon, selection of the two points follows the principle of "needling tendon to treat tendon disease." The third reason of selection of the two points is that they are connected with the urinary bladder channel and they are therefore effective for stiffness of the neck.

6) Mumps (parotitis and inflammation of sub-auricular gland)

a. Bleed the ear back.
b. Prick point *Sihuawai* (77.14) to cause bleeding.
c. Prick *Sanchong* (77.07) to cause bleeding.

Delayed treatment of mumps may lead to testitis and give rise to infertility. Some patient who were infected by the disease when they were young, have aspermia. In the treatment of this disease, first bleed the ear back and then bleed point *Sanchong* (77.07) or *Sihuawai* (77.14). The herbal formula *Pu Ji Xiao Du Yin* (Universal Decoction for Disinfection) is very effective. It is also very good to use *San Huang Er Xiang San* (Powder of Three Yellow Drugs and Two Aromatic Drugs) for topical application.

7) Pain of the Shoulder and Neck

a. Needle *Shenguan* (77.18).
b. Needle *Shenguan* (77.18) and *Sihuashang* (77.08).
c. Needle *Chongzi* (22.01) and *Chongxian* (22.02).
d. Needle *Biguan* (ST31).

Shenguan (77.18) is a frequently used point for pain of the shoulder and back, especially when the pain of the neck is involved. It is often used in combination with *Sihuashang* (77.08) for better results. Further, for the pain of the shoulder and neck, *Chongzi* (22.01) and *Chongxian* (22.02) are also very effective.

It was more than 30 years ago when Master Tung would select *Shenguan* (77.18). At that time, there was not enough attention paid to sterilization. He needled the point through clothes. Later on, he gave sterilization to the point on the clothes and then inserted the needle into the point. After work, he soaked the used needles in alcohol for the night for sterilization. From 30 years ago when there was no sterilization of the needles to 20 years ago when the needles were sterilized in pressure cooker, to 15 years ago when practitioners started the use of disposable needles, there has been great progress in clean needle technique. If the patient cannot remove his clothes, select points which don't require taking off the clothes. One of the characteristics of Tung's acupuncture it often uses points on the arms and legs. It is therefore convenient, safe, and easier to avoid accusations of sexual abuse. Blood-letting on the back is very shallow and is therefore also very safe.

8) Neck Sprain

a. Needle *Chongzi* (22.01) and *Chongxian* (22.02).
b. Needle *Zhengjin* (77.01) and *Zhengzong* (77.02).
c. Needle *Muliu* (66.06).
d. Needle *Sshangbai* (22.03) and *Zhongbai* (22.06).

Neck sprain is a common disease. We often see cases in the clinic where there is a sudden attack with impaired neck rotation and pain referring to the shoulder and back. For the treatment, we first select either *Chongzi* (22.01) or *Chongxian* (22.02) and then needle *Chengjiang* (REN24). The therapeutic effect is very good. If the pain affects the neck, *Chongxian* (22.02) is better, and if the pain affects the shoulder, *Chongzi* (22.01) is better. If the pain affects both the neck and shoulder severely, select both points plus *Chengjiang* (REN24). Ask the patient to exercise their neck while stimulating the point with the needle for immediate and improved results. Patients who come to the clinic on the same day of an attack often get complete relief immediately following treatment. Even if the patients come to the clinic two to three days after attack, the pain can be relieved 80% in the first treatment. Other points that can support and assist including, *Zhengjin* (77.01) and *Zhengzong* (77.02). Moreover, the simultaneous use of *Muliu* (66.06), *Shangbai* (22.03) and *Zhongbai* (22.06) are also very effective. In the clinical practice, needling *Chongzi* (22.01) or *Chongxian* (22.02) are usually enough. As for herbal medicine, many physicians like to use *Gui Zhi Jia Ge Gen Tang* (Decoction of Ramuulus Cinnamomi and Radix Puerariae). But the therapeutic effect is not good enough since the formula is for the *taiyang* channel. Many patients with neck sprain have pain on the shoulder, especially at point *Jianjing* (GB21) which belongs to *shaoyang* channel. Therefore the treatment should cover *shaoyang* channel as well, therefore the formula must be modified. The therapeutic effect is improved by adding *Chaihu* (Radix Bupleuri). The pain at *Jianjing* (GB21) will not likely disappear without adding *Chaihu* (Radix Bupleuri). The results are improved further by adding drugs that dispel wind such as *Qianghuo* (Rhizoma seu Radix Notopterygii) and *Fangfeng* (Radix Ledebouriellae). One or two doses may completely cure a case. If the patient doesn't care for acupuncture, they can be quickly cured with herbal medicine. Combining acupuncture and herbal medicine provides the most reliable and expedient outcome.

3. Question: What is the location and indication for *Huagu* (55.02, 03, 04, 05)?

Answer: *Huaguyi* (55.02) is located between the great and second toes and is indicated in diseases of the face and neck; *Huagu'er* (55.03) is located between the second and third toes and is indicated in diseases of the shoulder and back; *Huagusan* (55.04) is located between the third and fourth toes and is indicated in pain of the waist; and *Huagusi* (55.05) is located between the fourth and fifth toes and is often used to treat sciatica. The indications for these points are more or less associated with holography. Once you understand holography, it is easy to understand the mechanism of their indications.

4. Question: What is the mechanism for the treatment of skin diseases?

Answer: Treatment of skin diseases is first based on the combined principles of "needling the skin for skin diseases and needle the muscle for muscular diseases." The location of skin is very extensive and the points located on big area are therefore often selected. Second, the points located on rich muscles such as *Quchi* (LI11), *Shousanli* (LI10), *Hegu* (LI4), *Sima* (88.17, 18, 19) and *Jianzhong* (44.06) are often related to *yangming* channels. Almost all these points are points of *yangming* channels, which have ample *qi* and blood and therefore are effective in regulating *qi* and blood, thus the therapeutic effect in treating skin diseases.

Tung's extraordinary points are not ordinary extra points which are separated from each other, rather, they are symmetrical points listed together with the points of the fourteen channels in parallel. They are also based upon systematic theory. I have spent a great deal of effort studying the *Neijing* (Yellow Emperor's Inner Classic), *Yi Jing* (The Book of Change) and many other classic canons of traditional Chinese medicine. This experience has helped me to develop and create effective theories based upon the application of Tung's extraordinary points. A good command of the points of the fourteen channels will help one to understand Tung's extraordinary points, similarly to the relationship between the *Shang Han Lun* (Treatise on Febrile Diseases) and *Wen Bing Tiao Bian* (Treatise on Differentiation and Treatment of Epidemic Febrile Diseases). If you have a good knowledge of *Shang Han Lun* (Treatise on Febrile Diseases) prescriptions, then you will be good at *Wen Bing* (Epidemic Febrile Diseases). However, *Wen Bing* (Epidemic Febrile Diseases) has its own theoretical system. In the treatment of febrile diseases, on the top of clearing heat, emphasis is mainly put on nourishing *yin*. While in *Shang Han Lun* (Treatise on Febrile Diseases), emphasis is less on nourishing *yin* and more on strengthening *yang*. The question is: which is the main contraindication? Historically, *Wen* Bing was a very small branch of practice. Only in the *Qing* Dynasty, did it become one of the major therapeutic systems in Chinese medicine. Tung's extraordinary points had similar circumstances. So also, Master Tung's system of extraordinary points was handed down for generations before he made it public. He contributed to the theory, quickening the development of the system and the therapeutic effects have been rapid and better.

5. Question: Would you like to talk something about the use of herbal prescriptions in treatment of headache?

Answer: Headache is a common disease in the clinic. There are various forms of acute and chronic headaches; however, they are generally divided into two categories, exogenous and endogenous. The exogenous headache is mostly caused by pathogenic wind. Since Chapter 5 of *Shu Wen* "Wind is liable to affect the upper part of the body first," headaches are often considered to be caused by pathogenic wind. When such headaches occur, the pathogenic wind often combines with cold blocking the channels and collaterals, heat disturbing the head, or damp suppressing the misting of *yang*. For headache due to wind, we can use *Ma Huang Gui Zhi Tang* (Decoction of Herba Ephedrae and Ramulus Cinnamomi) or *Jing Fang Bai Du San* (Antiphlogistic Powder of herba Schizonepetae and Radix Potentillae) according to the symptoms and signs of wind cold or heat; if the headache is intermittent with attacks due to exposure in wind and cold and severe pain during attacks, use *Chuan Xiong Cha Tiao San* (Powder of Rhizoma Ligustici Chuanxiong, to be taken together with tea) as the main prescription. In case of headache due to wind heat the attack of which is often induced by heat or sunshine, use modified *Sang Ju Yin* (Decoction of Folium Mori and Flos Chrysanthemi). In case of headache due to wind damp which is characterized by heaviness in the head like being wrapped by a piece of cloth, heaviness of the limbs and poor appetite, use *Qiang Huo Sheng Shi Tang* (Decoction of Notopterygium for Eliminating Damp) to dispel wind and eliminate damp.

The endogenous headache is usually caused by pathological changes of the liver, kidney and spleen, or disharmony of *qi* and blood. Pathomechanisms include dysfunction of the liver in maintaining free flow of *qi* due to excessive emotional changes. This leads to stagnation of the liver *qi* which transforms into heat, producing liver fire which travels upward attacking the head. Constitutional deficiency of liver and kidney *yin* may give rise to hyperactivity of the liver *yang* causing headache; Post-partum blood deficiency or massive bleeding due to any reason may lead to a failure of blood moving upward to nourish the brain; this gives rise to headache or dizziness. Headaches may also be cause by constitutional obesity or spleen dysfunction with regard to transformation and transportation may produce phlegm in the interior that prevents the clear *yang* from ascending. Further, blood stasis due to traumatic injury or prolonged headache may cause block the channels and collaterals and giving rise to headaches, which are characterized by repeated attacks in a fixed location. In case of headache due to wind and damp, use *Ban Xia Bai Zhu Tian Ma Tang* (Decoction of Rhizoma Pinelliae, Rhizoma Atractylodis Macrocephalae and Rhizoma Gastrodiae) with modification. For headaches due to liver *yang* uprising, use *Tian Ma Gou Teng Yin* (Decoction of Rhizoma Gastrodiae and Ramulus Uncariae cum Uncis) with modification. If the headache is due to blood stasis, use *Xue Fu Zhu Yu Tang* (Decoction for Removing Blood Stasis in the Chest). In my practice, I often use *Xuanfuhua* (Flos Inulae), *Daizheshi* (Ochra Haematitum), *Xiangfu* (Rhizoma Cyperi), *Heshouwu* (Radix Polygoni Multiflori), *Quanxie* (Scorpio) and *Jiangcan* (Bombyx Bytryticatus) combined with *Si Wu Tang* (Decoction of Four Ingredients) to treat headache as the sequela of traffic accident or cerebral concussion and have obtained good therapeutic effect.

Generally speaking, headaches with short duration and severe persistent attacks are usually caused by exogenous pathogenic factors. In this case, we should differentiate whether it is wind cold, wind heat or wind damp. If the duration is long and the headaches are mild and intermittent, then differentiate between deficiency of *yin* with hyperactivity of *yang*, deficiency of *qi* and blood, or phlegm damp and blood stasis. There are also many cases of headache with long duration and nausea and vomiting when the pain is severe, which is known as *jueyin* headache in Chinese medicine and it could be treated successfully with modified *Wu Zhu Yu Tang* (Decoction of Fructus Euodiae). There is another headache which is often induced by noise; it is known as “headache due to restlessness.” It can be treated effectively with *Bu Zhong Yi Qi Tang* (Decoction for Strengthening Spleen and Supplementing Qi) modified by *manjingzi* (Fructus Viticis).

I often treat headaches according to syndrome differentiation of diseased channels. *Yangming* headaches are often located in the front of the head and supraorbital area and should be treated with modified *Xuan Qi Tang* (Decoction of Selected Special Ingredients) from the book *Dong Huan Shi Xiao Fang* (Dong Huan’s Empirical Prescriptions); *shaoyang* headaches are often located on the temporal side of the head radiating to the ear, and I often treat it with modified *San Pian Tang* (Decoction for Treating Temporal Headache) of the book *Bian Zheng Lu* (Essential Collections of Syndrome Differentiation) written by Chen Shiduo. This prescription is very effective for migraine and trigeminal neuralgia; *jueyin* headaches are located on the vertex possibly radiating to the eyes (in severe case there might be nausea and vomiting) and is treated with *Wu Zhu Yu Tang* (Decoction of Fructus Euodiae) with modification; *taiyang* headaches are located at the occipital area radiating to the nape with local muscular tension. I often treat this kind of headache with *Yue Ju Wan* (Pills for Relieving Stagnancy) modified with *Shaoyao* (Radix Paeoniae), *Gancao* (Radix Glycyrrhizae), *Baijili* (Fructus Tribuli) and *Juemingzi* (Semen Cassiae).

In the treatment of headache, I often add some wind-dispelling drugs such as *Baizhi* (Radix Angelicae Dahuricae), *Chuanxiong* (Rhizoma Ligustici Chuanxiong), *Jingjie* (Herba Schizonepetae), *Gaoben* (Rhizoma Ligustici), *Qianghuo* (Rhizoma seu Radix Notopterygii), *Manjingzi* (Fructus Viticis), *Baijili* (Fructus Tribuli) and *Tianma* (Rhizoma Gastrodiae), because these drugs may bring other drugs directly up to the head to stop pain (among them Chuanxiong is most commonly used). Since these drugs are pungent, warm, aromatic and dry, additional drugs for regulating blood should be added in the long time use or use of big dosage.

The Principle of the Open, Close and Pivot, and the Extraordinary Connections of *Zangfu*

If you are interested in the study on "the Four Designs and Eight Trigrams," it would be very helpful to your clinical practice. My studies on *Yi Jing* (The Book of Changes) and the Heaven Stems and Earth Branches have been very beneficial in my learning of Tung's extraordinary points. The theory of the five elements in particular is very closely related to traditional Chinese medicine.

Many of my students have gone deeply into studies on *Yi Jing* and some of them are outstanding. Some have become very famous in Taiwan and Japan. Since it is helpful to the clinical practice, I have also written some books. The study on *yin-yang* and the eight trigrams is very helpful to the clinical practice. For instance, the theory of the open, close and pivot is very closely related to the theory of *Yi Jing*. To help you more easily understand the theory of this theory, here I'd like to talk about the relationship between *Yi Jing* and the meridians.

In acupuncture, the location, running direction, nature determination and listing order of the meridians are all closely related to the theory of *Yi Jing*.

1. The Old Eight Trigrams and the Locations of *Zangfu* and Meridians.

The book "*Xi Ci*" says: "*Taiji* gives rise to transformation and produces the two forms, namely *yin* and *yang*. The primeval pair produce the four symbols, from which are derived the eight trigrams." This is the source of the old eight trigrams which is illustrated as follow (Illustration 1):

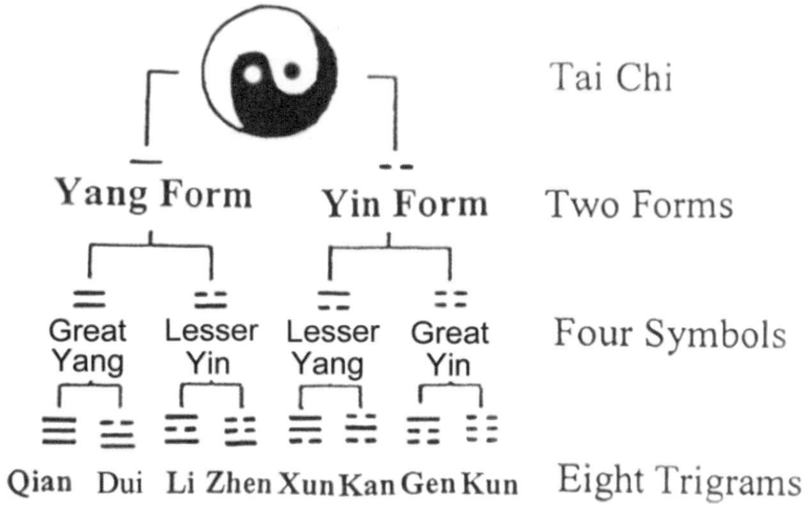

Illustration 1 — The Old Eight Trigrams

Then, based upon what is said in the book *Shuo Gua* (Talk on the Eight Trigrams): "The heaven and the earth (*Qian* and *Kun*) fix the location; the mountain and the marsh (*Gen* and *Dui*) ventilate *qi*; the thunder and the wind (*Zhen* and *Sun*) fight with each other; and the water and the fire (*Kan* and *Li*) are incompatible," the eight trigrams are located as follows:

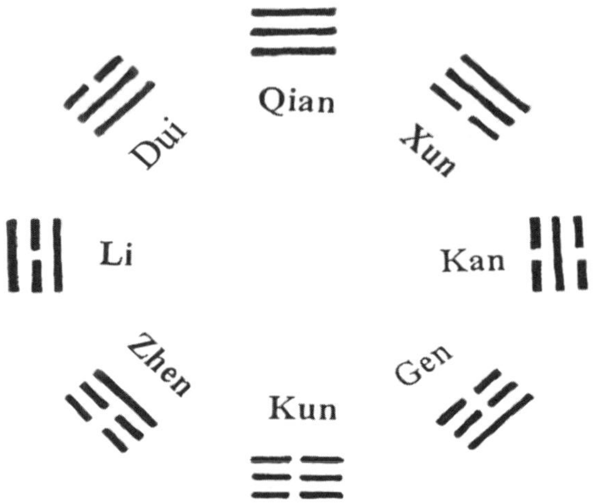

Illustration 2 — The Orientation of the Eight Trigrams

In the correspondence of *zangfu* to the eight trigrams, the trigram *Qian* corresponds to *Taiyang* (*yang* within *yang*) and is the extreme of *yang*. It dominates DU meridian that governs all the *yang* meridians. *Kun* corresponds to *Taiyin* (*yin* within *yin*) and is the extreme of *yin*. It dominates REN meridian that governs all the *yin* meridians. The other *zangfu* organs pertain to the rest of the trigrams according to their nature (see Illustration 3). The trigram *Dui* pertains to metal, the lung and large intestine also pertain to metal, and the lung and large intestine therefore correspond to *Dui*. The trigram *Li* pertains to fire, the heart and small intestine also pertains to fire. The heart and small intestine therefore correspond to *Li*. The trigram *Xun* pertains to wood and dominates wind, and the liver and gallbladder also pertain to wood. The liver and gallbladder therefore correspond to *Xun*. The trigram *Kan* pertains to water, the kidney and urinary bladder also pertain to water. The kidney and urinary bladder therefore correspond to *Kan*. The trigram *Gen* pertains to earth, the spleen and stomach also pertain to earth. The spleen and stomach therefore correspond to *Gen*. The pericardium and *Sanjiao* correspond to the trigram *Zhen* since it is the fire of the dragon and thunder and the pericardium and *Sanjiao* are the minister fire. Thus, the left three, *Dui*, *Li* and *Zhen*, are *yang* trigrams and dominate the hand meridians; the right three, *Xun*, *Kan* and *Gen*, are *yin* trigrams and dominate foot meridians. Thus, the following correspondence is formed:

1) The lung and large intestine (*Dui*, marsh) correspond to the spleen and stomach (*Gen*, mountain); 2) The heart and small intestine (*Li*, fire) correspond to the kidney and urinary bladder (*Kan*, water); 3) The pericardium and *Sanjiao* (*Zhen*, thunder) correspond to the liver and gallbladder (*Xun*, wind); 4) The DU meridian (*Qian*, heaven) corresponds to REN meridian (*Kun*, earth).

In addition to the REN and DU extraordinary meridians that form a circle, the 12 regular meridians have formed three small systems: the system of the lung, large intestine, spleen and stomach, the system of the heart, small intestine, kidney and urinary bladder and the system of the pericardium, *Sanjiao*, liver and gallbladder. The fact is that the 12 regular meridians form a major circulatory system under which there are 3 minor circulatory systems. Each trigram corresponds to one zang and one *fu* organs that pertain to yin and yang respectively and are externally-internally related to each other.

Dui (metal) LU, LI ☱	**Qian (metal)** DU ☰	**Xun (wood)** GB, LV ☴
Li (fire) HT, SI ☲		**Kan (water)** UB, KD ☵
Zhen (wood) PC, SJ ☳	**Kun (earth)** REN ☷	**Gen (earth)** ST, SP ☶

Illustration 3

2. THE OLD EIGHT TRIGRAMS AND THE NATURE OF THE SIX MERIDIANS

The names of *Taiyin* (Greater *Yin*), *Shaoyin* (Lesser *Yin*), *Taiyang* (Greater *Yang*) and Shaoyang (Lesser *Yang*) first appeared in the book *Yi Jing*, and *Jueyin* and *Yangming* in the book *Neijing* (The Yellow Emperor's Inner Classic). *Tai* (greater) and *Shao* (lesser) imply quantity and changes, which were used by the ancient people to understand the world. It influenced the book *Neijing* and its theory was used to study the human body. With the theory, the trunk is divided into three parts: the chest, back and lateral aspect, and the four limbs are also divided into three parts: the medial, lateral and middle. *Yangming* and *Jueyin* were put forward in the *Neijing* probably according the theory of *yin* and *yang* and local anatomical characteristics.

The natural occurrence of the six meridians in *Taiyang*, *Shaoyang*, *Taiyin*, *Shaoyin*, *Jueyin* and *Yangming* is more easily understood with the theory of *Yi Jing*. Now let's unfold this in the order of the old eight trigrams: *Qian*, *Dui*, *Li*, *Zhen*, *Xun*, *Kan*, *Gen* and *Kun* (see Illustration 4). *Qian* dominates DU meridian and *Kun* dominates REN meridian. The two are both extraordinary meridians and they do not pertain to any *zangfu* organs. The others are listed according to the *yang* trigrams (*Dui*, *Li* and *Zhen* with *zang* in the front) and *yin* trigrams (*Xun*, *Kan* and *Gen* with *fu* in the front) (the order contains balance of *yin* and *yang*). Then connect the *zang* and *zang*, *fu* and *fu* that are classified into the same trigrams. The result is that the lung and spleen are connected as *zang* organs and they correspond to *yin* trigrams; the large intestine and stomach are connected as *fu* organs and they correspond to *yang* trigrams; the heart and kidney are connected as *zang* organs; the small intestine and urinary bladder are connected as *fu* organs; the heart and pericardium are connected as *zang* organs; the *Sanjiao* and gallbladder are connected as *fu* organs. Finally list all the mentioned above according to the order of *yin* and *yang* on the right side (see Illustration 4 and 5). These illustrations can be seen in many books. However, there has been no more exploration and development.

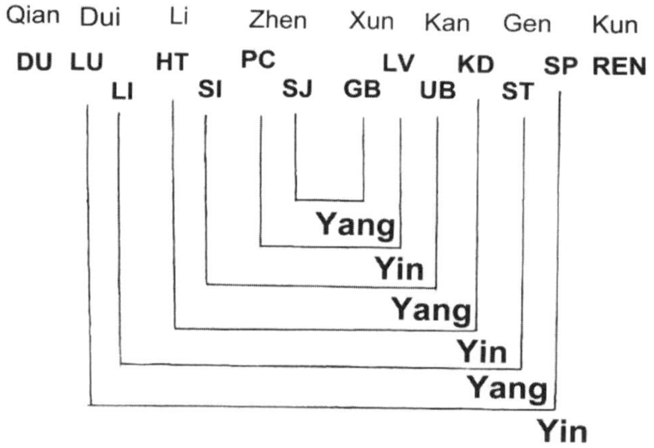

Illustration 4

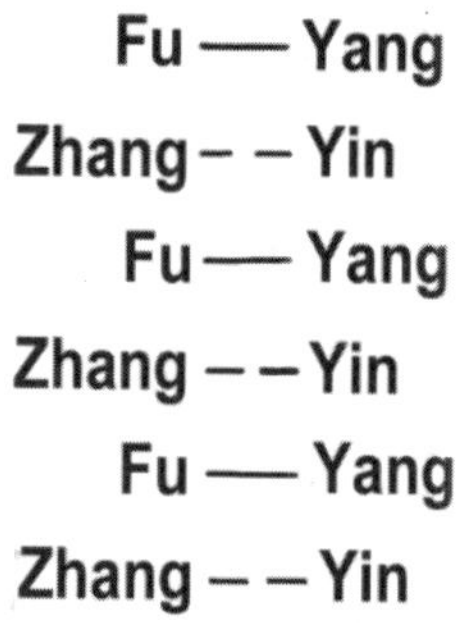

Illustration 5

When we explore the theory deeply, we have found it is very much related to the nature determination of the *zangfu* organs. This divination symbol exactly shows the fire (☲) is in the upper and water (☵) in the lower, like the human body with the heart in the upper and the kidney in the lower. The heaven and earth take *Qian* and *Kun* to fix the locations while the human body takes the fire and water to fix the locations. This divinatory symbol (Illustration 5) has six trigrams. According to the *qi* of *yin* and *yang*, earth and heaven in ascending and descending, *yang qi* increases when it descends and the uppermost *yang* is *Shaoyang*, and then *Taiyang*. The lowest *yang* trigram comes from merging of two *yang* is thus called *Yangming*. *Yin qi* decreases when it ascends. The lowest *yin* trigram is *Taiyin*, and then *Shaoyin*. The uppermost yin comes from mergence of two vanished *yin* and is thus called *Yueyin*. In this way the three *yin* and three *yang* are formed (see Illustration 6). Attach the *yin-yang* properties of the six trigrams to the Illustration 4, and the *yin-yang* properties of the *zangfu* organs are thus determined. That is, the lung and spleen are *Taiyin*, the large intestine and stomach are *Yangming*, the heart and kidney are *Shaoyin*, the small intestine and urinary bladder are *Taiyang*, the liver and pericardium are *Jueyin*, and *Sanjiao* and Gallbladder are *Shaoyang* (see Illustration 7).

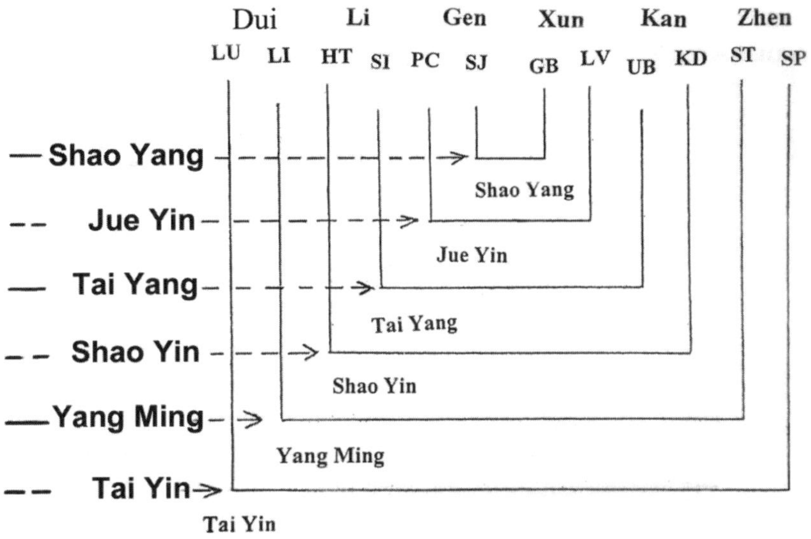

Illustration 6

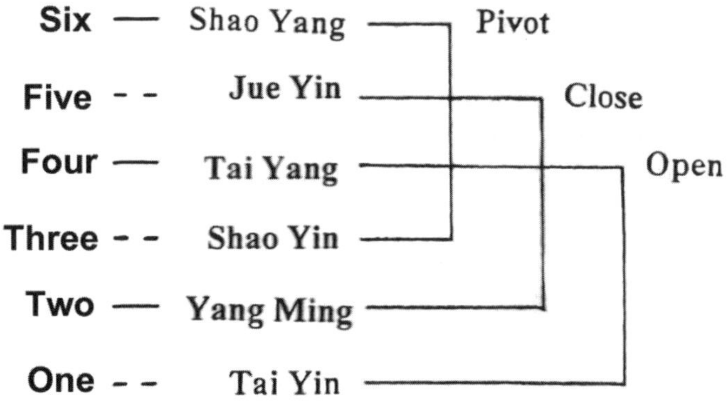

Illustration 7 — The Open, Close and Pivot of the Six Meridians

3. Open, Close and Pivot, and the Running Directions of the Meridians (As Well as Extraordinary Connections of *Zangfu*)

According the theory of *yin-yang* in inter-dependence, the theory of open, close and pivot of three *yin* and three *yang* meridians was put forward in the *Neijing* (*Yellow Emperor's Inner Classic*). It says in Chapter 6 of *Suwen* (Essential Questions): "In regard to the three *yang* meridians, *Taiyang* is the open, *Yangming* is the close and *Shaoyang* is the pivot; In regard to the three *yin* meridians, *Taiyin* is the open, *Jueyin* is the close and *Shaoyin* is the pivot." The concept of open and close originates booking the *Yi Jing*: "The close corresponds to *Kun*. The open corresponds to *Qian*. One open and one close form a change. Constant change gives rise to transformation."

According to the *Yi Jing*, the interrelationships of six divinatory symbols have certain correspondences. There is a correspondence between the first and the fourth, the second and the fifth, and the third and the upper (sixth). It can be seen that such correspondences exist in the opposite divinatory symbols and do not exist in the two that are the same in nature. The correspondence indicates dynamic harmony and unity of the two opposite aspects in one thing. Moreover, in the double divinations, the first and the fourth divinatory symbols occupy the same position, so do the second and fifth, and the third and sixth. This is because the first divinatory symbol is in the lower position of the lower divination, and the fourth divinatory symbol is in the lower position of the upper divination; the second divinatory symbol is in the middle position of the lower divination, and the fifth divinatory symbol is in the middle position of the upper divination; the third divinatory symbol is in the upper position of the lower divination, and the sixth divinatory symbol is in the upper position of the upper divination.

In the above introduced three *yin* and three *yang* symbolized by fire and water, *Taiyin* and *Taiyang* are in the lower and outmost position of the upper and lower divinations, pertaining to "Open;" *Yangming* and *Jueyin* are in the middle position of the lower and upper divinations, pertaining to "Close;" and *Shaoyang* and *Shaoyin* are in the upper position of the upper and lower divinations, all pertaining to "Pivot." This kind of correspondence (one *yin* and one *yang* that are in the same position, as shown in Illustration 7) indicates the harmony and unity between the first and fourth, second and fifth, and third and sixth divinatory symbols in the nature and movement, and this theory has been applied to explain the physiological activities and pathological changes.

Among the three *yin* and three *yang*, the first divinatory symbol of the lower divination *Taiyin* and the first divinatory symbol of the upper divination *Taiyang* occupy the outmost position, and therefore dominate "Open," including the urinary bladder meridian of foot-*taiyang*, the small intestine meridian of hand-*taiyang*, the lung meridian of hand-*taiyin* and the spleen meridian of foot-*taiyin*. When the pathological cold invades the human body, it affects *Taiyin* first, occupies the outmost position. Cold is a yin pathogenic factor and is liable to affect the lower part, and foot-*taiyang* is therefore affected first. That is why the urinary bladder meridian is discussed first in the book *Shang Han Lun* (Treatise on Attack by Cold). Heat is a *yang* pathogenic factor, and is liable to injure *yin* first. Since pathogenic *yang* often comes from the upper and it therefore affects the lung meridian of hand-*taiyin* first. Since *Taiyin* and *Taiyang* are often injured first by exogenous pathogenic factors, they are therefore considered as "Open." The upper divinatory symbols of both the upper and lower divinations are the places where changes happen. The upper divinatory symbols of both the upper and lower divinations *Shaoyang* and *Shaoyin* are all called as places of "Pivot." *Shaoyang* is located between the exterior and interior and their syndrome is characterized by alternation of chills and fever. However, this syndrome could have predominance of either the exterior or the interior. For example, *Xiao Chai Hu Tang* (Minor Decoction of Radix Bupleuri) is indicated in *Shaoyang* syndrome, but *Chai Hu Gui Zhi Tang* (Decoction of Radix Bupleuri and Ramulus Cinnamomi) is used for *Shaoyang* syndrome with predominance of the exterior, and *Da Chai Hu Tang* (Major Decoction of Radix Bupleuri) and *Chai Hu Jia Long Mu Tang* (Decoction of Radix Bupleuri plus Os Draconis and Choncha Ostreae) are used for *Shaoyang* syndrome with predominance of the interior. *Shaoyin* syndrome has the tendency of transformation into either cold or heat syndrome. When it transforms into a cold syndrome, we should use *Si Ni Tang* (Decoction for Resuscitation) and *Zhen Wu Tang* (Decoction for Warming *Yang* and Eliminating Water). When it transforms into a heat syndrome, we should use *Huang Lian E Jiao Tang* (Decoction of Rhizoma Coptidis and Colla Corii Asini), etc. *Yangming* and *Jueyin* are all middle divinations and imply the significance of "Close." In case of attack by cold when the *yang* goes to its extreme and affects *Yangming*, it gives rise to severe condition with such manifestations as floccitation and failure to recognize people; when the *yin* goes to its extreme and affects *Jueyin*, it gives rise to syncope. In case of febrile diseases, when the pathogenic heat goes into the pericardium meridian of hand-*jueyin*, it gives rise to coma; when it goes into the foot-*jueyin* meridian, it stirs up the internal wind. All these are critical conditions at the late stage of a disease that has affected the "Close" layer, manifesting the mental symptoms.

Then, how do "Open," "Pivot" and "Close" affect the meridians? Try to make a loose fist (see Illustration 8) like *Taiji*, you may find "Open," "Pivot" and "Close" are connected one another. Let's look at *Shaoshang* (LU11) and *Shaoze* (SI1) first. One is from *Taiyin* meridian and the other is from *Taiyang* meridian, they are both listed as "Open." *Guanchong* (SJ1) is a point on the *Shaoyang* meridian and *Shaochong* (HT9) is a point on the *Shaoyin* meridian, they are listed together as "Pivot." *Zhongchong* (PC1) is a point on the *Jueyin* meridian and *Shangyang* (LI1) is a point on the *Yangming* meridian, they are listed together as "Close." Thus there forms the law of movement through "Opening," "Pivoting" and "Closing." From the outmost *Taiyang* to move inward, it comes to *Shaoyang* and finally reaches *Yangming*. When *yang* vanishes, yin starts to grow in the order of *Taiyin*, *Shaoyin* and finally *Jueyin*. When the fingers are extended, the interrelationships of the "Open," "Pivot" and "Close" are as shown in Illustration 9.

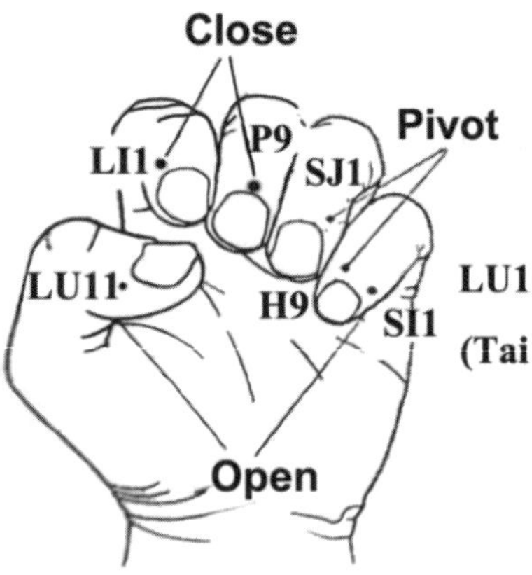

Illustration 8

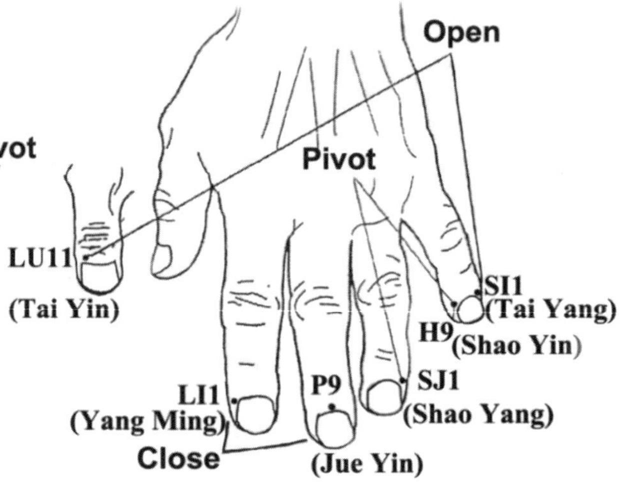

Illustration 9

Extending the sole of the foot, it becomes curved, *Taiyang* is neighbored with *Taiyin*, and *Jueyin* is neighbored with *Yangming*. Once one Japanese practitioner took *yongquan* (KI1) to do a temperature test, he used *neizhiyin* (medial *zhiyin*) that is located between *Zhiyin* (BL67) and *Zuqiaoyin* (GB44) to replace *Zhiyin* (BL67). In this way, *Shaoyang* and *Shaoyin* are also closely neighbored (see Illustration 10).

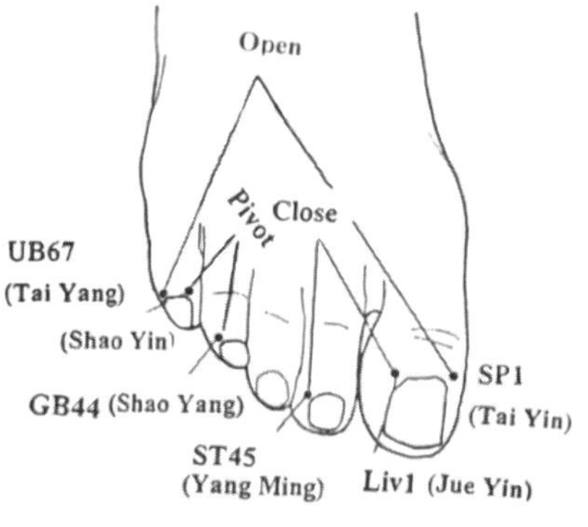

Illustration 10

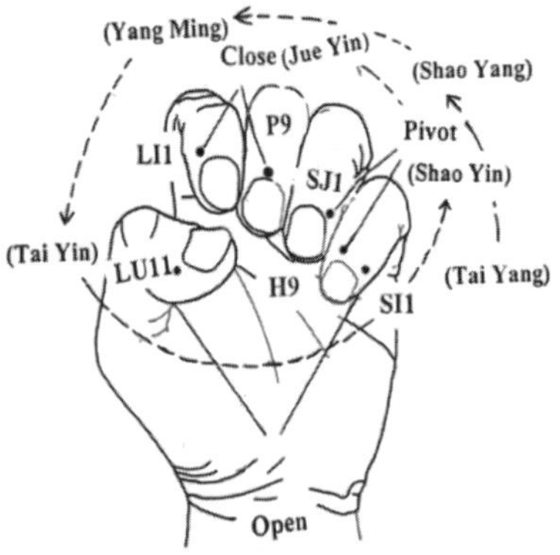

Illustration 11

These concepts are the bases for the meridian courses and distributions locations in the *Neijing* (Yellow Emperor's Inner Classic) (see Illustrations 9 and 10). They conform to what is in Chapter 10 of *Suwen* (Essential Questions): "*Yangming* is anterior to *Taiyin*," and "*Shaoyin* is posterior to *Taiyin*, and *Jueyin* is anterior to *Shaoyin*." The three *yang* meridians are on the *yang* aspect of the body, and the three *yin* meridians are on the *yin* aspect of the body. Then, according to *yang* determinants (*Dui*, *Li* and *Zhen* derived from *Taiyang* and *Shaoyang*), the lung and large intestine (*Dui*), heart and small intestine (*Li*), and pericardium and *Sanjiao* (*Zhen*) meridians are distributed on the upper limbs. According to the *yin* determinants (*Xun*, *Kan* and *Gen* derived from *Taiyin* and *Shaoyang*), the liver and gallbladder (*Xun*), kidney and urinary bladder (*Kan*), and spleen and stomach meridians are distributed on the lower limbs (see Illustrations 1 and 2). Besides, according to the principle of *yin* ascending and *yang* descending, the meridians originate from or terminate at the tip of finger. For example, the *Taiyang* meridian runs along the lateral side of *yang* aspect of the small finger, and *Shaoyang* meridian runs along the midline of the ring finger. On the analogy of this, other meridians are distributed following the same way.

The clockwise distribution of the "Open," "Pivot" and "Close" on the fist conforms to the transmission of diseases of the six meridians introduced in *Shang Han Lun* (Treatise on Attack by Cold), that is, from *Taiyang* to *Shaoyang*, *Yangming*, *Taiyin*, *Shaoyin* and finally to *Jueyin*. (see Illustration 11)

Every time we discuss the theory of "Open," "Pivot" and "Close," there is a question about *Shaoyin* or *Jueyin* as the "Pivot." There is no such sentence stating that the "*Jueyin* is the pivot" in *Nei jing* (Yellow Emperor's Inner Classic). Later physicians made the *Jueyin* a pivot based upon its interior-exterior relationship to the *Shaoyang*. Moreover, the *Jueyin* syndrome may have alternation of chills and fever, and they took *Jueyin* as a pivot incorrectly. It has been previously introduced in this book that "*Shaoyin* serves as the pivot and *Jueyin* as the close." The details were listed by taking the sequence of meridians as an example. To make it more clearly, I'd like to give you further explanation using the locations of the *Shaoyin* and *Jueyin*.

According to the classic literature and symptoms and signs, *yang* deficiency of *Shaoyin* (heart and kidney) is critical. It's easy to understand this according to the classical theory. However, if we read classical literature such as the *Shang Han Lun* carefully, it may be found that the dying syndromes appear more in *Jueyin* than in *Shaoyin*. That is to say, the *Jueyin* disease is more critical than *Shaoyin* disease. The critical cold syndrome of *Shaoyin* is often complicated with syncope and spasm of *Jueyin*. For instance, "when fading pulse resulted from attack by cold (due to *yang* deficiency of *Shaoyin*) lasts for 7-8 days, there appears constant restlessness (syncope of *Jueyin* known as viscera shock (*Zang Jue*)." From this, we can see *Jueyin* is affected after *Shaoyin*. The Chapter 3 of book *Wen Bing Tiao Bian* (Treatise on Differentiation and Treatment of Epidemic Febrile Diseases) says: "When pathogenic heat goes deeply into either *Shaoyin* or *Jueyin*, treatment should be focused on activating the pulse." The author Wu Jutong gave an annotation regarding this: "Since pathogenic heat greatly consumes *yin*, *Shaoyin* (kidney) stores essence and *Jueyin* relies on sufficiency essence of *Shaoyin*, the two meridians may all help restore the pulse. They have the same origin." It clearly points out that *Shaoyin* is in front of *Jueyin* and gives influence to *Jueyin*. For this reason, *Shaoyin* becomes the pivot.

4. The Later Eight Trigrams and the Circulation (order) of Meridian System

The order of circulation in the meridian system is familiar to the practitioner. However, it is still necessary to devote time and energy to the study of the abstract meridians. I seriously studied the *Yi Jing* (Book of Changes) at Beijing University where I obtained my Ph.D. degree, with doctoral studies on the *Shang Han Lun* (Treatise on Fabrile Diseases), I also took a doctoral level studies on meridians and collaterals at the University of Chinese and Western Medicines. Here I'd like to share some of those experiences.

We mentioned the old eight trigrams have influenced the location, nature and direction of the meridians. Besides, the listing order of the meridians is also related to the later eight trigrams. Let's look at the old eight trigrams and the illustration of *Luo Shu Jiu Gong Tu* (Illustration of Luo Shu) (see Illustrations 12, 13 and 14), in which the sum of all the numbers on a straight line in all directions is 15.

In the medical book excavated from *Ma Wang Dui* tomb, the meridians were not inter-connected. In the book *Yin Yang Shi Yi Jiu Mai* (The Eleven Yin and Yang Meridians for Moxibustion) and the book *Shou Zu Shi Yi Jiu Mai* (The Eleven Hand and Foot Meridians for Moxibustion), the meridians were not listed in fixed order. However, in *Lingshu* (Spiritual Pivot), the order of the meridians in circulation was already completed. Since the circulation theory was derived from the influence of *Yi Jing* (Book of Changes), the order of the meridians in circulation is closely related to the later eight trigrams, in which the key number is 9. The divinatory locations of the later trigrams are listed below: the upper is *Li*, the lower is *Kan*, the upper left is *Xun*, the left is *Zhen*, the lower left is *Gen*, the upper right is *Kun*, the right is *Dui* and the lower right is *Qian*. Since the Ren and Du meridians are not involved in the circulation of the 12 regular meridians, they are isolated from the 12 regular meridian

Xun (wood) Earth within wood **LV** ☴ Chen, si	**Li (fire)** **HT, SI** ☲ Wu	**Kun (earth)** Earth within fire **PC, SJ** ☷ Wei, shen
Zhen (wood) **GB** ☳ Mao		**Dui (metal)** **LI** ☱ You
Gen (earth) Earth within water **ST, SP** ☶ Yin, chou	**Kan (water)** **UB, KD** ☵ Zi	**Qian (metal)** Earth within metal **LU** ☰ Xu, hai

Illustration 12

systems. Try to list the positions of *zangfu* organs according to the properties of the five elements in the later eight trigrams. *Kan* and *Li* pertain to water and fire, and therefore the kidney and urinary bladder that pertain to water are listed in the position of *Kan* (1), and the heart and small intestine that pertain to fire are listed in the position of *Li* (9). Both metal and wood have two positions each in the later trigrams. Since both liver and gallbladder pertain to wood, they are located in the positions of *Zhen* and *Xun*. The lung and large intestine pertain to metal and they are located in the positions of *Dui* and *Qian*. However, the liver pertains to the wood of *yin* nature, and the gallbladder pertains to the wood of *yang* nature. According to the divinatory number of the later trigrams (the number of Luo Shu, the origin of *Yi Jing*, see Illustrations 13 and 14), the wood of *yang* nature, the gallbladder, is fixed in the position of *Zhen* (3), and the wood of *yin* nature, the liver, is fixed in the position of *Xun* (4). According to the same principle, lung, the metal of *yin* nature, is fixed in the position of *Qian* (6), while large intestine, the metal of *yang* nature, is fixed in the position of *Dui* (yang number of 7). Such distribution conforms to the distribution of the meridians on the hand in Illustration 4: in the hand meridians (*yang* determinants) *zang* are in the front; in the foot meridians (*yin* determinants) *fu* are in the rear. The earth has two divinatory positions with the spleen and stomach fixed respectively in *Gen* and *Kun*; however, the pericardium and triple energizer do not have stable positions. According to the theory of *Jiu Xing Liu Nian* (Nine Stars and Fortune), when it comes to the number "5," *Yang* will be fixed in the position of 2 and *yin* in the position of 8. The other elements metal, water, wood and fire do not have such parasitism. The spleen and stomach meridians are distributed in the lower part of the body, pertaining to *yin*, and are therefore parasitized in the position of 8, while the pericardium and triple energizer are parasitized in the position of 2 which is *Kun*. *Kun* is the earth in the fire. The pericardium and triple energizer contain minister fire and are positioned in *Kun*, conforming to its five-element property. According to the order from 1 to 9 mentioned above (position 5 is replaced by position 2 and 8), the order of internal organs in circulation is as follow: 1. urinary bladder and kidney – 2. pericardium and triple energizer – 3. gallbladder – 4. liver – 6. lung – 7. large intestine – 8. spleen and stomach – 9. heart and small intestine – 1. urinary bladder and kidney .... This form of circulation is exactly in accordance with the circulation of the 12 regular meridians.

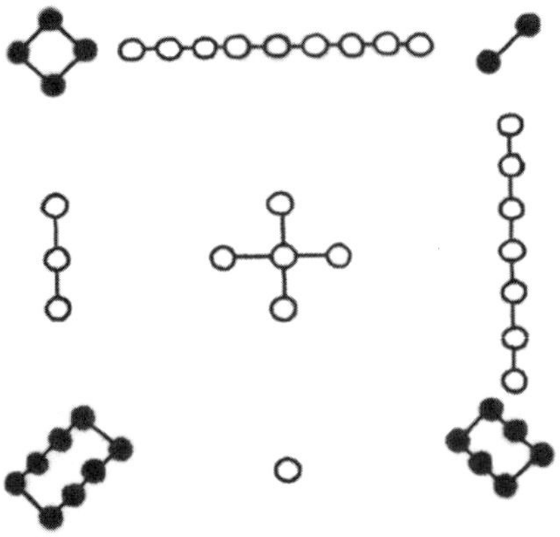

Illustration 13 Luo Shu

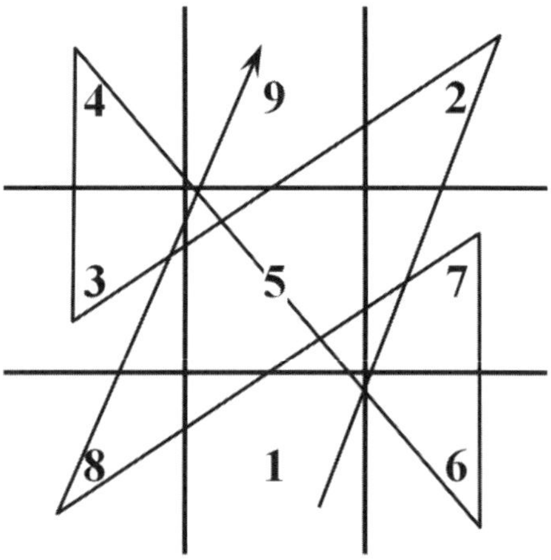

Illustration 14

In Chinese medicine, the theory of "correspondence between heaven and man" was derived from observation of the heaven and earth. Here, "heaven" means nature, the heaven and earth. In this theory, the physiological circulation inside the human body is in accordance with the circulation and change in heaven and earth. Based upon this, we can understand the mechanism of the meridians and collaterals.

The theory of "Open," "Pivot" and "Close" expounds the law of three *yin* and three *yang* in movement of separation and combination, inter-dependence, inter-transformation and the meridian *qi* in ascending and descending. It is essential in the application of *Shang Han Lun* (Treatise on Fabrile Diseases). It also guides the treatment of epidemic febrile diseases, making the therapeutic effect significant in the treatment of general miscellaneous diseases. Since imbalance of *yin* and *yang* is the general pathogenesis in *Shang Han Lun* (Treatise on Fabrile Diseases), it is essential to regulate the "Open," "Pivot" and "Close" of three yin and three yang so as to regain the balance.

From the above we can see that *Taiyang* and *Taiyin* are closely linked, belonging to the same category as do the *Shaoyang* and *Shaoyin*, and the

Yangming and *Jueyin*. It is stated in both *Suwen* (Essential Questions) and *Lingshu* (Spiritual Pivot): "*Taiyang* is the open, *Shaoyang* is the pivot and *Yangming* is the close; *Taiyin* is the open, *Shaoyin* is the pivot and *Jueyin* is the close." Based upon this, *Taiyang* and *Taiyin* are inter-correspondent, so are *Shaoyang* and *Shaoyin*, and *Yangming* and *Jueyin*. In this way, *yin* corresponds to *yang* and hand corresponds to foot. These correspondences are illustrated as follows:

Three Yang	**Taiyang (Open)**		**Shaoyang (Pivot)**		**Yangming (Close)**	
	Foot UB,	**Hand SI**	**Foot GB,**	**Hand SJ**	**Foot ST,**	**Hand LI**
Same Energy Attraction (Matching of the Hand and Foot channels)	|	|	|	|	|	|
	Hand LU,	**Foot SP**	**Hand HT,**	**Foot KI**	**Hand PC,**	**Foot LR**
Three Ying	**Taiyin (Open)**		**Shaoyin (Pivot)**		**Jueyin (Close)**	

Illustration 15

There exist extraordinary connections between the lung and urinary bladder, spleen and small intestine, heart and gallbladder, kidney and triple energizer, and liver and large intestine. In addition to the five *zang* organs, the pericardium is also connected with the stomach. Thus, the six *zang* and six *fu* organs are all connected, forming the extraordinary connections between the *zang* and *fu* organs. With the application of such theory, the treatments of the internal and miscellaneous diseases are very effective.

For over 30 years, I have used this method to treat many diseases with Chinese herbs and acupuncture and obtained extremely good therapeutic results, with acupuncture in particular.

The theory of "Open," "Pivot" and "Close," and the extraordinary connections of *zangfu* organs is the core of Tung's acupuncture. As is known to everyone, this theory is derived from *Yi Jing*, which emphasizes symmetry and balance. Tung's acupuncture also attaches importance to symmetry and balance. The following is the introduction to its clinical application and further elaboration of the theory of the extraordinary connections of *zangfu*.

5. The Extraordinary Connections of the *Zangfu*

1) The Lung and the Urinary Bladder

The disturbance of urinary bladder *qi* in transformation and dysfunction of the urinary bladder in control is related to the regulatory function of the lung. Dysfunction of the lung *qi* in dispersing and descending may lead to dysfunction of the bladder in storing and discharging urine. It is the *qi* of the lung that functions to regulate and control the bladder. "*Qi* transformation helps and controls urination." It is stated in Chapter 7 of the book *Jin Kui Yao Lue* (Essentials from the Golden Cabinet) that, "In case of deficiency of the lung with spit and no cough, the patient is not thirsty and there must be enuresis and frequent urination. This is because deficiency in the upper fails to control the lower. When there is cold in the lung, the patient will have vertigo and profuse spit. For the condition, *Gan Cao Gan Jiang Tang* (Decoction of Glycyrrhizae and Rhizoma Zingiberis) should be used to warm the cold." It is a deficiency syndrome with the lung failing to control the bladder. Dysfunction of the lung *qi* may also lead to water retention in the lung, giving rise to upward rebellion of the lung *qi* and resulting in asthma. Treatment is given to clear heat and promote the function of the bladder so as to cure asthma. In return, dysfunction of the bladder *qi* can be removed by regulating the lung; this is the method known as "removing the cover of a teapot to let the tea flow out." As Dr. Wu Jutong said, "Open the upper sluice gate, transform the lung *qi* and disperse the upper so as to promote urination in the lower." Dr. Zhu Danxi also said: "The lung is located in the upper *Jiao* and the urinary bladder in the lower *Jiao*. When the upper *Jiao* is blocked, the lower *jiao* is obstructed." *Ma Huang Tang* (Decoction of Herba Ephedrae) is therefore often used to help open the upper and benefit the lower so as to promote urination as well as to control frequent urination of the senior and child enuresis. In addition, needling point *Lieque* (LU7) can treat frequent urination and polyuria. Needling point *Yinlingquan* (SP9) can promote urination as well as frequent urination. Needling *Yuji* (LU10) can treat backache along the distribution of the bladder meridian. Needling the back-*shu* points can treat asthmatic breathing. All these are due to the extraordinary connection between the lung and spleen (*Taiyin*), and the urinary bladder (*Taiyang*).

In the application of Tung's extraordinary points, *Chongzi* (22.01) and *Chongxian* (22.02) located on the lung meridian are often selected to treat backache along the bladder meridian. The disorders of the uterus are also related to the bladder meridian. In *Shang Han Lun* (Treatise on Fabrile Diseases), there is the syndrome of blood retention the manifestations of which are "*Taiyang* disease ... heat accumulation in the bladder ... the patient looks maniac ... acute pain the lower abdomen." In case of the syndrome of blood retention of the bladder meridian, there often appear maniac symptoms. Many ladies with blood retention in the uterus may also have psychotic symptoms such as dysmenorrhea, amemorrhea and heat retention in the uterus, for which *Tao He Cheng Qi Tang* (Decoction of Peach Kernel for Activating *qi*) with modification is often used. It is also mentioned in *Jin Kui Yao Lue* (Essentials from the Golden Cabinet) that *Gui Zhi Fu Ling Wan* (Pills of Ramulus Cinnamomi and Poria) is often used to treat diseases with blood retention in the uterus. Both of the two prescriptions have the ingredient *Guizhi* (Ramulus Cinnamomi), which is the major herb for the urinary bladder meridian. From this example we can understand the significance of the selection of *Chongzi* (22.01) and

Chongxian (22.02) that can be used to treat hysteromyoma, and this therapeutic effect is closely related to the extraordinary connection between the lung and the urinary bladder. The therapeutic effect of point *Fuke* (11.24) located on the lung meridian, which can treat gynecological diseases, uterine diseases in particular, is also based upon the theory of extraordinary connection of *zangfu*.

2) The Spleen and the Small Intestine

The spleen dominates transformation and transportation, including the reception and transforming function of the small intestine. The small intestine relies on the warming function of the kidney *yang* to transform food, while the function of the small intestine in separating the clear from the turbid offers the material foundation to the spleen function in transforming *qi* and blood, ascending the clear and descending the waste. The spleen dominates ascending, prefers dryness and dislikes damp; correspondingly, pathogenic damp is liable to injure the spleen. The small intestine dominates descending, prefers warmth and dislikes cold, and pathogenic cold is therefore liable to consume the *yang qi* in the small intestine. Thus, the spleen and small intestine work closely together in coordination. Since the time of Neijing, disorders of the small intestine and disorders of the spleen and stomach have never been clearly separated. As stated in Chapter 22 of *Suwen* (Essential Questions): "When spleen is ill due to deficiency, there appear abdominal fullness, boryborygmus and indigestion." *Shang Han Lun* (Treatise on Fabrile Diseases) also says: "In *taiyin* disease, there appear abdominal fullness, vomiting, poor appetite, diarrhea and abdominal pain." Though it is the disease of the spleen, it can also be considered as the pathological change of the small intestine in reception and transformation. Therefore, in case of diseases of the small intestine, we often treat both the spleen and small intestine. When there is cold in the small intestine, we warm the middle *jiao* and dispel cold; When there is heat in the small intestine, we clear heat from the small intestine and purge the spleen; When the small intestine is slow in absorption with boryborygmus and diarrhea, we strengthen the spleen functions of transforming and transporting with additional drugs to eliminate damp. This is the method: solidify the stool by promoting urination; it is accomplished by treating both the spleen and the small intestine. Clinically, abdominal dull pain which is alleviated by warmth and pressure, watery and loose stool and poor appetite are often seen in gastro-duodenal ulcer and dysfunction of the small intestine in absorption. In Chinese medicine, it is differentiated as *yang* deficiency of the spleen and stomach and is treated with *Huang Qi Jian Zhong Tang* (Decoction of Radix Astragali ser Hedysari for Strengthening the Spleen) or *Fu Zi Li Zhong Tang* (Decoction of Radix Aconiti Praeparata for Regulating the Middle *Jiao*). Another example is the application of *Huang Tu Tang* (Decoction of Baked Yellow Soil) in *Jin Kui Yao Lue* (Essentials from the

Golden Cabinet) to treat hematochezia. Dr. Wu Jutong considered that bleeding after defecation is due to cold damp in the small intestine which is different from bleeding before defecation due to damp heat in the large intestine. Since the etiological root is in the small intestine, *Huang Tu Tang* is therefore used to warm the spleen and stop bleeding, the example of the spleen and small intestine being treated simultaneously.

In acupuncture treatment, *wangu* (SI4) is often used for obesity. In ancient classical literature, it is often selected to treat jaundice due to damp heat (see *Tong Xue Zhi Yao Fu* – Ode of Commonly Used Important Points, *Yu Long Ge* – Song of Jade Dragon and *Yu Long Fu* – Ode of Jade Dragon). *Wangu* (SI4) is the *yuan*-source point of the small intestine and can eliminate damp due to spleen deficiency. The Tung's extraordinary point *Ganmen* (33.11) is also located on the small intestine meridian and is indicated in hepatitis. All the ancient and contemporary physicians considered it is important that hepatitis should be treated by eliminating damp. In cases of *yang* jaundice due to acute hepatitis, emphasis of treatment should be placed on the *yangming*; while in case of *yin* jaundice in chronic hepatitis, the emphasis should be placed on eliminating damp. The small intestine is the organ of irrigation and has very strong ability to eliminate damp. An alternative example: the spleen point *Yinlingquan* (SP9) can be selected to treat periarthritis of the shoulder with remarkable effect. It is also due to the extraordinary connection between the spleen and small intestine.

3) The Heart and the Gallbladder

It is said in Chapter 8 of *Suwen* (Essential Questions): "The heart is the emperor organ and it houses mind .... The gallbladder is the upright organ and it helps to make decisions." The gallbladder is related to emotional activities and plays an important role in spirit, consciousness and thinking. The heart dominates blood and vessels. The gallbladder assists digestion. The heart dominates the emperor fire and the gallbladder dominates the minister fire. The gallbladder excretes bile and dominates ascending and descending in the triple energizer; it is therefore closely related to the formation of phlegm and damp. Dysfunction of the gallbladder often leads to hyperlipoidemia and cardiovascular diseases such as coronary heart disease, angina pectoris, myocardial infarction and arrhythmia. It is pointed out in the research of west medicine that the occurrence of coronary heart disease and angina pectoris is often related to the hyperlipoidemia, and cholecystitis, cholelithiasis and obstruction of biliary tract may all raise the blood lipids. Based on these concepts, we can treat heart disease by taking gallbladder into consideration; we often use *Xiao Chai Hu Tang* (Minor Decoction of Radix Bupleuri) and *Wen Dan Tang* (Decoction for Clearing Heat from the Gallbladder) to treat, coronary heart disease, angina pectoris and arrhythmia. There are many such clinical reports. The two herbal formulas are also very effective in treatment of insomnia. To treat biliary diseases by taking the heart into consideration, we often use *Gua Lou Jiu Bai Ban Xia Tang* (Decoction of Fructus Trichosanthis, Herba Allium and Rhizoma Peinelliae) to treat chronic cholecystitis with certain therapeutic effect. At present, the therapeutic effect of treating cardiac and biliary disease together is far better than considering one or the other alone. In acupuncture, needling point *Fengshi* (GB31) of the gallbladder meridian is very effective for insomnia, heart disease and cholecystitis. Needling point *Shenmen* (HT7) of the heart meridian is also very effective for deficiency of *qi* of the heart and gallbladder. Besides, the extraordinary point *Yanhuang* (11.23) located on the heart meridian is effective for yellow eyes. All these are examples of extraordinary connections of *zangfu*.

4) The Kidney and the Triple Energizer (*San Jiao*)

It is stated in Chapter 47 of *Lingshu* (Spiritual Pivot): "The kidney controls the triple energizer and the urinary bladder." There exist two systems in the triple energizer (*Sanjiao*).

The first system is that of *qi* activity dominated by the lung, spleen and the kidney. The *qi* activity in the upper energizer functions to disperse and distribute the body fluid and essential substance and this function relies on the lung. The *qi* activity in the middle energizer functions to transform the nutrient *qi* (*yingqi*), defensive *qi* (*wei qi*), and essential blood and this function relies on the spleen. The *qi* activity in the lower energizer dominates the anterior and posterior orifices and controls discharge of the waste and this function relies on the kidney, and the kidney is the original motive power of the *qi* activity in all the triple energizer.

The second system is that of ministerial and emperor fire of the triple energizer which is dominated by the heart, liver and kidney. The heart is the emperor fire located in the upper energizer. The liver is the minister fire located in the middle energizer while the kidney and *Mingmen* (vital gate) are the minister fire located in the lower energizer. Kidney is the organ that contains both water and fire and therefore both of the two systems originate from the kidney. During the course of diseases of the two systems, they can transform into each other usually in the late stages.

Prolonged illness of either system may eventually affect the kidney. This is because both systems originate from the kidney which contains *yin* and *yang*, water and fire, and serves as the general pivot of the whole body. Clinically, the triple energizer should be considered in the treatment of kidney diseases. Cold limbs due to shaoyin patterns result from kidney *yang* deficiency, the prescription *Si Ni Tang* (Decoction for Inducing Resuscitation) is indicated for this condition. However, it is formed with *Fuzi* (Radix Aconiti Praeparata) to warm the kidney *yang* in the lower energizer, *Ganjiang* (Rhizoma Zingiberis) to warm the spleen *yang* in the middle energizer, and *Gancao* (Radix Glycyrrhizae) to warm the heart *yang* in the upper energizer, treating the *yang* of all the three energizers.

There are many such formula examples in the book *Shang Han Lun* (Treatise on Fabrile Diseases). The basic principle of treatment is "treating the disease and protecting the patient." It means the physicians should consider the body constitution of the patient in order to avoid weaking the patient with the drugs. Many formulas of *Shang Han Lun* (Treatise on Fabrile Diseases) are modified by adding such herbs as *Gancao* (Radix Glycyrrhizae), *Shengjiang* (Rhizoma Zingiberis) and *Dazao* (Fructus Ziziphi Jujubae) to protect and strengthen the anti-pathogenic *qi*. Moreover, *Gui Zhi Tang* (Decoction of Ramulus Cinnamomi) should be used only after taking *Ma Huang Tang* (Decoction of Herba Emphedrae); further, *Da Cheng Qi Tang* (Major Decoction for Clearing Heat with Purgation) cannot be used repeatedly even when there still remain symptoms of exterior patterns. All these measures are for protecting the anti-pathogenic *qi* of the patient. This is different from the western medicines where strong drugs are sometimes used and they badly weaken the body constitution of the patient before the disease is controlled.

Another principle often used in TCM, acupuncture, is "two-way regulation." For instance, needling point *Neiguan* (PC6) to slow down the heartbeat in case of tachycardia and speed up the heartbeat in case of bradycardia; needling *Zusanli* (ST36) can treat both hyperperistalsis and bradystalsis of the stomach. The two-way regulatory function of acupuncture is obvious and safe. Many formulas in *Shang Han Lun* (Treatise on Fabrile Diseases) also have two-way regulatory functions. For instance, in *Si Ni San* (Power for Treating Cold Limbs), *Chaihu* (Radix Bupleuri) can ascend *qi* and *Zhishi* (Fructus aruantii Immaturus) can descend *qi*. Through the ascending and descending functions, the formula effectively regulates the *qi* activity. Besides, *Shaoyao* (Radix Paeoniae) and *Gancao* (Radix Glycyrrhizae) can regulate blood, thus the formula functions to regulate both *qi* and blood in ascending and descending. Another example is *Gui Zhi Tang* (Decoction of Ramulus Cinnamomi) in which *Guizhi* (Ramulus Cinnamomi) and *Shengjiang* (Rhizoma Zingiberis) can warm the *yang* and regulate defensive *qi*, and *Shaoyao* (Radix Paeoniae), and *Dazao* (Frictis Ziziphi Jujubae) can nourish yin and harmonize nutrient *qi*, thus the formula has two-way regulatory function for both *yin* and *yang*, and *Ying* (nutrient *qi*) and *Wei* (defensive *qi*).

The third principle in TCM is "considering the body as an integrated whole in treatment." For example, *Si Ni Tang* (Decoction for inducing Resuscitation) is mainly used to warm the kidney *yang*, and in fact, it warms *yang* of all the three energizers. Another example is *Gui Zhi Jia Hou Po Xing Ren Tang* (Decoction of Ramulus Cinnamomui plus Cortex

Magnoliae Officinalis and Semen Armeniacare Amarum), which is used to treat asthmatic breathing. However, in that prescription, *Xingren* (Semen Armeniacae Amarum) is for regulating lung *qi* in the upper energizer, *Houpo* (Cortex Magnoliae Officinalis) is for regulating the *qi* in the middle energizer and *Guizhi* (Ramulus Cinnamomi) balances and regulates the *qi* in the lower energizer. Though the formula is used to treatment asthmatic breathing, it regulates the *qi* in all the three energizers.

Now let's talk more about the extraordinary connection of the kidney and triple energizer. The five-*Shu* points *Guanchong* (SJ1), *Yemen* (SJ2), *Zhongzhu* (SJ3), *Zhigou* (SJ6) and *Tianjing* (SJ10), and *Yangchi* (SJ4) are all related to the water (kidney). In the treatment of nephritis, Master Tung often used *Zhongbai* (22.06) and *Xiabai* (22.07). The two points were also used to treat edema. Besides, *Zhongzhu* (SJ3) is often selected to treat lower back pain. Another example is the extraordinary point of Master Tung: *Huanchao* (11.06) is often needled to treat infertility. This point is located on the triple energizer meridian and it functions through the extraordinary connection of *zangfu*.

5) The Liver and the Large Intestine

The liver maintains the unrestrained and free-going condition for the flow of *qi*, and it also assists urination and defecation. The transportation of the large intestine greatly relies on the function of the liver in maintaining free-flow of *qi*. In his medical record of treatment of hypochondriac pain, constipation and abdominal distention, Dr. Wu Jutong emphasized liver function in regulating urination and defecation, which is based upon the liver meridian winding around the external genitalia and the extraordinary connection of the liver and large intestine. For example, the form of dysentery where the herbal formula *Wu Mei Tang* (Decoction of Fructus Mumo) is indicated results from prolonged damp heat. Here, stagnation of the liver transversely invades the spleen and dysfunction of the liver in maintaining free flow of *qi* gives rise to dysentery with tenesmus. The type of dysentery that is treated with *Bai Tou Wong Tang* (Decoction of Radix Pulsatillae) is caused by deficiency of the earth that gives rise to stagnation of the wood, and in return, it makes the stagnation of the wood even worse. As a result, accumulation of damp heat in the intestine occurs. Treatment can obtain therapeutic results by dispersing the wood and regulating the liver. *Bai Tou Weng Tang* here works to clear heat and eliminate damp from the *yangming* (large intestine) and disperse the *qi* stagnation of the liver so as to cure dysentery. Moreover, *Si Ni San Jia Jiu Bai Tang* (Decoction for Treating Cold Limbs modified by Allium Tuberosum Rottier) can also be used to treat dysentery. The two formulas are also effective for diseases of external genitalia since such diseases are often caused by damp heat in the liver meridian. In acupuncture, needling *Quchi* (LI11) can treat hypertension due to liver *yang* hyperactivity and various kinds of vertigo. The extraordinary point *Linggu* (22.05) located on the large intestine meridian is effective for vertigo. Point *Mu* (11.17) on the large intestine meridian can treat hernia of the large intestine. And the points *Dajian* (11.01), *Xiaojian* (11.02), *Waijian* (11.04), and *Fujian* (11.03) located on the large intestine meridian can all treat hernia. Besides, needling *taichong* (LR3) of the liver meridian can treat diarrhea with abdominal pain. All these are examples in which the theory of extraordinary connection of *zangfu* is used.

6) The Pericardium and the Stomach

A common clinical picture is the patient with myocardial infarction caused by an upward attack of the stomach *qi* after overeating. Since some patients with angina pectoris due to coronary heart disease also have obvious symptoms of the upper digestive tract, the formula for chest *bi* can treat stomachache simultaneously, it is a treatment known as the "simultaneous treatment for both the heart and stomach." This is because the stomach is connected with the pericardium, and excessive heat in the stomach may go upward attacking the pericardium giving symptoms such as disturbance of the mind. In this case, *Da Cheng Qi Tang* (Major Decoction for Clearing Heat with Purgation) is used to purge the excess heat from the stomach. When the stomach is cured, the pericardium will be calm. It is stated in chapter "Middle Energizer" of *Wen Bin Tiao Bian* (Systematic Differentiation of Warm Diseases), "In the *yangming* warm disease, there is constipation, … the pathogenic heat invades the pericardium, leading to unconsciousness and delirium, obstruction of the mind and thirst. For the condition, *Niu Huang Cheng Qi Tang* (Decoction of Calculus Bovis for Clearing Heat) should be used;" also, "In case of stomach disease with dysentery, delirium, excessive or slippery and rapid pulse, *Xiao Cheng Qi Tang* (Minor Decoction for Clearing Heat with Purgation) should be used." Further, it is said in chapter "*Jueyin*" of the *Shang Han Lun* (Treatise on Attack by Cold), "In case of dysentery with delirium and dry stool, *Xiao Cheng Qi Tang* (Minor Decoction for Clearing Heat with Purgation) should be used." In cases of *yangming* and *jueyin* being diseased simultaneously, use purgatives to clear heat for constipation, but also use cooling drugs to help induce resuscitation such as *Niu Huang Qing Gong Wan* (Pills of Calculus Bovis for Clearing Heat to Inducing Resuscitation) and *Zi Xue Dan* (Pills of cool drugs for Inducing Resuscitation). The simultaneous use of both the cool drugs such as *Niuhuang* (Calculus Bovis) and the heat-clearing purgatives are also used. *Cheng Qi Tang* (Decoction for Clearing Heat with Purgation) is often used to treat epidemic dysentery with unconsciousness, delirium and convulsion due to toxic heat, known as "treating dysentery by promoting bowel movement and protecting anti-pathogenic *qi* with purgation;" this carries the patient through the crisis. Needling point *Neiguan* (PC6) of the pericardium meridian is very effective for stomachache (where the stomach meridian travels) and knee joint pain. The stomach point *Zusanli* (ST36) is also very effective for stuffiness in the chest due to heart disease. Master Tung often used *Tongguan* (88.01), *Tongshan* (88.02) and *Tongtian* (88.03) to treat heart disease. All these points are located on the stomach meridian, indicating the extraordinary connection of the pericardium and stomach.

Concluding remarks

Guided by the theory of the open, close and pivot, personally, I have explained the extraordinary connection of five *zang*, and supplemented the extraordinary connection of the pericardium and the stomach, making the theory more complete. The clinical application of the theory has improved the therapeutic effect for the miscellaneous diseases, especially for acupuncture treatment. At present, points are usually selected from the same-named meridians (for instance, select points of the hand-*yangming* meridian to treat the foot-*yangming* meridian, points of hand-*taiyang* meridian to treat foot-*taiyang* meridian, etc.); or the externally-internally related meridians (such as the hand-*yangming* and hand-*taiyang*). Points from the same-named meridians, the points of hand and foot, the upper and lower, are selected mainly to dredge the meridians (for instance, select points of the hand-*yangming* meridian to treat the foot-*yangming* meridian, points of hand-*taiyang* meridian to treat foot-*taiyang* meridian, etc.); while the points of the externally-internally related meridians, points of *zang* and *fu*, yin and yang, are selected mainly to maintain balance (for instance, select points of the hand-*yangming* meridian to treat the foot-*yangming* meridian, points of hand-*taiyang* meridian to treat foot-*taiyang* meridian, etc.). Based on the extraordinary connection of *zangfu*, points are selected from both *zang* and *fu*, hand and foot, *yin* and *yang* meridians (taking the extraordinary connection of the lung and urinary bladder as an example, the lung meridian is a hand-yin meridian and the urinary bladder meridian is a foot-*yang* meridian), functioning in both dredging the meridians and maintaining balance, thus the remarkable therapeutic results. This is the most important part, the core of the theory of Tung's extraordinary points.

Chapter Two

The Four Limbs and Trunk

1. Diseases of the Upper Limbs

1) Numbness of the Fingers

a. Needling *Shenguan* (77.18) and *Fuliu* (K7) has specific effect.
b. Needling *Huoju* (66.11) is effective.
c. Needle *Jiuli* (88.26, 27).
d. Needle *Mudou* (66.07) and *Muliu* (66.06).
e. Needle *Wuhu* (11.27) on the opposite side.
f. Pricking *Shuangfeng* (DT.05) to cause bleeding is effective.

Symmetrical methods are useful for diseases of the four limbs, they will be introduced in detail later. To treat numbness of the fingers, the first point is *Shenguan* (77.18). The second point *Huoju* (66.11) is also very effective. The third point is *Jiuli* (88.26, 27). These points are useful for mild finger numbness. A few treatments may cure the condition if it is not related to cervical problems. Examination of the cervical vertebrae is necessary to rule out cervical complication.

When numbness of the fingers is due to problems of cervical vertebrae, in addition to *Shenguan* (77.18) and *Huoju* (66.11), bleed *Shuangfeng* (DT.05), which is lateral 1.5 *cun* to the 2nd cervical vertebra. Include the other 6 points below with the distance of 1 *cun* between each other, with seven points in total. With an aging patient population the incidence of cervical bone spurs is increasing as a result, more patients are suffering from numbness of the fingers. Other common sites for bone spurs include the lumbar vertebrae, knees and heels. In my many years clinical practice, the most common conditions I have treated are bone spurs. In addition to spurring numbness may be caused by poor circulation due to high cholesterol. Generally, *Shenguan* (77.18), *Huoju* (66.11) or *Jiuli* (88.26, 27) are good enough for simple numbness of the fingers. If the numbness is due to bone spurs, additional points should be selected. In Tung's acupuncture, *Minghuang* (88.12) is often selected to treat bone spurs of the cervical and lumbar vertebrae; *Sihuazhong* (77.09) and *Sihuaxia* (77.11) are often used to treat bone spurs of the knee joint and heel. When needling *Sihuazhong* (77.09) and *Sihuaxia* (77.11), insertion of the needle should be close to the border of tibia, known as "needling the bone for bone diseases" in order to obtain therapeutic effect.

At present, many patients with knee pain receive good and fast therapeutic effect with acupuncture. However, more severe cases often involve bone spurring. In this case, it should be insert the needle along the border of the bone. Otherwise, the result will be poor. The therapeutic effects are improved if *Neiguan* (PC6) and *Taichong* (LR3), or *Xinmen* (33.12) and *Taichong* (LR3) are combined. Knee pain caused by bone spur may be cured quickly by selecting these points.

The causes of bone spurring are many. The first is incorrect posture, or inquire about softness of the bed and ergonomic factors for computer workers. Lack of exercise may be a cause as can injuries. Even though there is no pain and no treatment right after injury, there may still be formation of bone spurs over time. Other factors may include invasion by wind cold or frequent squatting for extended periods of time. I have one special acupuncture method for bone spur of cervical and lumbar vertebrae. Needle *Renzhong* (DU26), *Houxi* (SI3), *Sugu* (BL65) and *Fengshi* (GB31) for good therapeutic effect. *Renzhong* (DU26) on the *DU* meridian dredges the meridian. *Houxi* (SI3) is one of the eight confluent points and is connected with the *DU* meridian and thus indicated in diseases of the *DU* meridian. The urinary bladder meridian travels on both sides of the *DU* meridian and is thus indicated in the diseases of the *DU* meridian, *Sugu* (BL65) is an effective choice. *Fengshi* (GB31) is the point located on the shaoyang meridian that dominates bone and is thus indicated in bone diseases. It is better to needle *Houxi* (SI3) and *Sugu* (BL65) along the border of the bones and *Fengshi* (GB31) deeply enough to touch the bone. The above four points are the best points for treatment of bone spur. In severe case, bleed *Weizhong* (BL40) once every 10 days to two weeks, in order to improve responsiveness and therapeutic outcomes.

In the past years, I have treated many cases of shoulder and arm pain and numbness of the fingers due to bone spur of cervical vertebrae. Here is mini case. In 1985, I had a patient named Mr. Zheng who was the father-in-law of an acupuncturist in Los Angeles. He was suffering from left shoulder and cubital pain and numbness of the left hand for over 6 months. He went back to Taiwan to visit his family and came to my clinic during the spring festival. I treated him with the points including *Fengshi* (GB31), *Shenguan* (77.18) and *Fuliu* (KI7). He received treatment 2-3 times per week with blood-letting at *Weizhong* (BL40) once every two weeks. I further prescribed the herbal formula *Ge Gua Shao Cao Tang* (Decoction of Radix Puerariae, Fructus Chaenomelis, Radix Paeoniae Rubra and Radix Glycyrrhizae Praeparata) which was made by me for bone spur of cervical vertebrae. The ingredients include *Gegen* (Radix Puerariae), *Mugua* (Fructus Chaenomelis), *Chishao* (Radix Paeoniae Rubra), *Baishao* (Radix Puerariae Alba), *Zhicao* (Radix Glycyrrhizae Praeparata), *Qinjiao* (Radix Gentlanae Macrophyllae), *Qianghuo* (Rhizoma seu Radix Notopterygii), *Sigualuo* (Retinervus Lufffae Fructus), *Weilingxian* (Racis Clematidis) with modifications. The treatment lasted for less than five weeks and then all the symptoms disappeared.

In 1981, I published an article entitled, *Experience in Acupuncture Treatment of Neurological Symptoms with Picked Points* in the annual symposia of Taipei Municipal Association of Traditional Chinese Medicine. In the article, there is a section "Experience in Treatment of 7 Cases of Hyperplasia of Cervical Vertebrae with Immediate Effect," in which I described the acupuncture treatment and selection of points in details with case examples. Here I'd like to give one example. Not long after the treatment of Mr. Zheng I mentioned above, there came Mr. Huang who was suffering from stiffness and pain of the neck, nape, back and scapula as well as numbness of the fingers. Examination at the hospital revealed hyperplasia at C5 and C6. I needled *Shenguan* (77.18), *Fuliu* (KI7), *Fengshi* (GB31) and *Houxi* (SI3). Sometimes I used *Renzhong* (DU26) and *Shugu* (BL65) instead of *Shenguan* (77.18) and *Fuliu* (KI7). The patient also received bleeding therapy to *Weizhong* (BL40) once every 2 weeks. At the same time he also took herbal decoction of Modified *Ge Gua Shao Cao Tang* (as introduced above). He was cured in 32 days.

The most effective method that I have used for bone spur is bleeding *Weizhong* (BL40). Bleeding therapy can move the blood and disperse blood stasis, thus regulating blood circulation. Bleeding promotes metabolism and improves the general health condition. Some people may even have improvement of the career promotions after bleeding *Weizhong* (BL40). This is because bleeding improves blood circulation and gives rise to better facial complexion and the mind that gives others better impression, and thus better career.

Here are some true examples. One professor was promoted after he received bleeding treatment at *Weizhong* (BL40) for his hemorrhoid. Another patient was an ambassador and was due to retire soon. After bleeding treatment he was promoted to minister. One professor was very famous and he was nominated for academician of the Central Academy the year before but didn't pass the examination of credentials. Then he came to me to receive bleeding treatment for his hemorrhoid the second year and he passed the examination after that. Another patient was a university president. He was going to be retired soon. But he was promoted as the chairman of the educational committee after receiving bleeding treatment. It may have been a coincidence; however it may be useful to hear about these correlations since there is no harm.

6. Question: How does a doctor give bleeding treatment in oral cavity for facial paralysis?

Answer: Use three-edged needle to prick the mucus membrane of the inner wall of oral cavity to cause bleeding (demonstration). This method is very helpful in clinical practice. Without it, the cure may take seven days instead of three days. After bleeding, have the patient rinse the mouth with saline water for sterilization and to avoid infection on one hand, and give certain stimulation on the other for recovery. Ear apex bleeding on the diseased side is also very good for facial paralysis, and it can be used in alternation with oral cavity bleeding to avoid repeated injury of the same point.

7. Question: What is the standard method of the cure for facial paralysis?

Answer: This is a good question. I have treated many patients with facial paralysis in Taiwan and have accumulated very rich experience. When the mouth starts to deviate, the eye cannot close generally and the mouth cannot whistle either. There is often food retention around the gums. After treatment for certain period of time, the food retention disappears. Further, assess the therapeutic effect by asking the patient to whistle before and after treatment. The sound of whistle indicates great progress after treatment. The ability of the patient in closing eye suggests the cure of the disease and the course of treatment could be finished. Often, the patient looks fine after treatment. However, they cannot completely close the eyes; in this case needle *Hegu* (LI4) on the healthy side. As mentioned in the ancient medical classic[1], "*Hegu* (LI4) is indicated in the diseases of the face and mouth." Ask the patient to close the eye as much as possible while manipulating the needle, and gradually the patient will be able to close the eye. In severe cases, the mouth deviates downward. Some patients have the deviation on both sides; in these cases, give traction by needling *Dicang* (ST4). For downward deviation, needle *Chengjiang* (REN24) for better and faster results. However, the stimulation of the traction shouldn't be too strong. Facial paralysis is not a difficult disease to cure. But if the duration of the disease is more than 2 months, the improvement will be slow and the course of treatment will be long, and early treatment is therefore advisable.

8. Question: What are precautions of bleeding therapy?

Answer: The precautions are as follows:

1. **Preparation**. If the patient takes a standing position for bleeding, place some drape sheets under his /her feet. If the patient bends over for bleeding, place some drape sheets (paper) under the location to be bled. For example, if *Weizhong* (BL40) is to be bled, put some papers under the knee; if *Taiyang* (Extra) is to be bled, place a bucket on the ground to let the blood drop into the bucket. All these preparations must be done before treatment.

2. **Pay attention to the weather**. This is also important for other aspects of treatment. Good weather may allow more bleeding with improved therapeutic results. If the weather is cloudy, the blood vessels contract

[1] "Si Zong Xue Ge" (Song of the Four General Points)

and bleeding will be less. Therefore, bleeding treatment should be given generally when the weather is fine to all the chronic cases except acute condition.

3. **Food-intake of the patient is important**. It is not advisable to give bleeding when the patient is either full or hungry. When the patient is hungry, the blood becomes thicker and it will affect the volume of the bleeding. Do not have bleeding treatment long after eating. Besides, the patient is liable to have fainting when hungry.

4. **Thickness of the needle and needling technique**. Though the three-edged needle is thick and looks terrifying, its therapeutic effect is good. Besides, the needling technique is even more important. To avoid too deep insertion when the technique is not good enough, hold the tip of the needle with fingers first and then prick the point. In bleeding therapy, it requires the insertion of the needle tip only. Since the surface of the three-edged needle is very smooth, autoclaving sterilization is good enough. But now disposable three-edged needle is commonly used. It is important that the tip is sharp enough and that the three blades are smooth, problems of increased pain and inefficient outcomes occur when the tip is dull and the blades are rough. If the tip and three blades are sharp enough, slight pricking may easily cause bleeding. Otherwise there is possibly no bleeding but injury of the skin only. It is therefore necessary to check the tip and three blades before needling. Besides, the volume of bleeding is also related to the technique and the flow of air in the pricked point. If the insertion is too shallow and the air flow in the point is too little, bleeding will be less. The pricked area of three-edged needle is much larger than that of a filiform needle. Slight pricking may cause much bleeding. Pricking with the depth of 0.1 *cun* may give rise to a lot of bleeding. Poor technique will not cause enough bleeding but long wound.

How do we cause heavy bleeding? I'd like to talk about this in detail. If a practitioner's skill is sufficient, just pricking the point slightly will cause bleeding. With lower skill, there will be more tissue injury with little or no bleeding; under these circumstances, prick the blue vein. When there is bleeding, there will be no pain, and when there is no bleeding, there will be pain. If there is no bleeding after pricking the vein, just prick another vein nearby. It is just like opening milk can that needs two drilled hole to let milk flow out.

Further, some areas have no vein on such as the back. To cause bleeding to occur more easily, first press and massage the local area to cause local congestion. Thumb-pressing may also be used when bleeding point *Weizhong* (BL40) and *Chize* (LU5). It may reduce the pain caused by pricking. When bleeding *Taiyang* (Extra) with no local obvious vein, we could ask the patient to tighten the collar first to cause congestion at the point for ease and a larger amount of blood. When bleeding the *Jing*-Well points such as *Shaoshang* (LU11) or *Shangyang* (LI1), make it congested first. If not, even squeezing after pricking the point will not cause enough bleeding. If the finger root of the thumb or index finger is pressed to make congestion first and then bleed the point, more blood will flow out.

5. **Time for bleeding**. The appropriate time for bleeding therapy is essential and affects the amount of blood and efficiency of bleeding therapy. For example, when *Taiyang* (Extra) is bled at 11:00 am when the weather is fine, the therapeutic effect would be the best. Especially when getting close to mid-noon, more *yang qi* exists in the vein and the blue vein is clearer such as in case of migraine. If we prick such blue vein at point *Taiyang*, there could bleed 40-50 drops of blood. Generally, every 10 drops are equal to 1 c.c. Bleeding *Taiyang* (Extra) treats many diseases with excellent results, especially diseases of the face and neck such as migraine, trigeminal neuralgia, or even asthma. The depth of insertion is about 0.1 *cun*. When it bleeds to certain drops, the bleeding will stop spontaneously. To cause heavy bleeding, just prick with the needle against the blue vein. Generally speaking when the patient's facial complexion is rosy and moist, it would be more difficult to find the blue vein. In this case, just tighten the collar to cause local congestion at the point and then bleed the point. If the bleeding is still not enough, just squeeze it. However the amount of bleeding available by squeezing is limited and it is advisable to prick the point long enough after causing congestion. In general, when there are more blue veins, the bleeding will be easier and doesn't require squeezing, and the blood even sprays out, leading to good therapeutic effect.

The above are the principle and method of bleeding *Taiyang* (Extra). For lower back pain and bone spur of spinal vertebrae, it is better to give bleeding in the afternoon, following the theory of Midnight-noon Ebb Flow. After bleeding, the use of Acupuncture may make the therapeutic effect even better. As we know, the ebb and flow of the circulation in the 12 regular meridians follow certain time regularity, so does the circulation of the *REN* and *DU* meridians. The flow circulating in the 12 regular meridians arrives at the small intestine meridian of hand-*taiyang* during the period of 1:00-3:00 pm and the urinary bladder meridian of foot-*taiyang* during the period of 3:00-5:00 pm. Both the hand and foot *taiyang* meridians travel on the posterior aspect of the human body, and therefore best result could be obtained when bleeding is given in the afternoon for sciatica and hemorrhoids. However, bleeding *Jing*-well points like *Shaoshang*

(LU11) are emergency points and have nothing to do with the time since there is no blue vein in the local areas. When treating backache and lumbago, bleeding *Weizhong* (BL40) is the best. If no blue vein is found at the point, bleeding may be given on the back and lower back. Pain of the leg can be treated by bleeding certain areas of the back and or lower back too. To bleed the back or lower back, there is no strict requirement regarding time. Though the amount of bleeding is not as much as that in pricking a blue vein, we can increase the bleeding by squeezing or cupping. Generally, the patients without much exposure of the blue veins do not have a large amount of bleeding during these procedures. When bleeding the oral cavity, it is not necessary to find blue veins and 7-8 drops of bleeding would be enough. Just ask the patient to open the mouth, prick the mucous membrane at the level of mouth angle. Blood-letting is usually given to the diseased side in case of facial paralysis.

2) Pain of the Index Finger

a. Needling *Wuhuyi* (*Wuhu* 1), the first point of *Wuhu* (11.27), may have special effect.
b. Needling *Sihuazhong* (77.09) may also have good effect.

In the treatment of index finger pain, we usually needle point *Wuhu* 1, the first point of *Wuhu* (11.27) on the healthy side. The point is also indicated in the pain of all the five fingers. *Sihuazhong* (77.09) is also good for the pain of the index finger. At present, many patients are suffering from the pain of finger joints, for which I often needle point *Wuhu* 1. I also select the point in treatment of finger pain due to rheumatoid arthritis. Best result could be obtained by the combination of acupuncture and herbal medicine in treatment of rheumatoid arthritis.

The most commonly used herbal prescription is *Gui Shao Zhi Mu Tang* (Decoction of Ramulus Cinnamomi, Radix Paeoniae and Rhizoma Anemarrhenae). Rheumatoid arthritis is known as *Wan Bi* or *Wang Bi* (stubborn Bi syndrome). *Gui Shao Zhi Mu Tang* modified by *Quanxie* (Scorpio) and *Wugong* (Scolopendra) has very good therapeutic effect for rheumatoid arthritis. Many patients with swelling and deformity of finger joints came to my clinic for treatment. If the condition is not too severe, this prescription may help the patient completely recover. Acupuncture is often taken mainly for the control of pain. Master Tung also often selected *Tongguan* (88.01) and *Tongshan* (88.02) to treat the disease.

9. Question: How effective is acupuncture in the treatment of *yin* deficiency? Please explain it by taking Parkinson's disease as an example.

Answer: Generally, acupuncture has very good analgesic effect. It is also very effective for insomnia due to deficiency of *yin*. But some *yin* deficiency syndromes are not very well treated with acupuncture. For instance, Parkinson's disease due to *yin* deficiency is not so easy to treat. The therapeutic effect is slow and the duration of treatment is long. We have already introduced a method for treating Parkinson's disease, that is to needle *Qianhui* (1010.05) and *Houhui* (1010.06), or *Qili* (A.01) and *Jiuli* (88.26, 27), or *Shangsanhuang* (88.12, 13, 14) and *Xiasanhuang* (77.18, 19, 21) alternatively. Since Master Tung only used above acupuncture method to treat the disease without herbs, the therapeutic effect was slow. If scalp acupuncture or the four-gate points (*Hegu*, LI11 and *Taichong*, LR3) were added, the result would be better. Therefore, the best result could be obtained by using Tung's extraordinary points and the points of the fourteen meridians plus Chinese herbal medicines that can nourish *yin* and dispel wind. To treat tremor due to wind, the best medicine is *Lingyangjiao* (Cornu Antelopis). Many doctors have used it but now are mostly using *Shanyangjiao* (Goat Horn) instead. The formula for the disease is *Tian Ma Gou Teng Yin* (Decoction of Rhizoma Gastrodiae and Raulus Uncariae cum Uncis) or *Ding Zhen Wan* (Pills for Calming Tremor). The commonly used medicines are *Shanyangjiao* (Goat Horn), *Muli* (Concha Ostreae), *Guiban* (Plastrum Testudinis) and *Biejia* (Carapax Trionycis). They are quite effective. There is a saying "use sedative drugs to dispel wind" in Chinese medicine. All the above drugs have sedative function.

The patients of tetanus and convulsion are often treated with such moving drugs as *Quanxie* (Scorpio) and *Wugong* (Scolopendra). In treatment of arthritis, these drugs are also used to dispel wind. In severe case of pain, *Quanxie* (Scorpio) and *Wugong* (Scolopendra) have an excellent analgesic action. They are therefore often added to the prescriptions in the treatment of severe trigeminal neuralgia, intercostal neuralgia, herpes zosters and sciatica. In the treatment of severe sciatica, *Du Huo Ji Sheng Tang* (Decoction of Radix Angelicae pubescentis and Ramulus Loranthi) is often modified with the two drugs, the best drugs for wind following the principle "treating the abnormality in movement with moving drugs."

The effect of acupuncture alone in the treatment of Parkinson's disease is slow. Further, the combination of acupuncture and herbal medicine has a better therapeutic effect.

Timely treatment is important in serious diseases. Take the injury of spinal nerved due to traffic accident as an example. The therapeutic effect is more remarkable when treatment is given within the first six months. If there is delay, the therapeutic effect will be slow and poor. Upper nerve damage is usually very difficult to treat. However, early treatment with the combination of both acupuncture and herbal medicine can still obtain certain therapeutic effect. No matter how serious the injury is, acupuncture can obtain therapeutic effects. While it can be difficult, the key is the early treatment.

3) Soreness of the Hand

a. Needling *Cesanli* (77.22) and *Cexiasanli* (77.23) on the healthy side.

Select *Cesanli* (77.22) and *Cexiasanli* (77.23) on the healthy side to treat soreness and numbness of the hand. Further, *Waiguan* (SJ5) of the fourteen meridians is also very effective because the *yangwei* meridian is connected with the five fingers. Generally, unilateral soreness of hand is treated by needling *Waiguan* (SJ5) on the healthy side. If both hands are involved, the point is needled bilaterally; alternate the exercise of each hand during needle manipulation. Alternatively, needle the points on the more severe side because needling the point unilaterally will treat both sides. Needling *Shenguan* (77.18) on the healthy side is also very effective. If there is wrist joint pain, needle *Cesanli* (77.22) on the healthy side plus *Wangu* (SI4) on the healthy side and *Houxi* (SI3) on the diseased as guiding point.

4) Tenosynovitis

a. *Wuhu* 1 (11.27) is very effective.
b. *Cesanli* (77.22) is effective.

Tenosynovitis at the radius often results from overuse leads to strain, giving rise to wrist pain. It is important to consider the types of work that cause this disease. Typical scenarios include writers and mothers who carry children in their arms for extended periods of time. A few years ago, I was affected with tenosynovitis due to overuse of my wrist and fingers while rushing to write a manuscript. The clinical manifestations included dysfunction of the fingers when moving with large amplitude, with pain of the thumb. Needling point *Wuhu* 1 (11.27) on the opposite side is very effective. However, it can be more effective if a point on the diseased side is selected as a guiding point. Usually a few treatments will cure the disease. Tenosynovitis is often not easy to cure; however, with this method, one may obtain very good therapeutic results. During the treatment, the patient should avoid too much exercise of the wrist and fingers and take a good rest, especially when the patient has a bone spur. Periarthritis of the shoulder however, requires more exercise.

10. Question: In the case of bone spur, what other patient centered methods should be used in addition to rest?

Answer: Control of the body weight is essential to the patient of bone spur, especially the bone spur of the knee joint and heel. Obesity can aggravate the pathology. However, acupuncture over time may assist the reduction of body weight. The best method to reduce body weight is slow eating. Nine in every ten obese patents eat meals fast. Nine in every ten thin people eat their meals slowly. Therefore, the first thing, I ask such patients to eat slowly to eighty percent of his/her fill. If they avoid overeating and greasy food while controlling intake, they can lose weight. If herbal medicine is used in combination, the therapeutic effect will be improved.

Regarding the use of Chinese herbs for weight loss, there are two obesity types: excess and deficient. The deficiency type often has profuse sweating. In case of obesity of excess type, *Fang Feng Tong Sheng San* (Powder of Radix Ledebouriellae for Promoting Defecation) is often used. In case of obesity of deficiency type, *Fang Ji Huang Qi Tang* (Decoction of Radix Stephaniae Tetrandrae and Radix Astragli seu Hedysari) is often used. Most obese people have *yang* deficiency, and for this reason, *Huangqi* (Radix Astragali seu Hedysari) is added. At the same time some *yin* tonics such as *Shudi* (Radix Rehmanniae Praeparata) and *Heshouwu* (Radix Polygoni Multiflori) should be added into the prescription in order to reduce the appetite and balance *yin* and *yang*. Moreover, *Heye* (Folium Nelumbinis) which ascends *yang*, will enhance the loss of weight. In acupuncture treatment of obesity, needling points of small intestine is the best because the chyliferous vessels of the small intestines are involved in the absorption of nutrition. Needling the *yuan*-source point *Wangu* (SI4) and front-*mu* point *Guanyuan* (REN4) of the small intestine meridian plus *Liangqiu* (ST34) and *Gongsun* (SP4) can be very effective.

I have successfully used this method to treat obesity in Taipei. In 1998, I went to Tibet for benefit treatment on Tibetan Plateau. It could be very hard for me to go with my body weight. For this reason, I lost over 10 kilograms in 3 months with the treatment I gave myself. When I was in Tibet, I worked on the plateau over 4,000 meters above sea level, and treated over 100 patients per day. With *Sheng Mai San* (Pulse-activating Powder) I took daily, I was not feeling tired at all. *Sheng Mai San* has very good function to strengthen the heart. Use of the powder at the area of high elevation can help strengthen the heart and supplement *qi*.

5) Numbness of the Middle Finger

a. *Tongguan* (88.01) and *Tongshan* (88.02) are effective.
b. *Neiguan* (PC6) is very effective.

6) Pain of the Finger Joints

a. Needling *Wuhu* 1 (11.27) has special effect.
b. Needling *Renshi* (33.13) is effective.

7) Pain of the Wrist Joint

a. Needling *Cesanli* (77.22) and *Cexiasanli* (77.23) has special effect.
b. Needling *Wanshunyi* (22.09) and *Wanshun'er* (22.08) is very effective.

8) Dysfunction of the Shoulder in Lifting Arm

a. Needling *Shenguan* (77.18) on the opposite side has special effect.
b. Needling *Sihuashang* (77.08) (either of the two sides) is effective.
c. Needling *Sihuazhong* (77.09) of the diseased side is very effective.
d. Needling *Zuqianjin* (77.24) and *Zuwujin* (77.25) has special effect.
e. Needling *Huagu'er* (55.03) is effective.
f. Needling *Quling* (33.16) with elimination technique is very effective.

Tung's extraordinary points are often more effective than the points of the fourteen meridians for shoulder dysfunctions with impaired lifting of the arm. The best point is *Shenguan* (77.18) on the healthy side, while *Sihuashang* (77.08) on the healthy side and *Sihuazhong* (77.09) of the diseased side are also effective. For difficulty touching the scapula with the hand, *Zuqianjin* (77.24) or *Zuwujin* (77.25) on the healthy side may obtain therapeutic effect.

Please note that early treatment is ideal for good clinical outcomes. If the duration of the condition is more than three to four months, it can be very difficult and treatment will over a long period of time. However, in very late stages such as eight to nine months after the occurrence, the problem again becomes easier to treat. Treatment in the middle stage is the most difficult.

In periarthritis of the shoulder, the patient has difficulty raising the arm of the diseased side and touching the ear on the healthy side, neither can they push the arm backward; the pain often occurs unilaterally. It is more difficult to treat inability to push and raise the hand backward, which is known as "frozen shoulder." To treat such a case, bleed Tung's extraordinary point *Quling* (33.16) which is the same as *Chize* (LU5) of the fourteen meridians. Bleeding this point helps to loosen the tendons. This is because there is a major tendon beside point *Chize* (LU5) which follows the principle "needle tendons to treat tendon disease." To reiterate, for severe periarthritis of the shoulder, best results are achieved with blood-letting around point *Chize* (LU5). In mild cases, *Shenguan* (77.18) is sufficient. Additionally, if there is difficulty raising the arm against the back, use *Zuqianjin* (77.24) or *Zuwujin* (77.25).

Use the *shu*-stream point of the diseased meridian that passes through the area where the pain is located, and then add a guiding point to improve clinical outcomes. For example: when pain is located along the trajectory of the *yangming* meridian, needle *Sanjian* (LI3); if there is pain along the triple energizer (*Sanjiao*) meridian, needle *Zhongzhu* (SJ3); and if the pain is along the small intestine meridian, needle *Houxi* (SI3).

'Motortherapy' therapy will improve the therapeutic outcomes for periarthritis of the shoulder. Include the following mototherapeutic exercises:

a. **Standing and squatting exercise**. With one hand holding a chair on the side, do standing and squatting movement;

b. **Circular exercise** (clockwise and anti-clockwise). With the diseased arm, draw a circle in clockwise or anti-clockwise direction;

c. **Climbing a wall**. Put the palm against a wall and climb up with the fingers to the top and then slip down and then climb the wall again. All these exercises are helpful to the treatment of frozen shoulder.

9) Hand pain with Difficulty Holding an Object

a. Needle *Cesanli* (77.22) and *Cexiasanli* (77.23) on the opposite side.
b. Needle *Chongzi* (22.01) and *Chongxian* (22.02).
c. Needle *Shenguan* (77.18).

10) Sprain of the Shoulder Joint

a. Same treatment as that of difficulty in raising arm.
b. Needle *Jianzhong* (44.06).

11) Frozen Shoulder

a. Same treatment as that of difficulty in raising arm.
b. Needling *Jianzhong* (44.06) is also effective.

12) Shoulder Pain

a. Same as that of frozen shoulder.
b. Needle *Shenguan* (77.18) and *Jiuli* (88.25, 26, 27).

When there is difficulty holding an object, *Cesanli* (77.22) and *Cexiasanli* (77.23) on the healthy side are often selected. *Chongzi* (22.01) and *Chongxian* (22.02) are also effective. If *Shenguan* (77.18) is added, results are even better. All these points are very effective. The treatment of shoulder joint sprain is the same as that of periarthritis of the shoulder. *Jianzhong* (44.06) on the healthy side is also very effective for pain of the shoulder joint.

While acupuncture is very effective for periarthritis of the shoulder, the therapeutic effect is improved when Chinese herbal medicine is combined. The formula is *Juan Bi Tang* (Decoction for Treating Rheumatic or Rheumatoid Arthritis) or *Huang Qi Wu Wu Tang* (Decoction of Five Ingredients Including Radix Astragali seu Hedysari). If the left side is worse, add *Danggui* (Radix Angelicae Sinensis), and if the right side is worse, increase the dosage of *Huangqi* (Radix Astragali seu Hedysari). The same principle should be followed in the application of *Juan Bi Tang* (Decoction for Treating Rheumatic or Rheumatoid Arthritis), or *Huang Qi Gui Zhi Wu Wu Tang* (Decoction of Five Ingredients Including Radix Astragali seu Hedysari and Ramulus Cinnamomi). Periarthritis of the shoulder usually occurs for patients around the age of 50. However, it may also occur at ages 40 or 60. One reason is that senior patients often have deficiency of the liver and kidney yin, which can lead to weakness of the tendons and bones. I therefore often add *Luhancao* (Herba Pyrolae), or sometimes even *Qinjiao* (Radix Gentianae Macrophyllae) and *Sangzhi* (Ramulus Mori). *Qinjiao* (Radix Gentianae Macrophyllae) is very good for rheumatism of deficiency type and *Sangzhi* (Ramulus Mori) is also a very good herb for treating arthralgia. In the treatment of periarthritis of the shoulder, I often add *Qinjiao* (Radix Gentianae Macrophyllae), *Sangzhi* (Ramulus Mori) and *Luhancao* (Herba Pyrolae) into *Juan Bi Tang* (Decoction for Treating Rheumatic or Rheumatoid Arthritis). The dosage of *Shaoyao* (Radix Paeoniae) and *Gancao* (Radix Glycyrrhizae) may also be increased in order to capture the pain relieving function of *Shao Yao Gan Cao Tang* (Decoction of Radix Paeoniae and Radix Glycyrrhizae). In summary, acupuncture combined with Chinese herbal medicine is very effective in treatment of periarthritis of the shoulder.

13) Pain of the Acromion

a. Select point *Tongshen* (88.09), *Tongwei* (88.10) and *Tongbei* (88.11).
b. Select *Jiuli* (88.25, 26, 27) and *Cexiasanli* (77.23).
c. Needling *Shenguan* (77.18) is very effective.
d. *Chongzi* (22.01) and *Chongxian* (22.02) are also effective.

14) Pain of the Upper Arm

a. Needling *Cesanli* (77.22) and *Liuwan* (66.08) of the healthy side are effective.
b. Needling *Shenguan* (77.18) is very effective.
c. Needling *Xiyan* (Extra) is very effective.

d. Bleeding *Sihuazhong* (77.09) is very effective.
e. *Qili* (A.01) and *Jiuli* (88.25, 26, 27) are very effective.

Now let's discuss the pain of the acromian and upper arm which is an area that is typically not difficult to cure. *Shenguan* (88.17) is the best point, while *Jianzhong* (44.06) or *Yanglingquan* (GB34) on the healthy side may also be very effective. *Qili* (A.01) and *Jiuli* (88.25, 26, 27) also treat shoulder pain effectively. For pain at the acromian, *Shenguan* (77.18) or *Tongshen* (88.09) and *Tongwei* (88.10) are effective. For pain of the shoulder, upper arm and clavicle, use *Shenguan* (77.18) and *Chongzi* (22.01) since the indications for these two points are extensive. My preference is to select *Shenguan* (77.18) and *Zusanli* (ST36) to treat acromial pain.

11. Question: What are your thoughts about treatment based upon syndrome differentiation and the use of specific methods?

Answer: Treatment according to syndrome differentiation is characteristic of Chinese medicine and is the preferred method for treating difficult to treat miscellaneous diseases. However, syndrome differentiation can be used as a shield to hide one's knowledge. I would like to make an argument for specific treatment. For example in frontal headache, the solution is usually to needle *Yinlingquan* (SP9) or *Huoju* (66.11). This is simple and clear. However, some teachers intentionally or unintentionally hide their practical knowledge. They will recommend the selection of points or herbal formula based upon syndrome differentiation after inspection, auscultation and olfaction, inquiry and palpation, even though they use specific points and herbal formulas. This practice can obscure the transmission of clinical experience. In fact, acupuncture, like herbal medicine, also has points with special therapeutic effect for some diseases. Such specific drugs or acupuncture formulas are obtained from decades of clinical experience.

There is a law of 20% and 80% that exists throughout society and enterprise. In terms of economy in social systems, 20% of the population own 80% of the wealth and 80% of the population owns 20% of the wealth. In the clinic, 20% of the diseases have affected 80% of the patients. In Chinese medicine, 20% of acupuncture points are used to treat 80% of diseases while 80% of the points are used to treat 20% of the diseases. The same is true for Chinese herbal formulas.

Take gastropathy for example. Gastric ulcer is a common disease that is differentiated into five syndromes, among which deficiency of spleen and stomach *yang* is most commonly seen. According to my clinical experience and many clinical reports, the best and most effective formula for the condition is *Huang Qi Jian Zhong Tang* (Decoction of Radix

Astragali ser Hedysari for Strengthening Spleen and Stomach). This formula is almost a 'specific' for treating gastro-duodenal ulcer. In other words, 80% of the patients with gastric ulcer have this syndrome and the other four syndromes only exist in 20% of the population. Thus, the cure rate for *Huang Qi Jian Zhong Tang* when used to treat ulcer of the digestive tract is approximately 80% for the general population. The other 20% of patients are then treated according to syndrome differentiation, which takes time for inquiry regarding "cold and heat, sweating, head and body, chest, food-intake, bowel movement and urination, hearing function, drinking, old disease, and etiological factor … ." With such methods, one can only treat a few patients in one day.

It is also possible to diagnose diseases according to the main symptom. It may save time but requires rich clinical experience and diagnostic skills. Not all the doctors can do it easily. If we use specific formulas for some diseases, at least 80% of the patients may have very good effect. Though correct treatment is the most important, there are some principles in Chinese medicine to follow: The first is correctness and the second is rapidness. That is to decide the points or herbal formula quickly with no hesitance. Facing many patients, we do not have time to waste. The third is flexibility. TCM treatment is a kind of art. We can never rigidly adhere to one point or one formula in treatment. In acupuncture, we have specific points in the fourteen meridians as well as extraordinary points, and specific formulas in Chinese classical herbal medicine as well as empirical formulas based upon clinical experience. If we understand all these, we can still manage treatment without certain drugs. If we have at least two groups of points in mind, we will not always needle the same points in treatment causing repeated injury to the local tissues. Instead, we will be able to let the points have rest. There is another possibility; if we always needle the same points without change, the patient may treat him or her self at home with the same points after several treatments. Will that achieve the therapeutic effect?

15) Elbow Joint Pain

a. *Linggu* (22.05) has a special therapeutic effect.
b. *Huofuhai* (33.07) of the opposite side is very effective.
c. *Zhongjiuli* (88.25) is very effective.
d. *Sihuazhong* (77.09) also has special therapeutic effect.

Elbow joint pain is often caused by overuse syndromes and is typically medial or lateral epicondylitis. In tennis elbow (lateral epicondylitis), the pain is often located on the *yangming* meridian and we can needle *Quchi* (LI11) and *Shousanli* (LI10) on the healthy side. *Quchi* (LI11) should be punctured with the needle close to the border of the bone, following the principle of "needle the bone for bone disease." Point *Shousanli* (LI10) is located in both muscle and tendon tissues. *Huofuhai*

(33.07) is located adjacent to *Shousanli* (LI10) and also provides access to needling the tendon and muscle layers. Therefore *Quchi* (LI11) is punctured at the border of the bone, needling the bone to treat bone disease while *Huofuhai* (33.07) focuses on the tendon, treating those tissues. Further, *Linggu* (22.05) of the diseased side is selected as the guiding point for better result. Actually, point *Linggu* (22.05) is both guiding and therapeutic point, increasing the effectiveness. In this way, few treatments can cure a case.

Golf elbow (medial epicondylitis) presents with pain on the ulnar aspect of the elbow, on the course of hand-*taiyang* meridian. Needle *Xinmen* (33.12) on the healthy side; it is 2 *cun* or 3 fingers breadth away from the tip of the elbow. The point which is needled along the border of the bone was originally effectively used for spurring of the knee joint and coccygeal vertebrae. To treat golf elbow, we may needle *Xinmen* (33.12) on the healthy side and *Houxi* (SI3) or *Wanshunyi* (22.08) on the diseased side as the guiding point. The therapeutic effect will be very good.

12. Question: There is no reinforcing and reducing methods have been mentioned in Tung's Acupuncture book. What are the reinforcing and reducing techniques in the practice of Tung's acupuncture?

Answer: I also often used reinforcing and reducing methods in practice 30 years ago. Also, the detailed description of reinforcing and reducing techniques with either rotation of the needle or the direction along or against the course of meridian are addressed in my book *Zhen Jiu Jing Wei* (The Strategy of Acupuncture). Tung's acupuncture has its own characteristic methods including: active *qi* moving (*Dong Qi*) technique, point coupling (*Dao Ma*) technique, and point guiding (*Qian Yin*) technique which I created; here, Tung's extraordinary points are combined with the points of the fourteen. All these techniques are characterized by a two-way regulatory function that is generated by the use of distal points, *qi* induction and *qi* moving. The even method is sufficient when distal points are needled causing the reinforcing or reducing method to be generally unnecessary. Reinforcing and reducing methods are often used with the fourteen meridians because many local or *Ashi* points are selected. When the needles are inserted locally, the patient cannot move the diseased area, and fails to move *qi*, thus reinforcing or reducing method is necessary. Thirty years ago in mainland China, there were many texts addressing reinforcing and reducing techniques. Recently, there is more attention on the selection of distal points; as a result, the reinforcing and reducing techniques are less frequently emphasized. However, I do continue to use the respiratory reinforcing and reducing method.

However, let's look more deeply into this question since deep studies have identified two circulatory systems of the meridians. Discrepancies regarding reinforcing and reducing techniques continue. An area of question is the reinforcing and reducing methods that involve needling with or against the course of meridian. Chapter 10 of *Lingshu* (Spiritual Pivot) discusses the *qi* of the five-*shu* points running from the hands and feet to the heart, that is, from the distal aspect of the limbs to the heart. The *Lingshu* also discusses *qi* traveling from *Zhongfu* (LU1) to *Yunmen* (LU2), *Taiyuan* (LU9), *Chize* (LU5), *Yuji* (LU10), and finally to *Shaoshang* (LU11). However, the first acupuncture book to appear after the *Lingshu* (Spiritual Pivot) is the *Zhen Jiu Jia Yi Jing* (The Systematic Classic of Acupuncture and Moxibustion). It details the flow of lung meridian *qi* in only one direction, from *Shaoshang* (LU11) to *Yuji* (LU10), *Taiyuan* (LU9), *Jingqu* (LU8), and finally to *Chizi* (LU5). While these two books have disparate views, yet both affirm the movement of *qi* from the distal aspect towards the heart.

Chapter 10 of *Lingshu* (Spiritual Pivot) describes two different circulations of the 12 regular meridians: the concentric and the eccentric. The one that runs from hands and feet to the heart is concentric, and the one that runs from the chest to the hands and feet is eccentric. The identical description about the running directions in the two books are the three yang meridians of hand which run from the hand to the head and heart, and the three yin meridians of foot which run from the foot to the heart. The difference in the two books is that, in *Lingshu* (Spiritual Pivot), the three *yin* meridians of hand run from the chest to the hand, and the three *yang* meridians of foot run from the head to the foot; while in *Zhen Jiu Jia Yi Jing* (The Systematic Classic of Acupuncture and Moxibustion), they are all concentric. With so many contradictions regarding the direction of the meridians, how shall we perform reducing and reinforcing techniques by needling along and against the meridians? We can forget those that are contradictory, and follow those that are the same in the two books. However, my experience is that neither needling points along nor against the running directions nor needling with rotation is as effective as the active *qi* moving method.

Until now, the method of reinforcing and reducing that has no argument is the one with lifting and thrusting. It states in Chapter 76 of *Nanjing* (The Classic of Difficulties): "Take the *qi* from the *Wei* system for tonification and *Ying* system for elimination." It means, in case of tonification, take the *qi* in the *Wei* system and push the *qi* inward; and in case of elimination, take the *qi* in the *Ying* system and pull the *qi* outward. The needling techniques *Shao Shan Huo* (Heat-producing Needling) and *Tou Tian Liang* (Cold Heaven-penetrating Needling) are derived from the development of the lifting and thrusting methods. *Shao Shan Huo* consists of three thrusts and one lift and the emphasis is placed on thrust, whereas *Tou Tian Liang* consists of one thrust and three lifts and the emphasis is placed on the lift, to pull *qi* outward from the *Ying* system. *Tou Tian Liang* has the therapeutic effect of elimination and *Shao Shan Huo* has the therapeutic effect of tonification. But, how do we use this technique in the clinic? Take for example, a common disease such as gout with increasing morbidity in recent years. Generally, there appears redness, swelling and pain of the great or middle toe in gout. Needling the third point of *Wuhu* (11.27) may quickly stop pain. However, the pain often reoccurs soon after treatment because the treatment doesn't target the underlying condition, which is the uric acid. To treat the underlying condition, it is necessary to lower the uric acid. Otherwise the disease continues to recur. While one treatment can stop pain, more treatments are needed to lower the uric acid. Once the uric acid is low, the patient will not have attacks for a long period of time.

I usually select the third point of *Wuhu* (11.27) plus *Zusanli* (ST36) for gout. When needling *Zusanli* (ST36), insert the needle to a depth of 2 *cun* and retain the needle for 10 minutes. Then, manipulate the needle with strong stimulation and lift the needle one-third of the insertion. Retain the needle for another 10 minutes and then manipulate the needle with strong stimulation and lift the needle for another one-third of the insertion. This method is known as "taking the *qi* from the *Ying* system," which clears heat and reduces fire with good therapeutic effect for gout. The needle is retained for another 10 minutes and then manipulated with strong stimulation, and finally removed. In this way, the needle is first inserted directly to the layer of earth, then lifted to the layer of man; and finally to the heaven, and removed. One thrust and three lifts places the emphasis on lifting; this eliminates *qi* from the *Ying* system so as to clear heat from the blood. When the needle is removed from *Zusanli* (ST36), needles in the point *Wuhusan*, the third point of *Wuhu* (11.27) can still be retained in the point for few more minutes, and at the same time ask the patient to exercise the painful area. The patient may feel much relieved or no pain at all after one such treatment.

Let's explore skin diseases as another example. Many texts recommend *Quchi* (LI11) and *Xuehai* (SP10) or *Sanyinjiao* (SP6) for skin diseases. While these are commonly used points, the outcomes are often less than desired. Some texts recommend *Quchi* (LI11) as the main point for the upper part of the body, and *Xuehai* (SP10) for the lower part of the body. The therapeutic effect of *Xuehai* (SP10), *Quchi* (LI11) or *Fengshi* (GB31), are improved when using the eliminate *qi* from the *Ying* system method. In many skin diseases, the skin becomes red and itches when there is heat in the blood. In this case, *Quchi* (LI11) and *Fengshi* (GB31) can be needled to a depth of 2 *cun*. Then the needle is lifted one-third of the depth with strong stimulation 10 minutes later. Repeat this 3 times before the needle is removed. This type of reducing method often causes itching to quickly subside. While I have introduced in detail the reinforcing and reducing method with lifting and thrusting manipulation, I believe that you will develop even better and more effective reinforcing and reducing method in your own clinical studies.

There is detailed description about reinforcing and reducing method in the book *Zhen Jiu Jing Wei* (The Strategy of Acupuncture) I published 30 years ago. In recent years I have been revising and compiling the book and it is completed. A new book *Zhen Jiu Bao Dian* (The Treasure of Acupuncture and Moxibustion) is published in Taiwan and mainland of China, and Korea soon. The content of the book will be much richer and more profound than *Zhen Jiu Jing Wei* (The Strategy of Acupuncture). The book "The Strategy of Acupuncture" has been printed over 20 times with certain revision and served as the textbook of universities, the new book "The Treasure of Acupuncture and Moxibustion" will become the textbook of the doctoral studies.

16) Cramping of the Hand and Arm

a. Needle *Huoshan* (33.06) on the opposite side.

Now let's discuss cramping of the hand and arm. To treat this disease, we can needle point *Huoshan* (33.06) on the opposite side first. Second, we can needle *Quling* (33.16) which is *Chizi* (LU5) of the fourteen meridians and use the reducing method. It is also very good to needle *Waiguan* (SJ5) on the healthy side. If applying correspondence method, we can also needle *Boqiu* (77.04) or *Chengshan* (BL57).

I would like to introduce the correspondence method in detail. I went to the largest bookstore in Korea today where I found books that introduce the correspondence needling method but without details. Here I'd like to introduce the method briefly. There are several *Taijis* in the human body. The great *Taiji* takes the umbilicus as the core. The medium *Taiji* takes the knee and elbow as the core. And the minor *Taiji* takes the wrist and ankle as the core. All these form the basis of the correspondence method, which is a holographic model. Here, I will introduce the great *Taiji* and address the medium and minor *Taijis* later. A good command of *Taiji* correspondences will greatly help improve one's acupuncture skill, and can assist the selection of points without consideration of the meridians.

Since the *Song* dynasty, there have been 361 points in the fourteen meridians and the number has not been changed. Physicians have concentrated on the study of these points, greatly improving the level of acupuncture. Newer points discovered more recently have been taken as the extraordinary points. Many of Tung's extraordinary points are located on the fourteen meridians. We will use the points published by Master Tung for the first time in 1973 as the standard. There are many points that were added later, which are not recognized as Tung's extraordinary points. This prevents confusion in the system of Tung's extraordinary points.

What we should do is to continue our profound studies of the original Tung's extraordinary points, making a more consummate use of his system.

I have mentioned previously that there are several groups of effective points for each disease, and that each group must have one principal point. Though *Linggu* (22.05) and *Dabai* (22.04) are often selected together, however, we try to use only one of these points. In this way, we can deepen our understanding to the property and therapeutic effects of each point. At present, doctors often select many points for various diseases, selecting 5-6 points for each disease. If we treat one patient suffering from several diseases, we will have to select a large number of points. For this reason, I am going to write a book in 2-3 years, which will be published by Great Star Press in Korea. In the book I will talk about treatment with one needle, known as one needle therapy. For each disease, only one point is selected. For example, select *Quchi* (LI11) for hypertension. In the book, the mechanism and needling technique will be introduced in detail. *Quchi* (LI11) is the *He*-sea point of the large intestine meridian which has ample *qi* and blood, the point is therefore able to regulate *qi* and blood. It is stated in *Neijing* (Yellow Emperor's Inner Classic): "*He*-sea points are indicated for disorders of the *fu* organs." Based upon this statement we use *He*-sea points for the *fu* organs. In the book written by Tang Zonghai of *Qing* dynasty, it is mentioned that the liver is connected with the large intestine. To treat liver disease, we dredge the large intestine. It also says in Chapter 72 of *Suwen* (Essential Questions), "To reduce the wood (liver), needle the *He*-sea point of the hand-*yangming* meridian." This is *Quchi* (LI11), the *He*-sea point of the large intestine meridian, which should be needled for hyperactivity of liver *qi*. This point is effective for hyperactivity of liver *yang* and hypertension is mostly due to hyperactivity of liver yang. It may help lower both systolic and diastolic hypertension. Further, *Quchi* (LI11) is a very good point for vertigo. Chinese medicine holds that the liver is closely related to vertigo.

I'd like to take hiccup as another example. The most commonly used point for hiccup is *Jianshi* (PC5). It is the *Jing*-river point of pericardium meridian and pertains to metal according the theory of five elements. It is said in *Neijing* (Yellow Emperor's Inner Classic): "In case of pathological changes of voice, select *Jing*-river point." *Jing*-river point is a very effective point for abnormal change of the voice and hiccup is a type of abnormal voice. Then why do we have to select the *Jing*-river point of the pericardium meridian? It is because the pericardium is connected with the stomach through the extraordinary connections of the *zangfu*. Hiccup is related to the stomach *qi*. *Jianshi* (PC5) is the *Jing*-river point of the pericardium, which is connected with the stomach, and hiccup is a pathological change of the voice, this point is therefore effective for hiccup. If the condition is mild, it will be cured soon. If the condition is severe, it takes more treatments.

If all kinds of diseases are treated with selection of one point according to these principles, the therapeutic results will be more remarkable and bring the therapeutic function of the point into full play.

17) Tonic Spasm of the Hands

a. Needle *Quling* (33.16) with reducing method, and needle *Shenguan* (77.18).
b. Needle *Chongzi* (22.01) and *Chongxian* (22.02).

Tonic spasm of the hands relates to tendon problems. *Quling* (33.16), which is the same as *Chize* (LU5), is effective. It is the water point and the son point of the lung meridian. Needling this point with strong stimulation will reduce metal, causing the metal to not overact on the wood, thus curing disease of the tendons. There is also a large tendon beside *Chize* (LU5), we needle this point just at the border of the tendon, following the principle of "needle tendon to treat tendon disease." Further, *yanglingquan* (GB34) is the influential point of tendons and it is also an effective point for spasm of hands. Other points that relax the tonic spasm of the hands include *Chongzi* (22.01) and *Chongxian* (22.02). *Shenguan* (77.18) may also help for disorders of the palm, including tonic spasm of the hands.

2. Diseases of the Lower Limbs

1) Sciatica

a. *Linggu* (22.05) and *Dabai* (22.04) have a special effect.
   Biyi (1010.22) has a special effect.
b. Blood-let *Jinlin* (DT.09).
c. Bleed the blue vein at point *Weizhong* (BL40).

Sciatica is a common disease in modern society. When using the fourteen meridians, we need to understand the etiology and the diseased meridians. It often seems there are no specific points for the disease and local tender points are typically needled. However, in my experience, distal points of the fourteen meridians are also very good.

The point coupling (*Dao Ma*) technique is useful for both the fourteen meridian and the extraordinary points. The point coupling method employs two and occasionally three needles. For instance, in case of pain of the *taiyang* meridian, select *Wangu* (SI4) coupled with *Houxi* (SI3). If the pain goes along the *shaoyang* meridian on the lateral side of the leg, select *Waiguan* (SJ5) coupled with *Zhigou* (SJ6). In Master Tung's system of extraordinary points, sciatica is mainly treated with selection of *Linggu* (22.05) coupled with *Dabai* (22.04). The two points are the most effective ones for the pain on either *taiyang* or *shaoyang* meridian, and possibly pain on the medial aspect of the thigh. There is no comparison between the two points and the points of the fourteen meridians. After *Linggu* (22.05) and *Dabai* (22.04), *Biyi* (1010.22) is another effective point. In Tung's acupuncture, *Shouwujin* (33.08) and *Shouqianjin* (33.09) are also effective for sciatica.

The points that I use to treat various kinds of sciatica include *Linggu* (22.05) and *Dabai* (22.04). *Weizhong* (BL40) is bled to improve results when the sciatica is caused by a bone spur. Blood-letting therapy has very good therapeutic effect for complicated compressive sciatica. Needling *Linggu* (22.05) and *Dabai* (22.04) is enough for simple sciatica and sometimes guiding point (*Qian Yin*) is selected in combination on the diseased side when the condition is severe. The method is to select the guiding point from the diseased channel after needling *Linggu* (22.05) and *Dabai* (22.04), and 80-90% of the patients are completely cured. For example, in treatment of pain along the *taiyang* meridian, add point *Sugu* (UB65) of the urinary bladder meridian of foot *taiyang* as the guiding point. In case of sciatica with pain along the *shaoyang* meridian, we can select *Zulingqi* (GB41) as the guiding point. If the pain is located at the groin on the medial aspect of the thigh along the path of the liver meridian, we can select *Taichong* (LR3) as the guiding point. If the pain is on the anterior aspect of the thigh where the stomach meridian of foot-*yangming* travels, we can select *Menjin* (66.05) located on the stomach meridian as the guiding point. In summary, needling *Linggu* (22.05) and *Dabai* (22.04) in combination with a guiding point is most effective for sciatica. I have treated many patients of sciatica with this method. In the treatment, I mainly select *Shu*-stream point as the guiding point, because it is said in book *Nanjing* (The classic of Difficulties): "*Shu*-stream point is indicated in heaviness and pain of the body and joints." All these *Shu*-stream points are specific points for pain syndromes, functioning together with *Linggu* (22.05) and *Dabai* (22.04) for the upper and lower of the body, and thus the good therapeutic effect.

Following are herbal prescriptions for sciatica. In TCM, Chinese herbal medicine and acupuncture have the same theoretical foundation. This is an example of using the same treatment to address similar diseases. While *Linggu* (22.05) and *Dabai* (22.04) are specific for sciatica, and hemiplegia, *Du Huo Ji Sheng Tang* (Decoction of Radix Angelicae Pubescentis and Ramulus Loranthi) is also indicated in sciatica; it therefore must also be indicated in hemiplegia. Similarly, we use *Bu Yang Huan Wu Tang* to treat sciatica and hemiplegia, just like the above two points. TCM holds that to treat wind we need to treat blood first, because when the blood circulation goes back to normal, wind will disappear. Both of these formulas have the ingredients that treat blood. However, the herbs for regulating *qi* are indispensable. In *Bu Yang Huan Wu Tang*, *Huangqi*

(Radix Astragalicaser Hedysari) has a large dosage, and in *Du Huo Ji Sheng Tang*, *Renshen* (Radix Ginseng) is applied. The reason is that blood circulation relies on propelling function of *qi*.

When sciatica results from bone spur, the following acupuncture methods may obtain better therapeutic effect. Master Tung's first choice for treatment of bone spur of lumbar vertebrae was *Minghuang* (88.12). He secondly, needled *Sihuazhong* (77.09) and *Sihuaxia* (77.11) along the border of the bone for enhanced effect. According to my own experience, there is a group of points that can be selected they include *Renzhong* (DU26), *Houxi* (SI3), *Sugu* (UB65) and *Fengshi* (GB31). I previously mentioned this point set for numbness of the fingers. However, these points are also effective for sciatica and bone spurring of the lumbar vertebrae and the cervical vertebrae. If blood-letting is applied to *Weizhong* (BL40), the therapeutic effect will be even faster. The blood-letting therapy is given once every week or every 10 days.

2) Pain of Thigh

a. Needle *Sanchasan* (A.04) for a special effect.
b. Bleed point *Jinlin* (DT.09).
c. Needle *Qili* (A.01) and *Jiuli* (88.26).

Sanchasan (A.04) is the most effective and frequently used point for the treatment of thigh pain. The point is especially good when the thigh pain is due to fatigue since it alleviates soreness and pain but also eliminate fatigue after a long walk. Additionally, *Biyi* (1010.22) is effective for fatigue and *Jiuli* (88.25, 26, 27) is effective for pain of the thigh.

3) Cramping of Foot

a. Needling *Zhengjin* (77.01) is effective.
b. Needle *Cibai* (A.06).
c. Needle *Ganmen* (33.11).

In treatment of cramping of the foot, we can needle *Zhengjin* (77.01) according to the principle of "needle the tendon to treat tendon diseases." The second point is *Cibai* (A.06) and *Ganmen* (33.11) is effective as well. *Cibai* (A.06) is located 0.5 *cun* distal to the junction of the third and fourth metacarpal bones, and levels with point *Zhongbai* (22.06). It is a very good point for cramping as well as distension, pain and soreness of the leg. *Ganmen* (33.11) is located on the hand-*taiyang* meridian on the forearm, corresponding to point *Chengshan* (BL57) of the foot-*taiyang* meridian. It is also effective for cramping of the leg. In the points of the fourteen meridians, we often select *Chengshan* (UB57) on the healthy side to treat cramping of the leg.

4) Heel Pain

a. Needling *Linggu* (22.05) is very effective.
b. Needle the five points of *Wuhu* (11.27).
c. Bleeding *Weizhong* (BL40) has special therapeutic effect.

There are 10-20 specific points for heel pain, including the points of the fourteen meridians. Selecting only a few of them would be sufficient. In Tung's acupuncture, the most frequently used points are *Linggu* (22.05) and *Wuhu* (11.27), with the most commonly used point of the fourteen meridians being *Daling* (PC7). There is another effective point, *Jiaogengxue* that is 0.5 *cun* anterior to *Daling* (PC7) for heel pain. The point most frequently used by Master Tung is *Linggu* (22.05). According to holographic theory, it is located at proximal end of the second metacarpal bone, this corresponds with the leg and heel, and is therefore effective for heel pain. Heel pain often results from kidney deficiency or bone spur. To treat bone spur, we use the principles, "treat the bone for bone disease" and "treat the bone for kidney disease." Here, we needle point *Linggu* (22.05) along the border of the bone.

Baihui (DU20) and *Houhui* (1010.06) may also be needled for heel pain. This method is based on the correspondence between the vertex and the sole. I often select *Linggu* (22.05) and find it very effective. Further, *Sugu* (BL65) as a guiding point (*Qian Yin*) is also effective. It is the *Shu*-stream point of the urinary bladder meridian, needling this point along the border of the bone also employs the principle, "needle the bone to treat bone disease." Heel pain pertains to pathological changes in the kidney and bladder meridians. Moreover, heel pain can also be cured by needling *Sihuazhong* (77.09) and *Sihuaxia* (77.11) along the border of the bone. In herbal medicine, modified *Liu Wei Di Huang Wan* (Pills of Six Ingredients Including Radix Rehmanniae) may be used with large dosage of *Dihuang* (Radix Rehmanniae) 30g plus *Niuxi* (Radix Achyranthis Bidentatae) and *Weilingxian* (Radix Clematidis).

5) Soreness of Foot with Difficulty Walking

a. Needle *Cibai* (A.06) or bleed the blue vein at point *Weizhong* (BL40).
b. Bleed *Jingzhi* (DT.08).

Soreness of the foot with difficulty walking results from pathological changes of the leg. *Cibai* (A.06) has a special therapeutic effect for this. It is also good to bleed *Jingzhi* (DT.08) on the back. We can also bleed the blue vein at *Weizhong* (BL40) for leg pain. It is similar to bleeding *Chize* (LU5) for the arm pain. It treats pain of both the thigh and leg, but the thigh in particular. In case of soreness and pain of the thigh only, needling *Sanchasan* (A.04) is very effective. In severe case, bleed point *Jinlin* (DT.09). In case of soreness of both the thigh and leg, needle both

Sanchasan (A.04) and *Cibai* (A.06). Bleeding *Weizhong* (BL40) is given only when the pathological condition is severe.

6) Weakness of Legs

a. *Jianzhong* (44.06) and *Tongtian* (88.03) have a special effect.
b. *Muzhi* (1010.18) also has a good therapeutic effect.
c. *Shuijin* (1010.20) or *Shuitong* (1010.19) are also effective.

Jianzhong (44.06) and *Tongtian* (88.03) are very good for weakness of the legs. *Muzhi* (1010.18) is also every good. Needling *Shuijin* (1010.20) and *Shuitong* (1010.19) may tonify the lung and kidney effectively. In case of hemiplegia, needle *Muhuo* (11.10) for a good therapeutic effect. Further, *Muzhi* (1010.18) is effective for weakness of legs of senior patients.

7) Numbness of Legs

a. Needle *Sima* (88.17, 18, 19).
b. Needle *Jianzhong* (44.06).

Needling *Sima* (88.17, 18, 19) for numbness of the legs is effective. Besides, *Jianzhong* on the healthy side can also be selected. *Shenguan* (77.18) is also effective. In severe case, bleed *Shuangfeng* (DT.05). Bleeding this point may treat numbness of the hands and feet. If needling *Xiasanhuang* (77.18, 19, 21) is added on the leg, the therapeutic effect is even better.

8) Numbness of Toes

a. Needle *Xiasanhuang* (77.17, 19, 21).
b. Needle *Wuhusan*, the third point of *Wuhu* (11.27).
c. Bleed *Shuangfeng* (DT.05).

In the treatment of numbness of foot, we may needle *Xiasanhuang* (77.18, 19, 21), or needle *Renhuang* (77.21) and *Dihuang* (77.19) first and then needle *Shenguan* (77.18). *Shenguan* (77.18) is an important and effective point. Besides, the third point of *Wuhu* (11.27) is also effective. In severe case, bleed *Shuangfeng* (DT.05). If the numbness of toes is resulted from bone spur of spinal vertebrae, treat the bone spur.

9) Cold Pain of Legs

a. Needle *Muhuo* (11.10).
b. Needle *Jianzhong* (44.06) and *Jiuli* (88.25, 26, 27).
c. Bleed *Shuangfeng* (DT.05).
d. Needle *Tongtian* (88.03) and *Tongwei* (88.10).

Cold pain of legs is more common in senior persons. Point *Muhuo* (11.10) has very good therapeutic effect for the disease. Everybody knows how to use this point. Someone has compiled a book titled "Tung's Extraordinary Acupuncture Therapy," in which it is said *Muhuo* has four points: Muhuo1, Muhuo2, Muhuo3 and Muhuo4. It is stated that only Muhuo2 is most effective. Actually, Muhuo2 is the real point *Muhuo* (11.10). In the same book, point *Fuyuan* (11.22) is subdivided into Fuyuan1, Fuyuan2 and Fuyuan3, and point *Fuke* (11.24) into Fuke1, Fuke2 and Fuke3. However, only one or two of them are used in practice. It is just like drawing a snake and adding feet to it, giving more confusion to practitioners. The Tung's extraordinary are always simple and clear.

10) Cold Pain of Knees

a. Needle *Tongtian* (88.03) and *Tongshan* (88.02).
b. Needle *Jianzhong* (44.06).
c. Bleeding *Sanjin* (DT.07) is very effective.

Cold pain of knees often occurs in winter, and *Muhuo* (11.10) is very effective. *Jianzhong* (44.06) is also very good. *Tongshan* (88.03) and *Tongtian* (88.02) are also effective. Point *Neiguan* (PC6) of the fourteen meridians is also very effective. For knee joint pain including bone spur, chronic condition in particular, bleeding *Sanjin* (DT.07) is the best and has radical effect.

11) Knees Joint Pain

a. Needling *Jianzhong* (44.06) has special effect.
b. Bleeding *Sanjin* (DT.07) has special effect for chronic knee joint pain.
c. Needle *Zhongjian* (11.05).
d. Needle point *Dan* (11.13).
e. Needle *Xinmen* (33.12).
f. Needle *Muhuo* (11.10).
g. Needle *Sihuazhong* (77.09) and *Sihuaxia* (77.11) along the border of the bone.

There are many effective points for knee joint pain. According to my experience, point *Neiguan* (PC6) of the fourteen meridians is the best point. It is because there exists the extraordinary connection between the pericardium and the stomach. Via *Waixiyan* (ST36), the stomach meridian is closely connected with the knee joint. *Neiguan* (PC6) is the *Luo*-connecting point of the pericardium and is located between two tendons, it is very effective to treat spasm, pain and dysfunction of the knee joint in flexion and extension, since needling tendon can treat tendon disease. In Tung's acupuncture, *Jianzhong* (44.06) is a very good point for knee joint pain. Master Tung also often selected *Dan* (11.13) and *Zhongjian* (11.05) to treat knee joint pain. Besides, *Chongzi* (22.01) and *Chongxian* (22.02) are also indicated in knee joint pain.

The most effective point for knee joint pain introduced in the ancient medical songs such as *Zhou Hou Ge* (Song to Keep Up your Sleeve) and *Xi Hong Fu* (Ode of Xi Hong) is *Taichong* (LR3). *Tong Xuan Fu* (Ode of the Essentials of Understanding) and *Sheng Yu Ge* (Song More Precious than Jade) consider that this point can treat difficulty in walking. Besides, point *Xingjian* (LR2) located anterior to *Taichong* (LR3) is also another important point for swelling and pain of knee joints (see *Za Bing Xue Fa Ge* (Song of Points for Miscellaneous Diseases), *Tong Xuan Zhi Yao Fu* (Ode of the Essentials of Understanding)and *Sheng Yu Ge* (Song More Precious Than Jade)). Personally, I often select *Neiguan* (PC6) of the healthy side combined with *Taichong* (LR3) of the diseased side to treat knee joint pain, and have obtained very immediate effect. Both of the two points are therapeutic points. However, *Taichong* (LR3) on the diseased side serves as the guiding point as well. In selection of guiding points, the most commonly used are *Ying*-spring points and *Shu*-stream points, and the latter in particular, because "*Shu*-stream points are indicated in heaviness and pain of the body and joints." Better result can be obtained if *Taichong* (LR3) is selected in combination with *Neiguan* (PC6), one in the upper, and one in the lower, working together to regulate *qi*, thus complement each other. In recent years, we have select *Xinmen* (33.12) on the diseased side as the therapeutic point for knee joint pain; especially that caused by arthritis due to bone spur. In the treatment, *Taichong* (LR3) of the diseased side is taken as the guiding point to make the therapeutic effect better and faster. Knee joint is very liable to have bone spur and the knee joint pain in many cases is caused by spur. In this case, when the above method is combined with needling *Sihuazhong* (77.09) and *Sihuaxia* (77.11) along the border of the bone, the therapeutic effect could be even better. We can also needle *Xinmen* (33.12) and *Taichong* (LR3), and then bleed *Sanjin* (DT.07) once a week to speed up the cure.

I have been to many Korean restaurants here this time and some of them are very large. According to the local habit, everybody has to squad and sits down for meal and it is quite difficult for the patients with knee joint pain. The above method can help such patients with filiform needling only. If blood-letting therapy is added, the effect will be even better.

12) Ankle Sprain

a. Needling *Xiaojie* (A.05) has special effect.
b. Needle the fourth point of *Wuhu* (11.27).
c. Bleeding *Weizhong* (BL40) has special effect.

Now let's discuss ankle sprain. If you don't know the point *Xiaojie* (A.05), you can needle the fourth point of *Wuhu* (11.27). *Xiaojie* (A.05) is located on the radial side of the first metacarpal bone, at the junction of the white and dark skin (on the course of the lung meridian of hand-*taiyin*). To needle this point is with a fist in the direction towards *Chongxian* (22.02) or *Daling* (PC7). This point is very effective for ankle sprain of either medial of lateral side. Many athletes are liable to get ankle sprain. I have used this point to treat many of them, including basketball player, tennis player and gymnastic athletes successfully. If there is no redness and swelling, one treatment can cure the patient completely or at least 70-80%. If there is redness and swelling, it has immediate analgesic effect. In addition, we can grind red beans into powder that is mixed with egg white and then apply the paste on the local area. It can help eliminate swelling quickly. Or use the three-edged needle to bleed *Sihuawai* (77.14) first to subside swelling and then needle point *Xiaojie* (A.05).

13) Foot Pain

a. Needle *Jiuli* (88.25, 26, 27).
b. Needle the third and fourth point of *Wuhu* (11.27).

Here the foot pain mainly refers to the pain of the sole and dorsum of the foot. To treat such foot pain, we can needle *Jiuli* (88.25, 26, 27) on the opposite side. The point *Jiuli* corresponds to *Fengshi* (GB31). It is also effective to needle the third point of *Wuhu* (11.27). In case of leg pain, needling *Jiuli* (88.25, 26, 27) is effective. Besides, *Cibai* (A.06) is also effective.

14) Distending Pain of Legs (soreness and pain)

a. Needling *Cibai* (A.06) has extremely good effect.
b. Needle *Jianzhong* (44.06).
c. Bleeding *Jingzhi* (DT.08) is extremely good.

To treat distending pain or soreness and pain of the leg, we can needle *Cibai* (A.06) on the opposite side. It is also effective to needle *Jianzhong* (44.06) on the diseased side. In severe case, we can bleed *Jingzhi* (DT.08) on the back.

15) Soreness and Pain of Thigh

a. Needling *Sanchasan* (A.04) is effective.
b. Needle *Jianzhong* (44.06).
c. Needle *Qili* (A.01) and *Jiuli* (88.25, 26, 27).
d. Needle *Shuitong* (1010.19) and *Shuijin* (1010.20).
e. Bleeding the area around *Beimian* (44.07) is very effective.
f. Bleeding *Jinlin* (DT.09).

To treat soreness and pain of thigh, *Sanchasan* (A.04) may obtain the best result. It is also very effective to needle *Qili* (A.01) and *Jiuli* (88.25, 26, 27) on the opposite side. *Shuitong* (1010.19) and *Shuijin* (1010.20) are also effective points. Besides, it is also good to give blood-letting around point *Beimian* (44.07) or to *Jinlin* (DT.09) when the condition is severe.

16) Pain of Toes

a. Needle the third point of *Wuhu* (11.27).

Generally, it is quite effective to needle the third point of *Wuhu* (11.27) for simple pain of toes, including sprain, contusion and rheumatism. If it is caused by gout, *Wuhu* (11.27) on the opposite side is effective. However, the pain may come back after treatment due to uric acid. To avoid this, it is advisable to needle *Zusanli* (ST36) on the diseased side simultaneously, strengthening the earth to restrict the wood so as to speed the excretion of uric acid. The method of eliminating *ying* (nutrient) system should be adopted when needling *Zusanli* (ST36). That is to insert the needle directly to the earth with the depth of 2 *cun*. Then lift the needle 0.5-0.7 *cun* once every 10 minutes. Remove the needle after 30 minutes retention. It is an effective therapeutic method for gout, because TCM considers there is heat in the blood due to local redness and swelling. It is stated in *Nanjing* (The Classic of Difficulties): Take *qi* from the *ying* system for elimination. This method is applied to eliminate heat from the blood. (For tonification, we have to push *qi* inward, that is to push *qi* inward from the *wei* "defensive" system; for elimination, we have to eliminate *qi* from inside by lifting the needle).

I think there must be many patients of gout in Korea. Why? Because there is a lot of sea food here. I don't know whether Korean people eat internal organs of animals. But I do know Korean people drink a lot. So there must be a lot of gout patients. In herbal medicine, the formula *Dang Gui Nian Tong Tang* (Decoction of Radix Angelicae Sinensis for Pain Relief) is very effective for gout. In my early years, I often used this formula. In recent years, I often use *Shao Yao Gan Cao Tang* (Decoction of Radix Paeoniae and Radix Glycyrrhizae) combined with *Si Miao San* (Powder of Four Wonderful Drugs). Though the ingredients are less, it is still very effective for acute attack of gout. After acute attack, we need to strengthen the underlying condition (*ben*) for which I often use *Si Miao San* (Powder of Four Wonderful Drugs) combined with *Si Ling San* (Powder of Four Diuretic Drugs) with modification to reduce uric acid. The only difference between *Si Ling San* (Powder of Four Diuretic Drugs) and *Wu Ling San* (Powder of Five Drugs Including poria) is the use of *Guizhi* (Ramulus Cinnamomi). The two formulas combined together are very effective for decrease of uric acid and prevention of gout attack. During my lectures for Shanghai Association of Traditional Chinese Medicine and Shanghai Association of Acupuncture and Moxibustion in 1992, I was asked what gout was and how it was treated. The question shows that there were few cases of gout at that time. Many people had never heard of it. After many years passed, this disease has developed very fast in mainland of China. When I visited Shanghai again in 1999, many doctors there had already treated many case of gout. I think there must be many patients of gout here in Korea after so many years of development. The method I have introduced for treating gout is quite effective. In acupuncture treatment, needle the third point of *Wuhu* (11.27) and *Zusanli* (ST36). During acute attack, take *Shao Yao Gan Cao Tang* (Decoction of Radix Paeoniae and Radix Glycyrrhizae) combined with *Si Miao San* (Powder of Four Wonderful Drugs) or *Dang Gui Nian Tong Tang* (Radix Angelicae Sinensis for Pain Relief).

13. Question: How is twitching of the lower eyelid treated with acupuncture?

Answer: I have talked about this before. Here I'd like to talk about it again more in details. Twitching of the lower eyelid pertains to facial spasm. The points that I select most frequently are *Sanjian* (LI3) of the large intestine meridian and *Houxi* (SI3) of the small intestine meridian, because the distribution of the two meridians are closely related to the face. The small intestine meridian arrives at the outer and inner canthus, and needling *Houxi* (SI3) is therefore effective. According to the five elements, *Houxi* (SI3) pertains to wood, and tremor or twitching is related to liver wind, thus the point has the function to dispel wind, and is therefore effective for the wind symptom of the small intestine meridian. Besides, it is the *Shu*-stream point of the small intestine meridian and the *Shu*-stream point is indicated in heaviness and pain of the body and joints, it is therefore effective for pain on the distribution of the small intestine meridian such as trigeminal neuralgia. Why *Sanjian* (LI3) is selected? The location of point *Sanjian* (LI3) is close to *Dabai* (22.04)). According to the theory of holography, it corresponds to head and face. Moreover, it pertains to wood according to the theory of five elements, and is therefore indicated in liver wind. Thus it is effective for treating twitching of the face due to wind, and trigeminal neuralgia as well. In addition to the above two points, *Taichong* (LR3) of the fourteen meridians is also effective. It is a point of the liver meridian and liver dominates wind, the point is therefore effective to dispel wind. The liver meridian "enters the head at vertex and connects with the eye system. Its branch travels downward from the eye, passes the cheek and winds around inside of the lips." The liver meridian is closely connected with the eye and periocular tissues.

The most frequently used points by Master Tung are *Cesanli* (77.22) and *Cexiasanli* (77.23). The two points are located between the *shaoyang* and *yangming* meridians, and are therefore indicated in disorders of the two meridians, or wind disease of *yangming* meridian. Both *shaoyang* and *jueyin* meridians dominate wind, and the two points are therefore effective. It is also advisable to needle *Dabai* (22.04) and *Houxi* (SI3) together with the above two points to strengthen the therapeutic effect from both the upper part and lower part of the body. In this way, we needle few points and obtain better result. In herbal medicine, I personally often use *Shao Yao Gan Cao Tang* (Decoction of Radix Paeoniae and Radix

Glycyrrhizae) combined with *Zhi Jing San* (Powder for Eliminating Spasm). The prescription is very effective and can sometimes be modified with *Jiangcan* (Bombyx Batryticatus) and *Gouteng* (Ramulus Uncariae cum Uncis) for sedation and dispelling wind. Some doctors use *Zhen Gan Xi Feng Tang* (Decoction for Dispelling Liver Wind) combined with *Qian Zheng San* (Powder for Correcting Deviation of the Face) which is also effective. *Jiangcan* (Bombyx Batryticatus) and *Gouteng* (Ramulus Uncariae cum Uncis) have the sedative and wind-dispelling function. According to my own many years experience, *Shao Yan Gan Cao Tang* (Decoction of Radix Paeoniae and Radix Glycyrrhizae) combined with *Zhi Jing San* (Powder for Eliminating Spasm) plus *Jiangcan* (Bombyx Batryticatus) and *Gouteng* (Ramulus Uncariae cum Uncis) is very effective. If the pathological condition is more severe, add in *Zhimu* (Rhizoma Anemarrhenae) and *Gegen* (Radix Puerariae). *Zhimu* (Rhizoma Anemarrhenae) has strong sedative function and *Gegen* (Radix Puerariae) can stop spasm. It is mentioned in *Jin Kui Yao Lue* (Essentials from the Golden Cabinet) that *Ge Gen Tang* (Decoction of Radix Puerariae) is used for spasmodic diseases, and it is therefore indicated in cramping. Besides, to treat wind, we should treat the blood. Though *Shaoyao* (Radix Paeoniae) and *Gancao* (Radix Glycyrrhizae) have the function to mediate the blood, the therapeutic effect would be even better if *Danshen* (Radix Salviae Miltiorrhizae) is added in. It has the similar function of activating blood and dispersing blood stasis as *Si Wu Tang* (Decoction of Four Ingredients). In general, the method of using herbs for the disease doesn't go beyond the above principle. There is one thing that you have to pay attention to. For this disease, it is not advisable to puncture local points, nor use electric stimulation, or the condition may get worse.

14. Question: What are the points for lowering blood sugar in Tung's acupuncture?

Answer: Pathologically, diabetes is mostly resulted from deficiency of the spleen and kidney, and in some cases deficiency of the lung yin as well. Treatment is therefore focused on strengthening the spleen *qi* and nourishing the yin of the lung and kidney. In Tung's acupuncture, point *Xiasanhuang* (77.18, 19, 21) is therefore often selected because it can strengthen the spleen and kidney. When it tonifies the spleen, it strengthens the lung simultaneously. So the point is often used to treat diabetes. In application of points of the fourteen meridians, many doctors often select *Yangchi* (SJ4). Japanese acupuncturists also like to select this point. It is the *Yuan*-source point of the triple energizer meridian and has the function to strengthen the kidney and tonify *Yuan qi* (source *qi*) so as to lower blood sugar. Some doctors have selected *Chengjiang* (REN24) because it is the meeting point of *Ren* meridian and *yangming* meridians of hand and foot and has the function to regulate *qi* and blood. If the above two points are selected in combination with *Xiasanhuang* (77.17, 19, 21), it would be even better. A good herbal prescription for diabetes must have the function to supplement *qi* and nourish *yin*. Personally I often use *Shen Qi Mai Wei Di Huang Tang* (Decoction of Radix Codonopsis Pilosulae, Radix Astragali seu Hedysari, Radix Ophiopogonis, Fructus Schisandrae and Radix Rehmanniae). *Dangshen* (Radix Codonopsis Pilosulae) and *Huangqi* (Radix Astragali seu Hedysari) are used with large dosage up to 30 grams. Moreover, the use of *Maidong* (Radix Ophiopogonis) and *Wuweizi* (Fructus Schisandrae) also implies the function of the formula *Sheng Mai San* (Pulse-activating Powder). When *Xuanshen* (Radix Scrophulariae) is added in, it works together with *Maidong* (Radix Ophiopogonis) and Shengdihuang (Radix Rehmanniae), forming another formula *Zeng Ye Tang* (Decoction for Increasing Body Fluid), which is often used for deficiency of body fluid and thirst in warm and febrile diseases.

In case of severe thirst, we can increase dosage of *Zhimu* (Rhizoma Anemarrhenae) and *Tianhuafen* (Radix Trichosanthis). Why? We know it is stated in *Shan Han Lun* (Treatise on Injury by Cold) that, in use of *Xiao Chai Hu Tang* (Monor Decoction of Radix Bupleuri), *Tianhuafen* (Radix Trichosanthis) is added in after *Banxia* (Rhizoma Pinelliae) removed when there appears thirst; and in use of *Bai Hu Tang* (Decoction of White Tiger), *Zhimu* (Rhizoma anemarrhenae) is added in when there is severe thirst. Therefore, the two herbs have the best therapeutic result for lowering blood sugar in case of diabetes. In chronic diabetes, there must be blood stasis, for which *Danshen* (Radix Salviae Miltiorrhizae) should be added in to move the blood and disperse blood stasis.

3. Diseases of Chest and Abdomen

1) Pain of the Lateral Side of the Chest and Abdomen

a. Needle *Sima* (88.17, 18, 19) with point coupling technique.

2) Pleuritis

a. Bleeding *Sihuazhong* (77.09) first and then needle *Sima* (88.17, 18, 19).

3) Lateral Lower Abdominal Pain

a. Needle *Sima* (88.17, 18, 19), *Tongtian* (88.03) and *Tongwei* (88.10).
b. Needle *Menjin* (66.05) and *Huoju* (66.11).

4) Pleurisy (intercostals neuralgia)

a. Needle *Sima* (88.17, 18, 19).
b. Bleeding *Sihuazhong* (77.09).

Many points are indicated in chest pain. *Tongguan* (88.01) and *Tongshan* (88.02) are good points for pain in the middle of the chest.

Neiguan is also good. The pain on the side of the chest is mostly related to the lung, and point *Sima* (88.17, 18, 19) is very good. Generally, *Neiguan* (PC6) of the fourteen meridians is the best point for the pain from the abdomen to the chest. There is a saying in TCM: "Select *Neiguan* (PC6) for the chest." So is *Sima* (88.17, 18, 19). It also works effectively for the chest and abdomen, more for pathological changes of the chest and less for those of the abdomen. There are many points in the fourteen meridians that are indicated in diseases of the chest. In addition to *Neiguan* (PC6) often used for chest pain, the pain in the middle of the chest in particular, *Zusanli* (ST36) and *Gongsun* (SP4) are also effective for chest pain.

In treatment of pain on the lateral side of the chest, clavicular area and around the breast, *Liangqiu* (ST34) of the stomach meridian is the best. The extraordinary point *Menjin* (66.05) is also very effective, since the stomach meridian passes through the clavicular and breast area. It has been mentioned that *Sima* (88.17, 18, 19) is very effective for intercostals neuralgia. However, *Yanglingquan* (GB34) and *Zhigou* (SJ6) could be even better. *Yanglingquan* (GB34) is indicated more in costal pain and *Zhigou* (SJ6) more in pain of the costal cartilage. In case of hypochondriac pain, select both of them for better effect. It is mentioned in some ancient classics that either *Yanglingquan* (*Tong Xuan Fu*-Ode of the Essentials of Understanding and *Za Bing Xue Fa Ge*-Song of Points for Miscellaneous Diseases) or *Zhigou* (SJ6) (*Biao You Fu*-Ode to Elucidate Mysteries) is effective and combination of both points can obtain even better result. In treatment of diseases, it is advisable to select one point for many diseases, not many points for a single disease. Usually we select one point first. If it is not very effective, select another point, two points in maximum.

If the pain is located in many areas including the chest, costal area and abdomen, *Sima* (88.17, 18, 19) is generally enough. If treatment is bilateral, we should use six needles in total. It seems a lot of needles to be used. However, selection of this point implies holographic significance. Generally, *Simashang* (88.18) corresponds to the upper energizer, *Simazhong* (88.17) corresponds to the middle energizer and *Simaxia* (88.19) corresponds to the lower energizer. We could select the point according to the location of the pain. If the pain is on one side, needle the point unilaterally. If the pain is on both sides, needle the point bilaterally. After needle insertion, ask the patient to have some exercise during needle retention. This is so called active *qi* moving technique, which can guide *qi* to arrive at the painful area and serve as the best therapeutic method of pain syndrome. In case of unable to move, use massage or breathing method instead. For pain syndrome, points are mainly selected on the healthy side. If the pain is prolonged and severe, the time of needle retention can be longer. Try not to use many needles.

5) Abdominal Colic Pain (dry cholera)

a. Bleeding *Fuchao'ershisan* (VT.05).

In Tung's extraordinary points, there are many points in groups. Though each group has many points, not all the points are selected in treatment. Take abdominal colic pain as an example. We often select *Fuchao'ershisan* (VT.05), but not all the 23 points of *Fuchao* are needled. *Wuling* (DT.04) has 40 points, not all of them are needled. The use of those points is very selective. Blood-letting is often given to point *Fuchao* by taking the umbilicus as the center and needling the point one *cun* above, below and lateral to the umbilicus. In severe case, select another four point one *cun* above, below and lateral to the selected points respectively with action of the points expanding to all the four directions. With the pathological condition getting worse, more points are selected in the same way. In addition, bleeding point *Sihuazhong* (77.09) and *Sihuawai* (77.14) is also good for abdominal colic pain.

6) Stuffiness in the Chest

a. Needle *Huoshan* (33.06) and *Huoling* (33.05) simultaneously, and it is forbidden to needle the points bilaterally.
b. Bleeding *Sihuazhong* (77.09) is very effective.

To select few points for the same result, Dr. Tung often selected left points for male patients and right points for female patients in treatment. In another word, if the points are selected unilaterally, needle the points on the left side for male patients and right side for female patients. In case of stuffiness in the chest, Dr. Tung often needled *Huoshan* (33.05) and *Huoling* (33.05) unilaterally. In the points of the fourteen meridians, *Neiguan* (PC6) is the best. *Sima* (88.17, 18, 19) is also a very good point for stuffiness of the chest. In severe case, it is better to bleed *Sihuazhong* (77.09) and *Sihuawai* (77.14). Acupuncture is good enough for stuffiness in the chest without heart disease. In case of heart disease, needling *Neiguan* (PC6) and *Zusanli* (ST36) is very effective. If the condition is really severe, bleeding either *Sihuazhong* (77.09) or *Sihuawai* (77.14) is necessary. I once treated a senior lady patient named Liu, who was going to receive an operation for heart disease in 1986. I gave her treatment with acupuncture and blood-letting therapy for 4 months and everything of her was good. She is still alive and healthy 17 years after the treatment, and she is now 85 and has never received operation.

7) Lower Abdominal Pain

a. Needle *Menjin* (66.05).
b. Needle *Huoju* (66.11).
c. Bleed *Quling* (33.16).
d. Bleed *Sihuazhong* (77.09) and *Sihuawai* (77.14).

There are many effective points for lower abdominal pain. The most frequently used effective one is *Menjin* (66.05). It is located behind *Xiangu* (ST43), the *Shu*-stream point of the stomach, close to the bone. It has the property of both wood and earth. Needling this point along border of the bone makes the point has water property. It is therefore indicated in diseases of the spleen, liver and kidney. *Huoju* (66.11) is also indicated in lower abdominal pain, and in severe case, bleed *Chize* (LU5) or *Sihuazhong* (77.09). If the therapeutic result of *Huoju* (66.11) is not good, there could be some organic pathological change, for which we should bleed *Sihuangzhong* (77.09) and *Sihuawai* (77.14). It is important for the patient to have careful examination for clear diagnosis in this case.

8) Pain Around the Umbilicus and Lower Back Pain

a. *Wanshunyi* (22.09) and *Wanshun'er* (22.08).
b. *Zhongbai* (22.06) and *Xiabai* (22.07).

9) Distending Pain of the Large Intestine

a. Needle *Menjin* (66.05).
b. Needle *Changmen* (33.10).

In case of pain around the umbilicus and waist, we could needle *Wanshunyi* (22.09) and *Wanshun'er* (22.08) or *Zhongbai* (22.06) and *Xiabai* (22.07). For distension or pain in the large intestine, we can needle *Menjin* (66.05) first and *Changmen* (33.10) after. Many patients suffer from abdominal distention. In case of upper abdominal distention and pain, needling *Menjin* (66.05) is very effective; in case of lower abdominal distention and pain, needling *Linggu* (22.05) is very effective. Needling both *Menjin* (66.05) and *Linggu* (22.05) may have even better result. Simultaneous selection of the two points may harmonize the upper and lower, not only eliminating pain but also regulating the stomach and large intestine meridians. In addition to distention and pain caused by gastrointestinal dysfunction, the two points are also effective to the distending pain due to liver *qi* stagnation or disharmony between the liver and spleen. Because *Menjin* (66.05) is the wood point of the earth meridian, it can regulate the disharmony of the liver and spleen. *Linggu* (22.05) can regulate the liver meridian to arrest pain because the liver and large intestine have extraordinary connection, and therefore it can help disperse liver *qi* stagnation. This is the method to treat abdominal distention and pain in Tung's acupuncture. In the ancient classics such as *Yu Long Fu* (Ode of the Jade Dragon), *Za Bing Xue Fa Ge* (Song of Points for Miscellaneous Diseases), *Wo Yan Ling Xiao Ying Xue Ge* (Song of Effective Points of Wo Yan Ling), *Tong Xuan Zhi Yao Fu* (Ode of the Essentials of Understanding), and *Yi Zong Jin Jian* (The Golden Mirror of Medicine), point *Neiting* (ST44) is often selected for abdominal distention, because it is the water point of the stomach meridian, and can therefore strengthen both the spleen and kidney. When it is combined with *Zusanli* (ST36), the effect will be even better. It is mentioned in *Zhen Jiu Da Cheng* (The Great Compendium of Acupuncture) that, if *Sanyinjiao* (SP6) is added additionally, the effect will be extremely good.

10) Chest Injury Due to Heavy Blow

a. Needle *Sima* (88.17, 18, 19).
b. Bleed *Sihuazhong* (77.09) and *Sihuawai* (77.14).
c. For fresh injury, needle point *Jie* (88.28).

In Tung's acupuncture, *Sima* (88.17, 18, 19) is often selected for chest injury due to heavy blow. In case of fresh injury, including the fresh injury due to heavy blow, puncture *Jie* (88.28) first to regulate *qi* and blood, and it is very effective. Besides, it is also very good for the pain due to stagnation of *qi* and blood after injury caused by heavy blow. *Sima* (88.17, 18, 19) is very good for traumatic injury of the chest. For severe injury or internal injury of the chest, it is better to bleed *Sihuazhong* (77.09). Point *Jie* (88.28) is indicated in traumatic injury because it is located near *Liangqiu* (ST34), which is the *Xi*-cleft point of the stomach meridian. Stomach meridian is the one with ample *qi* and blood. *Xi*-cleft point is the place where *qi* and blood accumulate, and it therefore has the function to regulate *qi* and blood, and the *Xi*-cleft point of the stomach meridian in particular. Point *Jie* is not only located near *Liangqiu* (ST34) but also close to the tendon, which is dominated by the liver. The liver stores blood. Therefore it has very strong function to regulate *qi* and blood, thus very effective for stagnation of *qi* and blood due to traumatic injury.

11) Pain of the Chest and Abdomen Along the Ren Meridian

a. Needle *Shuixiang* (66.14).

Since the pain along the *Ren* meridian is sometimes on the chest and it is not so convenient to needle the points on the chest, we may needle the points of kidney meridians instead because the kidney meridian runs closely along both sides of the *Ren* meridian. I always try not to select local points but distal and less points for pain, mostly the specific points below the elbow and knee joints. This method is just like the classical therapeutic method in Chinese herbal medicine. Like Chinese herbal medicine, there also exist classical school of thought and school of current prescriptions in acupuncture. In Chinese herbal medicine, the classical school of thought mainly refers to the school of *Shang Han Lun* (Treatise on Fabrile Diseases) and *Jin Gui Yao Lue* (Essentials from the Golden Cabinet), which is characterized by few ingredients with large dosage in prescriptions. The school of thought of current prescriptions generally refers to the schools of thought that appeared later. They have more ingredients in one prescription and the dosage of each ingredient is small. In the application of classical prescriptions, the physician must grasp the chief manifestations. Most of the great physicians in different times in China belong to the classical school of medicine. They are good at using classical prescriptions to treat diseases. It is the same in acupuncture. The doctors of classical school of thought follow the treatment principles from *Lingshu* (Spiritual Pivot) and *Suwen* (Essential Questions) and they take the Five-*shu* points as the main points in treatment of diseases of the whole body, which are located below the elbow and knee joints.

Today we can see that the theory of the Five-*shu* points implies the view of holography, and they pertain to the five elements, namely the wood, fire, earth, metal and water, and the five *zang*, namely the liver, heart, spleen, lung and kidney respectively. They are the holographic points of the internal organs on the meridians. The essential in application of the Five-*shu* points is "seeking *qi* from the same element point" and "needling method of body correspondence." For example, in case of a liver disease complicated with kidney disease, we don't have to select points from both the liver and kidney meridians, and instead, we could just needle the water point of the liver meridian. The liver pertains to wood, and its water point is connected with the kidney, needling this point could treat both the liver and kidney simultaneously. If the stomach and the liver are diseased at the same time while the stomach is the main diseased one, we could needle the wood point of the stomach meridian, and this method is very effective for disharmony between the liver and stomach. Point *Taichong* (LR3) is also very good for regulating the liver and the spleen since it is the earth point of the liver meridian. It can treat disharmony between the liver and the spleen, dispersing the liver stagnation and regulating the spleen. *Yanglingquan* (GB34) is also a good point for dispersing the liver stagnation and regulating the spleen because it is the earth point of the wood meridian – the gallbladder meridian. It is therefore able to treat wood and earth simultaneously involved in the same disease. The wood dominates tendon and earth dominates muscle and it is therefore effective for diseases of both the tendons and muscles. According to the theory of the five elements, this point has the property of both the wood and the earth, and can treat diseases of both the muscles and tendons, and it is therefore an essential point for diseases of the motor system.

Now let's look at Tung's extraordinary point *Menjin* (66.05) which is located behind *Xiangu* (ST43). In ancient classics, the two points are overlapped. *Xiangu* (ST43) is the wood point of earth meridian, the stomach meridian, it is certainly able to treat disharmony of the wood and earth. Therefore we often select *Menjin* (66.05) to disperse the liver stagnation and regulate the spleen. This point also has the function to strengthen the spleen. If the kidney is involved, it is also effective since it is close to the bone. Needling along the border of the bone may affect the kidney. For instance, we often select the point to treat diarrhea before dawn, a kind of diarrhea due to deficiency of *yang* of both spleen and kidney. Diarrhea before dawn is mainly resulted from kidney *yang* deficiency. Point *Menjin* (66.05) can not only regulate the spleen and stomach in case of diarrhea but also be effective for renal diarrhea because of needling the point along the border of the bone. Such needling method is based upon the theory of "seeking *qi* from the same element point" and "the needling method of body correspondence," and is therefore highly effective. This theory has been introduced in details in my book *Zhen Jiu Wu Shu Xue Ying Yong* (Application of the Five-*shu* Points in Acupuncture). Please read this book if you want to know more about the theory.

In the school of current prescriptions, much more points are selected and most of the points are local tender points or adjacent points. Personally, I mainly select points of classical prescriptions and therefore I use less needles or herbs in one treatment but still obtain good results.

Now let's see the effect of point *Shuixiang* (66.14) in treatment of pain of the *Ren* meridian. *Shuixiang* (66.14) is located at the side of *Taixi* (KI3), and therefore needling *Taixi* (KI3) is also effective. *Taixi* (KI3) is the point of kidney meridian, a very effective point for diseases of the *Ren* meridian. It can treat the pain along the midline of the anterior aspect of the body, the *Ren* meridian. *Chengjiang* (REN24) is another effective point of pain of the *Ren* meridian. In case of pain of the *Ren* meridian, it can be selected in combination with *Shuixiang* (66.14). The two points work together as guiding points to each other. Needling *Shuixiang* (66.14) as the therapeutic point and *Chengjiang* (REN24) as the guiding point is very effective for pain of the *Ren* meridian on the chest.

In treatment, we should try to select one point to treat multiple diseases instead of selecting more points to treat one disease. For every disease, there are several specific points. We may select one of them in the treatment. However, better result can be obtained if they are used in combination. It doesn't mean good result is obtained only by combining several points together. Actually, every specific point is effective. Once you understand all these points, you will be more confident in treatment. You may use these single points either alternatively or in combination for better result. When you select these points alternatively, you don't have to use many needles. In general, you have to remember several specific points for each disease. You don't have to select all of them at the same time but use them in alternation.

12) Pain of Both Chest and Back

a. Needle *Sima* (88.17, 18, 19).
b. Needle *Chongzi* (22.01).
c. Needle *Shenguan* (77.18).
d. Needle *Shangbai* (22.03).

We have introduced the treatment of chest pain and back pain. If both the chest and back are painful, we can needle *Sima* (88.17, 18, 19), and if it is selected together with *Chengshan* (BL57), the therapeutic result will be even better. Actually, point *Sima* (88.17, 18, 19) is enough. Personally, I often select *Chongzi* (22.01) and *Chongxian* (22.02) to treatment pain of the chest and back by needling left points for right pain and right points for left pain. Besides, *Shenguan* (77.18) is also very effective for pain of both chest and back. *Shangbai* (22.03) is a good point too.

15. Question: How is acute abdomen treated?

Answer: In case of acute abdomen, the first possible disease is appendicitis. *Jin Gui Yao Lue* (Essentials from the Gold Cabinet) has many good formulas for appendicitis such as *Yi Ren Fu Zi Bai Jiang San* (Powder of Semen Coicis, Radix Aconiti Praeparata and Herba Patriniae) and *Da Huang Mu Dan Pi Tang* (Decoction of Radix et Rhizoma Rhei and Cortex Moutan Radicis). In acupuncture treatment, we can needle *Lanweixue* (Extra) which is located one *cun* below *Zusanli* (ST36). It is a very good point for appendicitis. During an acute attack, there may appear a reaction tender point there. In case of cholecystitis, needle *Dannangxue* (Extra) which is located one *cun* below *Yanglingquan* (GB34). During an acute attack, there may appear a tender point there. Cholecystits and cholelithiasis are included in acute abdomen. To treat such acute abdomen, there are some principles to follow: The first is deep insertion, the depth of insertion should be at least 2 *cun*; second, long duration of needle retention which could be up to 90 minutes or even longer; third, strong stimulation with continuous lifting, thrusting and rotating. The method is used for all kinds of acute abdomen including cholecystitis, cholelithiasis and appendicitis. These are the important principles to follow in the treatment of acute abdomen. If we don't have time to retain the needles, apply blood-letting to *Sihuazhong* (77.09) and *Sihuawai* (77.14). Blood-letting therapy is very good for diseases of the chest and abdomen, appendicitis in particular. It is also good for acute abdomen of gallbladder. I would like to emphasize the principles in the treatment of acute abdomen once more: deep insertion, long duration of needle retention and strong stimulation.

4. Diseases of the Lumbus and Back

Pain of the lumbus and back is the most frequently seen disease in clinic, lower back pain in particular. The therapeutic effect of acupuncture is even better than that of medication. There are many specific points for lower back pain in the fourteen meridians such as *Renzhong* (DU26), *Houxi* (SI3), *Zhongzhu* (SJ3), *Yanglao* (SI6), *Fuliu* (KI7), etc. There are also some very effective empirical formulas for lower back pain. For instance, *Tong Qi San* (Powder for Moving Qi) from *Yi Zong Jin Jian* (The Golden Mirror of Medicine) is a very effective representative formula for acute lumbar sprain. Its ingredients include *Muxiang* (Radix Aucklandiae),

Chuanshanjia (Squama Manitis), *Chenpi* (Pericarpium Citri Reticulatae), *Gancao* (Radix Glycyrrhizae), *Xiaohuixiang* (Fructus Foeniculi), *Zhigancao* (Radix Glycyrrhizae praeparata), *Heichou* (Semen Pharbitidis) and *Yuanhu* (Rhizoma Corydalis), etc. Personally, I often add in *Chaoduzhong* (Stir-fried Cortex Eucommiae) for better and faster result. In the clinical practice, the prescription is very effective without use of acupuncture. In mild case, the pain is controlled after taking one dose of the herbs. In sever case, the patient is 70-80% cure after taking the first dose of the herbs and the pain is completely controlled after taking another dose.

Neck sprain is also a kind of acute sprain, for which acupuncture is effective too and *Chongzi* (22.01) may help immediately stop pain. Besides, *Shangbai* (22.03) and *Zhongbai* (22.06) are also very effective. I also have a very effective herbal prescription modified *Gui Zhi Jia Ge Gen Tang* (Decoction of Ramulus Cinnamomi Modified by Radix Puerariae), which may quickly cure neck sprain. The ingredients are *Guizhi* (Ramulus Cinnamomi), *Shengjiang* (Rhizoma Zingiberis Resens), *Zhigancao* (Radix Glycyrrhizae praeparata), *Baishao* (Radix Paeoniae Alba), *Dazao* (Fructus Ziziphi Jujubae), *Gegen* (Radix Puerariae), *Qianghuo* (Rhizoma seu Radix Notopterygii) and *Chaihu* (Radix Bupleuri). Why is *Chaihu* (Radix Bupleuri) used here? It is because neck sprain causes not only the pain of the neck and back but also the pain at point *Jianjing* (GB21) where *shaoyang* meridian passes. Many people like to use *Gui Zhi Jia Ge Gen Tang* (Decoction of Cinnamomi Modified by Radix Puerariae). However, it is not good enough because it doesn't cover *shaoyang* meridian, on which point *Jianjing* (GB21) is located. Therefore the prescription modified by *Chaihu* (Radix Bupleuri) is more complete. *Gui Zhi Tang* (Decoction of Ramulus Cinnamomi) works for *taiyang* meridian, *Gegen* (Radix Pueriae) works for both *yangming* and *taiyang* meridian and *Chaihu* (Radix Bupleuri) is the herb for *shaoyang* meridian. The above herbs used together may work effectively for all the three meridians, including the pain of the neck, back and shoulder.

Tong Qi San (Powder for Moving Qi) is very effective for acute lumbar sprain. In case of chronic lumbago, most of the cases must have kidney deficiency and we have to strengthen the kidney then.

1) Backache

a. In case of unilateral backache, needling *Chongzi* (22.01) and *Chongxian* (22.02) may immediately arrest pain.
b. In case of bilateral backache, needle *Zhengshi* (77.03) and *Boqiu* (77.04).
c. Needling *Tongbei* (88.11) is also effective.
d. Needling *Sima* (88.17, 18, 19) has specific effect.

Chongzi (22.01) is the most effective point for backache. In the fourteen meridians, there is no point that can compare with this point in treatment of unilateral backache. In case of bilateral backache, it is also very effective to needle *Chongzi* (22.01) bilaterally. When the backache radiates to the shoulder, *Chongzi* (22.01) is very good; and when the backache radiates to the neck, *Chongxian* (22.02) is very good. If the pain covers all the back, neck and shoulder, needle both *Chongzi* (22.01) and *Chongxian* (22.02). If the condition is bilateral, needle *Chongzi* (22.01) on one side and *Chongxian* (22.02) on the other, or needle the two points of the left side for male patient and right side for the female, or needle the two point of on the opposite side of the worse side. It is not necessary to needle the two points bilaterally. Besides, *Zhengshi* (77.03) and *Boqiu* (77.04) on the lower limbs are also very effective. *Boqiu* (77.04) is located below *Chengshan* (BL57) that is a specific point for backache. In case of unilateral backache, needle the two points on the healthy side only, and in case of bilateral backache, needle the two points bilaterally.

In addition, *Tongbei* (88.11) is also a good point for backache. Point *Biguan* (ST31) of the stomach meridian of foot-*yangming* is also effective for backache. *Sima* (88.17, 18, 19) is also a good point for backache, as chest and back is related to the lung.

When the backache is located on the midline, close to the spinal vertebrae, needling *Sugu* (BL65) of the bladder meridian is very good. Personally, I often select *Zhongzhu* (SJ3) to treat backache along the spine. It has always been an important point for backache since ancient time, and introduced in *Zhou Hou Ge* (Song to Keep up Your Sleeve), *Sheng Yu Ge* (Song More Precious Than Jade) and *Xi Hong Fu* (Ode of Xi Hong). In the book *Za Bing Xue Fa Ge* (Song of Points for Miscellaneous Diseases) and *Wo Yan Ling Xiao Ying Ge* (Song of Therapeutic Effect of points of *Wo Yanling*), the point is even considered as the specially effective point for spinal pain behind the heart, the backache along the spine.

In general, there are many points that are effective for backache. They can be selected according to the pathological conditions.

2) Backache Radiating to the Lower Limb

a. Needling *Makuaishui* (1010.13) is very effective. In case of backache radiating to the leg, point *Makuaishui* (1010.13) is selected.

3) Pain of the Shoulder and Back

a. Needling *Chongzi* (22.01) and *Chongxian* (22.01) has special effect.
b. It is also very effective to select *Tongshen* (88.09), *Tongwei* (88.10) and *Tongbei* (88.11).

It is also very effective to needle *Biguan* (ST31) of the stomach meridian to treat pain of the shoulder and back. In addition to the above-mentioned Tung's extraordinary points, *Shenguan* (77.18) is also a frequently used effective point.

4) Deformity of the Back and Spine

a. Needling *Minghuang* (88.12), *Qihuang* (88.14) and *Tongtian* (88.03) is effective.

Deformity of the back and spine refers to scoliosis. Master Tung selected *Minghuang* (88.12), *Qihuang* (88.14) and *Tongtian* (88.03) to treat the disease. In the ancient classics, *Renzhong* (DU26), *Quchi* (LI11) and *Kunlun* (BL60) are often recommended for treatment of ankylosing spondylitis. Besides, moxibustion applied to *Pishu* (BL20) and *Ganshu* (BL18) is also very effective for scoliosis.

5) Spur of Spinal Vertebrae

a. Blood-letting *Weizhong* (BL40) is very effective. It would be even better if *Minghuang* (88.12) is selected in combination.
b. Needling *Jiuli* (88.25, 26, 27) and *Wanshunyi* (22.08) also has specific effect.
c. Needle *Sihuazhong* (77.09) and *Sihuafu* (77.10) along the border of the bone.

6) Tenderness of the Spinal Vertebra

a. Blood-letting *Weizhong* (BL40) is very effective. It would be even better if *Minghuang* (88.12) is selected in combination.
b. Needling *Jiuli* (88.25, 26, 27) and *Wanshunyi* (22.08) also has specific effect.
c. Needle *Sihuazhong* (77.09) and *Sihuafu* (77.10) along the border of the bone.

Spinal vertebrae consist of cervical vertebrae, thoracic vertebrae and lumbar vertebrae, and the cervical and lumbar vertebrae are most liable to have bone spur, for which the point most frequently selected by Master Tung is *Minghuang* (88.12). Besides, he also bled *Weizhong* (BL40) once a week. The therapeutic effect was very good. In addition, needling *Sihuazhong* (77.09) and *Sihuafu* (77.10) along the border of the bone is also very effective for cervical and lumbar bone spur. They are even better for bone spur of the knee joint and heel. My personal empirical points are *Jiuli* (88.25, 26, 27), *Wanshunyi* (22.08) and *Renzhong* (DU26). If they are used together with *Shugu* (BL65), the therapeutic result will be even better. It is a group of very effective points for spinal bone spur, including the spur of the cervical and lumbar vertebrae.

Degeneration of cervical and lumbar vertebrae is closely related to the kidney since "the kidney dominates bone." Growth of bone spur is related to kidney deficiency and *Wanshunyi* (22.08) has the function to tonify the kidney. There is another effective point *Zhongjiuli* (88.25) which is *Fengshi* (GB31) in the fourteen meridians for bone spur. It is stated in Chapter 10 of *Lingshu* (Spiritual Pivot): "*Shaoyang* dominates bone." Needling *Fengshi* (GB31) along the border of the bone has therefore double functions. *Fengshi* (GB31) is a point of *shaoyang* meridian and hence frequently selected for bone spur. According to my own clinical experience, it is even better than *Tianhuang* (88.13), *Minghuang* (88.12), *Sihuangzhong* (77.09) and *Sihuafu* (77.10). However, the most frequently used points of my own for cervical and lumbar vertebrae are *Renzhong* (DU26), *Wanshunyi* (22.08) or *Houxi* (SI3), *Zhongjiuli* (88.25) and *Shugu* (BL65). I have used these points to treat hundreds of such cases during last 35 years. In case of numbness of the hand due to bone spur of cervical vertebrae, we may bleed *Shuangfeng* (DT05) located on the side of the cervical vertebra for better result. Needling *Renzhong* (DU26), *Wanshunyi* (22.08) and *Fengshi* (GB31) can not only treat the *biao*, the numbness of the hand, but also treat the *ben*, the underlying condition.

In case of sciatica resulted from lumbar disc hernia, there may be pain of the thigh or groin, or pain along the bladder meridian. According to clinical experience, the pain along the bladder meridian is mostly resulted from sciatica. 20-30% of the sciatica patients may also have pain along the gallbladder meridian and others have pain of *taiyang* and *shaoyang* meridians, the pain of the *taiyang* meridian on the buttock and *shaoyang* meridian on the leg, or the pain of the hip on the upper and the posterior aspect of the leg on the lower. To treat such patient, we need to select many points of the fourteen meridians. However, in Tung's acupuncture, only *Linggu* (22.05) and *Dabai* (22.04) will be enough and effective for any meridians affected. The two points are effective for sciatica in general. If there is bone spur, blood-letting therapy should be used in combination for better and faster result, or needle *Renzhong* (DU26), *Wanshunyi* (22.08) and *Fengshi* (GB31) along the border of the bone in combination which has been introduced already.

In treatment of sciatica, *Linggu* (22.05) and *Dabai* (22.04) are often selected in combination with the point of the affected meridian as the guiding point. To select guiding point, we often needle the *shu*-stream point, since "*shu*-stream point is indicated in heaviness of the body and pain of the joints." So, *Taichong* (LR3) on the diseased side is selected as the guiding point when the pain is on the anterior aspect, *Zulingqi* (GB41) on the diseased side when the pain is on the lateral aspect and *Shugu* (BL65) on the diseased side when the pain is on the posterior side of the buttock, thigh and leg. The two principal points *Linggu* (22.05) and *Dabai* (22.04) are selected from the healthy side. This method is very effective even if sciatica is caused by bone spur. For faster result, needling along the border of bone or bleeding *Chengshan* (BL57) or *Weizhong* (BL40) once every 7-10 days can be adopted at the same time. There are many patients of sciatica in the clinic and the disease cannot be cured easily. This method can be used to treat both *biao* and *ben*, pathological changes of both nerve root and nerve trunk.

I have treated hundreds of cases of sciatica and some of them have made me deeply impressed. Few days before I went to lecture in Singapore in 1980, one senior gentleman who was a relative of the governor of Hongkong, Mr. Dong Jianhua, was suffering from sciatica due to bone spur of lumbar vertebrae. The pain was so severe that he couldn't stand up straight and had to walk with the help by others. He had difficulty to go to toilet. He couldn't receive operation because he was also suffering from heart disease. Originally he didn't believe Chinese medicine very much. One captain working for him used to suffer from sciatica and was cured by me, and tried hard to recommend me to him. During treatment, I needled *Renzhong* (DU26), *Shugu* (BL65), *Wanshunyi* (22.08) and *Fengshi* (GB31) once every other day and give him blood-letting. He was remarkably improved one week later. Since I was going to lecture in Singapore and could not continue the treatment, he asked to come with me to Singapore and stay with me in the same hotel. After telling him the unnecessary, I gave him the prescription of the points and let him ask other doctor to treat him selecting the same points. He then called me once a week about his condition, and I changed the prescription according to his condition given by the doctor. He was improved quickly and cured soon. When I passed Hongkong on the way back to Taiwan, he came to the airport to pick me and invited me to dinner in his house.

It is quite often to have cases with bone spur of spinal vertebrae, lumbar vertebrae in particular. It is not so difficult to treat. Here is another example. In 2002, a very famous gentleman, Mr. Wang came to my clinic for treatment. He had suffered from sciatica for 3 years and was treated by some doctors with poor effect. He was walking with the body deviated to 30-40 degree. After hearing I was back to the United States, he came to see me, hoping he would be cured in 3 months. He was prepared to come for treatment every day. I told him to come 3 times a week since he was living far away. It took 3 hours to come to my clinic. He insisted on receiving treatment 3 times a week. I needled *Renzhong* (DU26), *Shugu* (BL65), *Wanshunyi* (22.08) and *Fengshi* (GB31) for one treatment, and *Linggu* (22.05) and *Dabai* (22.04) on the healthy side for the other day. Besides, I gave *Weizhong* (BL40) blood-letting once every 10 days. With the treatment, his condition was getting better and better. He had an abrupt severe attack of acute pain one day 3 weeks later, but after that, the pain completely disappeared. After 4 weeks, he was completely cured and could walk normally, much faster than he expected. This method can be used to treat bone spur of both cervical and lumbar vertebrae with very good therapeutic result.

The method of needling along border of bone can also be used. That is to needle *Sihuazhong* (77.09) and *Sihuafu* (77.10) along the border of tibia, or needle *Tianhuang* (88.13) and *Minghuang* (88.12). Personally, I prefer the preceding method, the experience of my own. As for *Sihuazhong* (77.09) and *Sihuangfu* (77.10), I often use them to treat bone spur of the knee joint or heel. Regarding knee joint pain, a Korean patient came to see me in my hotel with the complaint of knee joint pain for 9 months and difficult squatting. I needled *Jianzhong* (44.06) and *Xinmen* (33.12) on the healthy side. She told me she was 80-90% cured the next day. She was completely cured after another treatment.

7) Acute Sprain of Spinal Vertebra

a. Needling *Zhengjin* (77.01) and *Boqiu* (77.04) is effective.
b. Bleeding *Weizhong* (BL40) has extremely good effect.
c. Needle *Qili* (A.01) and *Jiuli* (88.25, 26, 27).

In treatment of acute sprain of spinal vertebra, we can needle *Zhengjin* (77.01) and *Boqiu* (77.04). It would be even better if blood-letting is given to *Weizhong* (BL40) after. Master Tung often used *Qili* (A.01) and *Jiuli* (88.25, 26, 27). Needling *Renzhong* (DU26) and *Houxi* (SI3) of the fourteen meridians is also very effective. Selecting *Renzhong* (DU26) and *Wanshunyi* (22.08) is also good. For the pain of thoracic vertebrae, *Kunlun* (BL60) is the best point. The name *Kunlun*, has two explanations. One is that the point is located close to the highest bone of the body, malleolus, like Mountain *Kunlun* in China. The other is that the thoracic vertebrae occupy the highest position of the spine when ape-man crawls and thus the name. In fact, the bladder meridian travels along both sides of the *Du* meridian and has diverging meridian to connect with the *Du* meridian and *Kunlun* (BL60) is the *yuan*-source point of the bladder meridian, the point is therefore indicated in the pain of spinal vertebrae according to either the meaning of the point name or distribution of the meridian.

8) Lower Back Pain

a. Needling *Linggu* (22.05) and *Dabai* (22.04) is very effective.
b. Needling *Erjiaoming* (11.12) is very effective (towards the small finger).
c. Bleeding *Weizhong* (BL40) is very effective.
d. Needling *Majinshui* (1010.13) is very effective.
e. Needling *Shuijin* (1010.20) and *Shuitong* (1010.19) is effective.
f. *Xiasanhuang* (77.18, 19, 21) is also an effective point.

9) Lower Back Pain Due to Kidney Deficiency

a. Needling *Zhongbai* (22.06) combined with *Wanshunyi* (22.08) is very effective.
b. Needling *Shuijin* (1010.20) and *Shuitong* (1010.19) is effective.
c. Needling *Shenguan* (77.18) combined with *Fuliu* (KI7) is very effective.
d. Point *Majinshui* (1010.13) or *Makuaishui* (1010.14) is also effective.

10) Acute Lumbar Sprain

a. Needling *Majinshui* (1010.13) and *Shuitong* (1010.19) is effective.
b. Needle *Erjiaoming* (11.12).
c. Bleeding *Weizhong* (BL40) is extremely effective.

Now let's discuss lower back pain which is one of the most commonly seen diseases in the clinic. In various kinds of lower back pain, acute lumbar sprain is most commonly seen. I have mentioned the specially effective herbal prescription for acute lumbar sprain is *Tong Qi San* (Powder for Moving Qi), which is effective for almost all kinds of acute lumbar sprain, even a ninety years old lady patient was cured after taking 2 doses of the herbs, the prescription of which was sent to her by fax. In acupuncture treatment, Master Tung often selected point *Majinshui* (1010.13). The horizontal line at the lower border of the nose (the upper end of the philtrum) corresponds to the kidney and lumbus. The points on this line are generally indicated in the pain syndrome of the kidney and lumbus. *Majinshui* (1010.13) is almost at the same level with *Renzhong* (DU26), and is therefore indicated in the pain of the lower back. Master Tung also often needled *Erjiaoming* (11.12) on the middle finger subcutaneously towards the small finger. When I followed Master Tung, I found the point most frequently used by him for acute Lumbar sprain is *Erjiaoming* (11.12). In Master Tung's treatment of acute lumbago, two points were most frequently used and they were *Erjiaoming* (11.12) and *Majinshui* (1010.13). Clinically, the two points are not selected simultaneously, and either of the two is enough.

In severe case, we could just give blood-letting to *Weizhong* (BL40). The patient could stand up and walk out of the clinic himself without help after such treatment.

There are many case examples of acute lumbar sprain. Here is a story about the treatment. Early in 1975, one taxi driver took a patient to my clinic with severe acute lumbar sprain. After taking the patient into the clinic, the taxi driver was then waiting outside. The patient had obvious blue vein swelling up at the popliteal fossa. I then bled the blue vein and the patient immediately felt much relieved and walked out himself. Not long after, the taxi driver came to see me for his stomachache and I cured him. Since he was constitutionally asthenic and easily getting tired, I gave him few more treatments and his body constitution was greatly improved. After then he quit the job of taxi driver and started to learn acupuncture with great effort, passed examination and became a licensed acupuncturist in California in the United States of America. He is now practicing acupuncture in south Taiwan and having many patients with good reputation.

In the treatment of acute lumbar sprain, bleeding *Weizhong* (BL40) is the best. If the condition is mild, needling *erjiaoming* (11.12) or *Majinshui* (1010.13) will be enough. The two points are selected alternatively. A mild case could be cured in one treatment, and in severe case, it takes two or three times only.

Now let's see how to treat acute lumbar sprain with the points of the fourteen meridians. First, we need to differentiate the pain is in the middle or the two sides of the lower back. *Renzhong* (DU26) is very good for lower back pain in the middle, and *Houxi* (SI3) is very good for the lower back pain of the both sides. When the pain is located on the lateral side of the waist or the whole waist, *Zhongzhu* (SJ3) is very good. In fact, there are many points that are indicated in lower back pain. Some doctors use *Quchi* (LI11) and others use *Neiguan* (PC6) to treat lower back pain. *Zanzhu* (BL2) is located at the starting point of the bladder meridian and is therefore effective for lower back pain. Lower back pain is most closely related to the bladder meridian and *Shugu* (BL65) is another effective point of lower back pain.

Clinically I often select *Renzhong* (DU26) combined with *Linggu* (22.05) to treat acute lumbar sprain and have obtained good result. This is because point *Linggu* (22.05) has very good therapeutic effect to regulate and tonify the kidney. *Dabai* (22.04) and *Linggu* (22.05) have the function to strengthen the metal and water, tonify the kidney and *qi*, as "*bai*" (white) corresponds to metal and *qi*, and "*gu*" (bone) corresponds to the kidney. They are therefore very good points for treating sciatica. For the same reason, *Linggu* (22.05) is often selected to treat lower back pain.

There are also many points in Tung's acupuncture to treat lower back pain due to kidney deficiency. The first points are *Shuijin* (1010.20) and *Shuitong* (1010.19). The second point is *Erjiaoming* (11.12). Needling *Erjiaoming* (11.12) in the direction towards the small finger is effective not only for acute but also chronic lower back pain. Besides, bleeding *Weizhong* (BL40) is also very good. *Xiasanhuang* (77.21), *Majinshui* (1010.13), *Linggu* (22.05) and *Dabai* (22.04) are all very good point for lower back pain. In addition, *Biyi* (1010.22) is a good point too.

There are also many effective points for chronic lower back pain in the fourteen meridians. The first is *Renzhong* (DU26), the second is *Houxi* (SI3) and the third is *Zhongzhu* (SJ3). In addition, *Shugu* (BL65) and *Fuliu* (KI7) are all good points. Many people consider that *Fuliu* (KI7) is an important point of the kidney meridian and is therefore a very good point for chronic lower back pain, as it is the metal point, the mother point of the kidney meridian which has the function to tonify the kidney. Chonic lower back pain is often of deficiency type. Actually, it is also an important point for acute lumbar sprain. *Xi Hong Fu* (Ode of Xi Hong) says: "*Fuliu* (KI7) functions to eliminate *qi* stagnation from the lumbus." *Tai Yi Ge* (Song of Tai Yi), *Tong Ren Zhen Jiu Tu Jing* (Illustrated Classic of Acupuncture Points on the Bronze Man) and *Yi Zong Jin Jian* (The Golden Mirror of Medicine) all take it as a very effective point for acute lumbar sprain. Generally, kidney deficiency often gives rise to lower back pain, and the patient with kidney deficiency is more liable to be affected by acute lumbar sprain, point *Fuliu* (KI7) is therefore extremely good for such condition. Besides, many other points such as *Xiasanhuang* (77.18, 19, 21) on the leg, and *Shuijin* (1010.20) and *Shuitong* (1010.19) on the face are also very good point. In the treatment, if *Zhongbai* (22.06) or *Wanshunyi* (22.08) is selected in combination, it would be even better.

11) Pain of the Midline of the Spinal Vertebrae

a. Bleed *Weizhong* (BL40).
b. Needle *Zhengjin* (77.01) and *Zhengzong* (77.02).

We have introduced this disease before. In Tung's acupuncture, *Zhengjin* (77.01) and *Zhengzong* (77.02) are the most frequently used points. The two points are very good for the pain along the midline of the spinal vertebrae. In the fourteen meridians, Kunlun (BL60) is a very effective point, and it would be even better if Renzhong (DU26) is added as it is the point of Du meridian that is very effective for the pain of the spinal vertebrae. In severe case, bleeding Weizhong (BL40) is always the best.

12) Pain of Coccygeal Vertebrae

a. Needling *Xinmen* (33.12) has special therapeutic effect.
b. Needle *Zhenghui* (1010.01) and *Houhui* (1010.06).
c. Needle *Dadu* (SP2) and *Haibao* (66.01).

Now let's discuss the pain of the coccygeal vertebrae. There are many patients suffering from this disease. Some cases are very severe. The pain is worse when sitting on chair. Such pain is often caused by fall from chair or slipping down when walking or from stair with bottom hitting the ground. The condition could last long without cure. Acupuncture is very effective for the disease, Tung's extraordinary points in particular. The first point is *Xinmen* (33.12) and such clinical application of this point has never been mentioned before. It is my own clinical experience. It is very effective for the pain of coccygeal vertebrae. The second point is *Zhenghui* (1010.01) combined with *Houhui* (1010.06). It is also very effective. Besides, *Haibao* (66.01) is also good for cyccygeal vertebral pain.

Here I'd like to talk something wide of the topic. In February of this year (2003), I was giving lectures in Houston. The lecture hour ranges from 8:00 am to 9:00 pm. At the request of the students, my lecture didn't stop until 1:00 pm the next day. Every one was tired after listening to the lecture for almost 17 hours. Some students had to drive for another 4 hours for home. So, I needled point *Biyi* (1010.22) for everyone after the lecture was finished. Because the students had been listening to my lecture continuously for 3 days and they were even more tired than me. After my treatment, everyone went home full of energy. If you are feeling tired now, I can help you needle *Biyi* (1010.22) to give you a lift.

Here I'd like to give you some supplementation. Since the pain of the spinal vertebrae is located in the middle of the back, we do not have to needle the points bilaterally but unilaterally with selection of the points on the left side for the male and right side for the female. When the therapeutic effect is not good enough, we needle the points on the other side. In Tung's acupuncture, many points are forbidden to needle bilaterally. But according to my own experience, some of these points may have very good effect without any side effect when they are needled bilaterally. I will give you more explanation in the introduction to the related treatment. Of course, we usually try to needle the points of one side first, and needle the other side only when the therapeutic result is not good cnough.

Regarding the pain of coccygeal vertebrae, I have read an article published in a journal of the mainland of China, which was written on the basis of "Tung's Acupuncture" published in mainland, China. It is mentioned in the articles that *Zhenghui* (1010.01) and *Houhui* (1010.06) may have good therapeutic result in treatment of the pain of coccygeal vertebrae. I understand the two points are effective for the disease. However, *Xinmen* (33.12) is the best point according to my own clinical experience. I noticed that the above book has missed point *Xinmen* (33.12) in the introduction.

Yesterday I went to a bookstore where there were many medical books in Chinese. I found many books with introduction to the fourteen meridians. There were also some books of Tung's acupuncture and some of them have mistakes about points. For example, point *Dabai* (22.04) was quite wrong. Some other books had mistakes about point *Yemen* (SJ2) and *Sanchasan* (A.04). I read the book briefly and found almost half of the points were wrong. So when you buy the book you need to pay more attention.

Here is one thing that I want to emphasize that needling *Renzhong* (DU26), *Houxi* (SI3), *Shugu* (BL65) and *Fengshi* (GB31) for lower back pain in the afternoon is better than in the morning. As everybody knows that the 12 regular meridians have the theory of Midnight-noon Ebb-flow. In fact, the *Du* and *Ren* meridians also have Midnight-noon Ebb-flow. The flow order of the *Ren* and *Du* meridians is as follow: it comes to *Baihui* (DU20) from 11:00 am to 1:00 pm, *Renzhong* (DU26) from 1:00 pm to 3:00 pm, *Tiantu* (REN22) from 3:00 pm to 5:00 pm, *Tanzhong* (REN17) from 5:00 pm to 7:00 pm, *Zhongwan* (REN12) from 7:00 pm to 9:00 pm, *Guanyuan* (REN 4) from 9:00 pm to 11:00 pm, *Huiyin* (REN1) from 11:00 pm to 1:00 am, *Yaoshu* (DU2) from 1:00 am to 3:00 am, *Mingmen* (DU4) from 3:00 am to 5:00 am, *Jinsuo* (DU8) from 5:00 am to 7:00 am, *Shenzhu* (DU12) from 7:00 am to 9:00 am, and *Fengfu* (DU16) from 9:00 am to 11:00 am. From this we can understand that the flow of the *Ren* and *Du* meridians comes to *Renzhong* (DU26) from 1:00 pm to 3:00 pm, the flow of 12 regular meridians comes to the small intestine meridian from 1:00 pm to 3:00 pm, and the bladder meridian from 3:00 pm to 5:00 pm. In the treatment of lower back pain and bone spur, we often needle *Renzhong* (DU26) of the *Du* meridian, *Houxi* (SI3) of the small intestine meridian and *Shugu* (BL65) of the bladder meridian, and all these points are therefore advisably needled form 1:00 to 3:00 pm and from 3:00 pm to 5:00 pm for best therapeutic result for pathological changes of either the lumbar or cervical vertebrae. In case of kidney deficiency, treatment should be given from 5:00 pm to 7:00 pm since it is the time for flow of the kidney.

Here I'd like to introduce another 2 points for lower back pain: *Zhongbai* (22.06) and *Xiabai* (22.07). *Zhongbai* (22.06) is a very good point for acute and chronic lower back pain. *Xiabai* (22.07) is often selected in combination with *Zhongbai* (22.06) as a coupling point. Besides, *Xiabai* (22.07) is a very good point foe nephrosis or colic pain due to renal stone. There is one point below *Shangbai* (22.03) corresponding to point *Menjin* (66.05) on the dorsum of the foot, which could be called Hand-*Menjin*. This point is very effective for acute lumbar sprain and the effective rate goes up to at least 90%. Now we can see that *Linggu* (22.05), *Xiabai* (22.07), Hand-*Menjin* and *Wanshun'er* are almost located on the same level and they are all very good points for lower back pain. It implies the theory of holography. The combination of Hand-*Menjin* and *Xiabai* (22.07) is even more effective. With the extraordinary connection of *zangfu*, *Xiabai* (22.07) is connected with the kidney and is therefore a very good point for renal colic and renal stone. At the beginning, Master Tung used *Zhongbai* (22.06) and *Xiabai* (22.07) to treat nephrosis. Since the two points are located on the *shaoyang* meridian of hand, they are also very effective for biliary colic and biliary ascariasis, as the two same-named meridians are connected with each other. The therapeutic result might not appear right after insertion of the needle, it works with the needle retention going on.

16. Questions: You have mentioned the meridians listed in your table of open, close, and pivot transversely are the same-named meridians that are connected with each other. Can you give more explanation?

Answer: The theory of open, close and pivot is used to describe the law of the three *yin* and three *yang* meridians in separating, gathering, interdepending, intertransforming, and the *qi* of the meridians in ascending, descending, moving in and out. *Taiyang* is the open, including the hand and foot *taiyang* meridians; *shaoyang* is the pivot, including the hand and foot *shaoyang* meridians; and *yangming* is the close, including the hand and foot *yangming* meridians. In the same way, *taiyin* is the open, including the hand and foot *taiyin* meridians; *shaoyin* is the pivot, including the hand and foot *shaoyin* meridians; and *jueyin* is the close, including the hand and foot *jueyin* meridians. It shows that the *taiyang* meridians of hand and foot dominates open and have the same property and law of movement, the *shaoyang* meridians of hand and foot dominates and serves as pivot and have the same property and law of movement, and the *yangming* meridians dominate close and have the same property and law of movement, so do the other *taiyin* meridians of hand and foot, *shaoyin* meridians of hand and foot and *jueyin* meridians of hand and foot. The same named meridians are connected with each other and their correspondence could be referred to "*Taiji* Holographic and Correspondence" attached to this lecture.

Because of "the connection of the same-named meridian," they help each other and can be combined with each other in treatment. They have the passage to make the couple meridians connected with each other. For instance, the hand and foot *taiyin* meridians are connected with each other near point *Zhongfu* (LU1); the hand and foot *yangming* meridians are connected with each other at point *Yingxiang* (LI20); the hand and foot *shaoyin* meridians are connected with each other in the heart; the hand and foot *taiyang* meridians are connected with each other at point *Jingming* (BL1); the hand and foot *jueyin* meridians are connected with each other at point *Tianchi* (PC1); and the hand and foot *shaoyang* meridians are connected with each other at point *Tongziliao* (GB1).

The combination of points of the same-named meridians is often introduced in the ancient songs of acupoints. Here are some examples from the book *Bai Zheng Fu* (Ode of One Hundred Symptoms): "Treatment of deafness relies on *Tinghui* (GB2) and *Yifeng* (SJ17)." *Tinghui* (GB2) is the point of the gallbladder meridian and *Yifeng* (SJ17) is the point of *Sanjiao* meridian. These two meridians are same-named meridians; "In case of dislike of speaking and preference of lying flat, select *Tongli* (HT5) and *Dazhong* (KI4)." *Tongli* (HT5) is the point of the heart meridian and *Dazhong* (KI4) is the point of the kidney meridian. The two points are from the same-named hand and foot meridians of *shaoyin*; "For the eye disease, needle *Ganshu* (BL18) and *Shaoze* (SI1)." *Ganshu* (BL18) is the point of the bladder meridian and *Shaozi* (SI1) is the point of the small intestine meridian. They are from the same-named meridians, the hand and foot *taiyang* meridians. Besides, it is also said in the book *Xi Hong Fu* (Ode of Xi Hong): "In case of febrile disease with anhidrosis, needle *Dadu* (SP2) and *Jingqu* (LU8)," "Needling *Shousanli* (LI10) and *Zusanli* (ST36) may treat food retention and abdominal distention." The former two points are from the hand and foot *taiyin* meridians; and the latter the hand and foot *yangming* meridians. Such examples of both the ancient and modern times are numerous, enough to prove that selection of points from the same-named meridians in treatment is one of the commonly used practical methods.

Taiji Holography and Correspondence

Holographic acupuncture technique is derived from the theory of holography, which considers that a relative independent part of an organic body is the same as the whole in chemical structure pattern, and is the narrowed form of the whole in proportion. In another word, the local is the miniature of the whole. Such biological holographic phenomena can be seen everywhere. In Chinese medicine, the tongue diagnosis and pulse palpation are the very concrete phenomena. Besides, observation of the face is another example. All these show that each relative independent part is the miniature of the whole.

In fact, this theory is originated from *Taiji*. In the theory of *Taiji* and *yuan qi* (source qi) in *Yi-jing*, there is an important point of view, that is, the local may manifest the general. It is also an important point of view in tradition Chinese medicine: correspondence between heaven and man. It considers that human body itself is a small universe, and any local part of human body is a miniature organic structure of the whole body. In another word, the whole includes the local and the local manifests the information of the whole. Such thought has been applied in the field of Chinese medicine in diagnosis and practice and created a special TCM holographic medicine.

Early in the book "The annals of Lü's Family," it says: "Like all parts of the human body, all the things in the universe form the universal harmony in the world." The theory of *Taiji* was greatly developed after Song Dynasty. From the theory of *Taiji*, the thinking of holography was derived, saying that "each object is an organic integrity and an organic integrity is a universe." The Confucian scholars of Song Dynasty further pointed out that "man exists in the universe and there is a universe in man." The Confucian of Song Dynasty *Zhu Xi* clearly pointed out that "everything has a *Taiji*." As for the interrelationship between the universe and man, the human body is a small universe and is the holographic structure of the universe." Furthermore, each human body is an organic integrity and each local part of the body is a miniature of the whole body.

The *Taiji* of the human body takes the umbilicus as the core. This is because the acquired is based upon the congenital and the nutrition is supplied by the umbilical cord at beginning of life. The part of the body above the diaphragm is known as upper energizer, (*Shang Jiao*) that between the diaphragm and the umbilicus is known as the middle energizer (*Zhong Jiao*) and that below the umbilicus is known as lower energizer (*Xia Jiao*). However, according to the theory of holography that "one object is a *Taiji* and each local part of the object is a small *Taiji*," there are many miniatures of *Taiji* on the body.

1. THE MAJOR *TAIJI*

There is a *Taiji* in each of the upper and lower extremities. The upper extremity takes the elbow as its *Taiji* and the lower extremity takes the knee as its *Taiji*. Furthermore, there are correspondence and inverse correspondence respectively. Compare with the umbilicus, this could be considered as the holography of grade one. With the upper extremities naturally dropping down, there is a natural correspondence between the arm and the trunk: the upper arm corresponds to the chest (or back) and epigastrium; the elbow corresponds to the umbilicus (waist); the forearm corresponds to the lower abdomen (lumbosacaral area); and the hand corresponds to the external genitalia. For instance, we can select points of the forearm to treat diseases of the lower abdomen or lumbosacral area, and the points of the hand to treat diseases of the external genitalia (or in return, select points of the lower abdomen and lumbosacral area to treat diseases of the forearm). Based upon this theory, Master Tung used to needle the five points of the hand including *Dajian* (11.01) to treat hernia.

When the upper extremity and the trunk are placed inversely, there is also a correspondence (known as inversive correspondence between the arm and trunk) as follow: the hand (wrist) corresponds to the head (neck); the forearm corresponds to the chest (back) and epigastrium; the elbow corresponds to the waist; the upper arm corresponds to the lower abdomen (or lumbosacral region); and the shoulder corresponds to the external genitalia. For instance, we cam select points of the forearm to treat diseases of the chest and epigastrium (such as *Neiguan*, PC6 and *Huochuan*, 33.04 and *Huoling*, 33.05 to treat palpitation and stuffiness in the chest); we can also select the points of the upper arm to treat diseases of the lower abdomen (on the contrary, we can select points of the chest, epigastrium and lower abdomen to treat diseases of the forearm and upper arm). That's why Master Tung often selected *Tianzong* (SI11) and *Yunbai* (44.11) at the shoulder to treat vaginal diseases in gynecology and points of the finger are often selected to treat diseases of the headache nowadays. With the same principle, selecting points of the fingers to treat diseases of the head is now very popular.

When the lower extremity and the trunk are placed in sequence (the sequence between the foot and the trunk), there is the correspondence as follow: the thigh corresponds to the chest (back) and epigastrium; the knee corresponds to the umbilicus (waist); the leg corresponds to the lower abdomen (lumbosacral region); the foot corresponds to the external genitalia. In case of diseases of the chest and back, needle the points on the thigh. For diseases of the lower abdomen, needle the points on the leg. On the contrary, for diseases of the thigh and leg, we can needle the points of the chest and abdomen.

Clinically, we often select point *Sima* (88.17, 18, 19) on the thigh to treat the lung, and *Santong* (88.01, 02, 03) to treat the heart. Personally, I often select *Menjin* (66.05) to treat dysmenorrhoea, *Dadun* (LR1) and *Yinbai* (SP1) to treat uterine bleeding, *Fuliu* (KI7) to treat lumbosacral pain and *Sanyinjiao* (SP6) to treat lower abdominal pain, etc.

When the lower extremities and the trunk are placed inversely, there is a correspondence as follow: the foot corresponds to the head; the ankle corresponds to the neck; the leg corresponds to the chest (back) and epigastrium; the knee corresponds to the umbilicus (waist); and the thigh corresponds to the lower abdomen (lumbosacral region).

If there is illness in the chest and epigastrium, needle the points on the leg. For diseases of the lower abdomen, needle the points of the thigh. On the contrary, the points of the chest and epigastrium are indicated in diseases of the thigh and leg. Master Tung used to selected *Zhengjin* (77.01) and *Zhengzong* (77.02) to treat disorders of the neck, and I personally often select *Zulinqi* (GB41) to treat migraine, *Xiangu* (ST43) to treat *Yangming* headache and *Shugu* (BL65) to treat occipital headache.

According to the above correspondence, the fingers and toes may correspond to the vertex where *Baihui* (DU20) and *Shenting* (DU24) are located, and this is why the *Jing*-well points can be used to treat mental disorders and acute apoplexy in emergency management. For instance, *Lidui* (ST45) and *Yinbai* (SP1) are often used to treat frequent nightmare, and *Dadun* (LR1) and *Shaoshang* (LU11) collectively known as ghost points to treat depressive psychosis. Wrist and ankle correspond to the neck. In addition to *Zhengjin* (77.01) which is indicated in stiffness of the neck, points around the wrist and ankle are also often selected to treat neck disorders. For example, *Lieque* (LU7) is indicated in stiffness and pain of the neck.

The above correspondence is tabled as follow:

Location in Correspondence	**Head**	**Chest and Epigastrium (Back)**	**Umbilicus**	**Lower Abdomen (Waist)**	**External Genitalia**
Correspondence Between Upper Extremity and Trunk	Shoulder	Upper Arm	Elbow	Forearm	Hand
Inverse Correspondence Between Upper Extremity and Trunk	Hand	Forearm	Elbow	Upper Arm	Shoulder
Correspondence Between Lower Extremity and Trunk	Hip	Thigh	Knee	Leg	Foot
Inverse Correspondence between Lower Extremity and Trunk	Foot	Leg	Knee	Thigh	Hip

Illustration 1

This kind of correspondence also exists between the upper and lower extremities. In correspondence, the elbow corresponds to the knee, the shoulder corresponds to the hip, the upper arm corresponds to the thigh, the forearm corresponds to the leg and the hand corresponds to the foot. For instance, shoulder points (such as *Jianzhong*, 44.06) can be selected to treat diseases of the hip. *Quchi* (LI11) or *Chize* (LU5) can be selected to treat diseases of the knee. On the contrary, points of the hip can be used to treat diseases of the shoulder and points of the knee can be used to treat diseases of the elbow. Personally, I often select *Xiaojie* (A.05) to treat ankle pain and it is the treatment following the same principle.

In the inverse correspondence of the upper and lower extremities, there is the correspondence as follows: the shoulder corresponds to the foot; the upper arm corresponds to the leg; the elbow corresponds to the knee; the forearm corresponds to the thigh and the hand corresponds to the hip. For example, we can select points on the shoulder to treat ankle diseases, and points of the forearm to treat thigh diseases. On the contrary, we can select points on the foot to treat diseases of the shoulder, and points of the thigh to treat diseases of the forearm. Master Tung often selected *Linggu* (22.05) and *Houxi* (SI3) on the hand to treat sciatica. Personally, I often select *Zhigou* (SJ6) and *Waiguan* (SJ5) to treat soreness and pain of the thigh.

The above correspondence is tabled with illustration as follow:

The Correspondence between Upper Extremity and Trunk | **The Correspondence between Lower Extremity and Trunk**

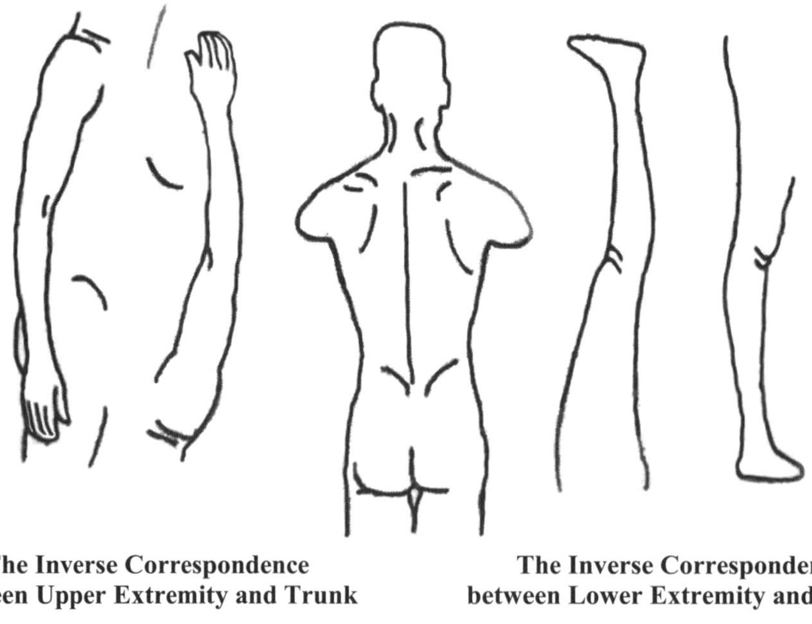

The Inverse Correspondence between Upper Extremity and Trunk | **The Inverse Correspondence between Lower Extremity and Trunk**

Illustration 2

However, the most frequently used in clinic is the consequent correspondence of the upper and lower extremities. This method is based on the theory of congenital eight diagrams in *Yi-Jing* (Book of Changes). (see Chapter One: The Principle of the Open, Close and Pivot, and the Extraordinary Connections of *Zangfu*, pp. 57-77).

The Correspondence between Upper Extremity and Lower Extremity

Shoulder	Upper Arm	Elbow	Forearm	Hand
Hip	Thigh	Knee	Leg	Foot

Since the lung and large intestine correspond to the spleen and stomach, they are often used to treat each other in treatment. But selecting points from the same-named meridians is the most frequently used one. That is, the lung meridian of hand *taiyin* and the spleen meridian of foot *taiyin* are used to treat each other, so are the large intestine meridian of hand *yangming* and the stomach meridian of foot *yangming*, the heart meridian of hand *shaoyin* and the kidney meridian of foot *shaoyin*, the small intestine meridian of hand *taiyang* and the urinary bladder meridian of *foot taiyang*, the pericardium meridian of hand *jueyin* and the liver meridian of foot *jueyin*, and the *sanjiao* meridian of hand shaoyang and the gallbladder meridian of foot *shaoyang*.

Here are some examples. Diseases of the meridian of hand-*taiyin* can be treated through needling the points of spleen meridian of foot-*taiyin*. The pain at *Shaoshang* (LI11) can be treated through needling *Yinbai* (SP1) and vice versa; the pain at *Yuji* (LU10) can be treated through needling *Taibai* (SP23) and vice versa; the pain at *Taiyuan* (LU9) can be treated through needling *Shangqiu* (SP5) and vice versa; the pain at *Chize* (LU5) can be treated by needling *Yinlingquan* (SP6) and vice versa. The treatment of diseases of the hand-*yangming* and foot-*yangming* meridians can also follow the same principle. The pain at *Xiangu* (ST43) can be treated through needling *Hegu* (LI4); the pain at *Yangxi* (LI5) can be treated through needling *Jiexi* (ST41); and *Shousanli* (LI10) and *Zusanli* (ST36) can be used in the same way. The heart meridian of hand-*shaoyin* and the kidney meridian of foot-*shaoyin* are the same. The pain at *Tongli* (HT5) can be treated by needling *Taixi* (KI3) and vice verse. So are the *taiyang* meridians. The pain at *Houxi* (SI3) can be treated by needling *Shugu* (BL65) and vice versa. In this way, the correspondent points can be selected to treat each other.

The following are some more examples: *Zhongzhu* (SJ3) and *Zulingqi* (GB41) can be selected to treat each other, and *Waiguan* (SJ5) and *Xuanzhong* (GB39) can also be selected to treat each other. The general pattern to follow is to select *Jing*-well point for *Jing*-well point, *Ying*-spring point for *Ying*-spring point, *Shu*-stream point for *Shu*-stream point,

He-sea point for *He*-sea point, or finger tip for toe tip, wrist for ankle, and elbow for knee (see Illustration 3).

The application of such correspondence between the hand and foot can even be enlarged to the treatment of not only the diseases of the upper and lower limbs but also the internal diseases or other diseases. For example, *Hegu* (LI4) and *Taichong* (LR3) are all indicated in eye diseases; *Zhongzhu* (SJ3) and *Zulingqi* (GB41) are all indicated in ear diseases; *Lieque* (LU7) and *Zhaohai* (KI6) are all indicated in throat diseases; *Neiguan* (PC6) and *Sanyinjiao* (SP6) are all indicated in diseases of the heart and chest; *Shousanli* (LI10) and *Zusanli* (ST36) are all indicated in gastro-intestinal diseases; *Weizhong* (BL40) and *Quchi* (LI11) are all indicated in diseases of the lower back; *Shenmen* (HT7) at and wrist and *Dazhong* (KI4) at the ankle are all indicated in dementia; *Yinxi* (HT6) and *Fuliu* (KI7) are all indicated in night sweating; *Zhizheng* (SI7) of the small intestine meridian of hand-*taiyang* and *Feiyang* (BL58) are often selected together to treat vertigo; *Yuji* (LU10) and *Gongsun* (SP4) are all indicated in stomach diseases and infantile malnutrition; *Shaoze* (SI1) can promote lactation and *Zhiyin* (UB67) can correct malposition of fetus, and they are all indicated in gynecological diseases; and *Xuanzhong* (GB39) and *Waiguan* (SJ5) are all indicated in neck sprain, etc. Such application will make acupuncture treatment more flexible and convenient.

The correspondence between the same-named meridians of hand and foot is listed as follow:

The Lung Meridian of Hand-Taiyin	**The Spleen Meridian of Foot-Taiyin**
Shaoshang (LU11)	Yinbai (SP1)
Yuji (LU10)	Taibai (SP3)
Taiyuan LU9)	Shangqiu (SP5)
Lieque (LU7)	Sanyinjiao (SP6)
Chize (LU5)	Yinlingquan (SP9)
The Large Intestine Meridian of Hand-Yangming	**The Stomach Meridian of Foot-Yangming**
Shangyang (LI1)	Lidui (ST45)
Hegu (LI4)	Xiangu (ST43)
Yangxi (LI5)	Jiexi (ST41)
Shousanli (LI10)	Zusanli (ST36)
Quchi (LI11)	Dubi (ST35)
Zhouliao (LI12)	Liangqiu (ST34)
Binao (LI14)	Futu (ST32)
Jianyu (LI15)	Biguan (ST31)
The Heart Meridian of Hand-Shaoyin	**The Kidney Meridian of Foot-Shaoyin**
Shaofu (HT8)	Rangu (SP2)
Shenmen (HT7)	Zhaohai (KI6)
Tongli (HT5)	Taixi (KI3)
Shaohai (HT3)	Yingu (KI10)

The Small Intestine Meridian of Hand-Taiyang	The Bladder Meridian of Foot-Taiyang
Shaoze (SI1)	Zhiyin (BL67)
Qiangu (SI2)	Tonggu (BL66)
Houxi (SI3)	Shugu (BL65)
Wangu (SI4)	Jinmen (BL63)
Yanggu (SI5)	Shenmai (BL62)
Yanglao (SI6)	Kunlun (BL60)
Zhizheng (SI7)	Chengshan (BL57)
Xiaohai (SI8)	Weizhong (BL40)
Naoshu (SI10)	Chengfu (BL36)
The Pericardium Meridian of Hand-Jueyin	**The Liver Meridian of Foot-Jueyin**
Zhongchong (PC9)	Dadun (LR1)
Laogong (PC8)	Taichong (LR3)
Daling (PC7)	Zhongfeng (LR4)
Ximen (PC4)	Ligou (LR5)
Quze (PC3)	Ququan (LR8)
The Sanjiao Meridian of Hand-Taiyang	**The Gallbladder Meridian of Foot-Shaoyang**
Guanchong (SJ1)	Zuqiaoyin (GB44)
Zhongzhu (SJ3)	Zulingqi (GB41)
Yangchi (SJ4)	Qiuxu (GB40)
Waiguan (SJ5)	Xuanzhong (GB39)
Sidu (SJ9)	Yanglingquan (GB34)
Qinglengyuan (SJ11)	Fengshi (GB31)
Jianliao (SJ14)	Huantiao (GB30)

Illustration 3

2. THE MEDIUM *TAIJI* (HOLOGRAPHY GRADE 2)

The medium *Taiji* is also known as holography grade 2. It takes the wrist and ankle as the core (*Taiji*), covering the fingers and toes, and the forearm and the middle section of the leg.

It is listed as follow:

Correspondent Location	Head	Chest and epigastrium (back)	Umbilicus	Lower abdomen (lower back)	External genitalia
Hand	Finger	Palm	Wrist	Forearm (distal part)	Forearm (middle part)
Foot	Toe	Dorsum of foot	Ankle	Leg (distal part)	Leg (middle part)

Illustration 4

The application of the theory was often used in ancient acupuncture (see Acupuncture Songs). Many of the applications are related to holography.

The examples are listed as follow:

Guanchong (SJ1)	**Ear**	Qiaoyin (GB44)
Dagukong (Extra)	**Eye**	Xingjian (LR2)
Erjian, Sanjian (LR2, 3)	**Throat**	Taichong (LR2), Taibai (SP3)
Laogong (PC8)	**Heart and Chest**	Yongquan (KI1)
Yuji (LU10)	**Stomach**	Gongsun (SP4)
Wangu (SI4)	**Waist and Navel**	Zhongfeng (LR4), Kunlun (BL60)
Neiguan (PC6)	**Lower abdomen**	Sanyinjiao (SP6)
Erbai (Extra)	**Anus**	Chengshan (BL57)

Illustration 5

In the correspondence of medium *Taiji* (holography grade 2) introduced above, *Taixi* (KI3) corresponds to the kidney and is therefore often selected to treat renal colic. *Shuiquan* (KI 5) corresponds to *Tianshu* (ST25) at the navel, and is therefore often used by ancient doctors to treat delayed menstruation (*Tianshu* ST25 is also the point of indication in *Bijing* – amenorrhea). *Zhigou* (SJ6) and *Chengshan* (BL57) correspond to the sacracoccygeal area and are therefore indicated in constipation and coccygeal pain.

According to the holography of grade 1 and 2 that often appears in classical literature, the application of points for common diseases are listed as follow:

Location of disease	**Most Commonly Used Point**
Head and face	Hegu (LI4)
Eyes	Hegu (LI4), Taichong (LR3)
Throat	Shaoshang (LU11), Hegu (LI4), Zhaohai (KI6), Taichong (LR3)
Chin	Yanggu (LI5), Xiaxi (GB43)
Neck	Chengjiang (REN24), Houxi (SI3), Sugu (BL65)
Chest	Daling (PC7), Neiguan (PI6), Yongquan (KI1), Jianshi (PC5)
Hypochondrium	Zhigou (SJ6), Yanglingquan (GB34), Wangu (SI4)
Abdomen	Zusanli (ST36)
Navel	Yinlingquan (SP9), Ququan (LR8), Zhongfeng (LR4)
Urinary Organs	Yinlingquan (SP9), Sanyinjiao (SP6) Dadun (LR1)
Women's Diseases	Sanyinjiao (SP6)
External Genitalia	Sanyinjiao (SP6), Dadun (LR1)
Anus	Chengshan (BL57), Baihui (DU20), Erbai (Extra)
Shoulder	Zhongzhu (SJ3), Zhigou (SJ6)
Waist (Lower Back)	Weizhong (BL40), Kunlun (BL60)

Illustration 6

3. THE MINOR *TAIJI*

In case of subdivision of the hand, arm, foot and leg, each part is related to the whole body and can be used to treat diseases of the whole body. According to the theory of holography, any minor part of the body, including the head, is a miniature of the whole and has the points corresponding to the different parts of the body respectively.

For instance, the radial side of the second metacarpal bone can be divided into small regions respectively corresponding to the head, upper energizer, middle energizer, lower energizer and external genitalia. Starting from the root of the finger to the root of the palm where the trapezium is, there locate the points respectively corresponding to the head, neck, upper limb, lung, liver, stomach, duodenum, kidney, waist, lower abdomen, leg and foot. The ulnar side of the fifth matacarpal bone also has the same correspondence.

Regarding to the division of small parts, from metacarpophalangeal joints (head) to carpimetacarpal joints is originally divided into 3 parts, the upper, middle and lower (see Illustration 7). The upper part corresponds to the head, heart and lung. The middle part corresponds to the spleen, stomach, liver and gallbladder. The lower part corresponds to the kidney, bladder and lower limbs. Later, the 3 parts were developed into 11 points. Their locations are as follows: the midpoint between the point Head, and Leg and Foot is Stomach; the midpoint between Stomach and Leg and foot is Waist; the midpoint between the Head and Stomach is Heart and Lung; the distance between Head, and Heart and Lung is divided into 3 equal parts: connecting point of the upper one-third and middle one-third is Neck; the connecting point of the middle and lower one-third is Upper Limb; the midpoint between Stomach, and Heart and Lung is Liver. The distance between Liver and Waist is then divided into 3 equal parts, the connecting point between the upper and middle one-third is Duodemum; the connecting point of the middle and lower one-third is Kidney; the midpoint between Waist and Leg and Foot is Hypogastrium (see Illustration). The division of other parts of the body such as upper arm, forearm, thigh and leg also follows the same principle.

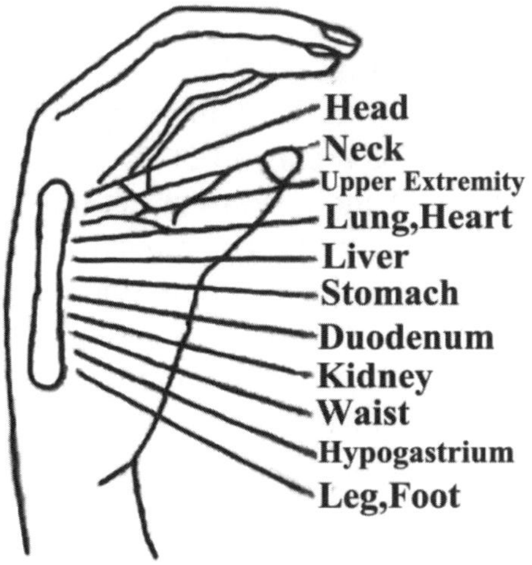

Illustration 7

However, I have to point out that: 1. Each point should be considered as a small area that includes the corresponding locations and organs. For example, point Head includes head, eyes, ears, nose, mouth and teeth, etc.; point Neck includes neck, throat, thyroid gland, trachea, etc.; point Leg includes leg and knee; and point Foot includes foot, ankle and toe. 2. The terminal end of each part is the starting point of another part that can be selected to treat diseases of both parts. Besides, each part also has both consequent and reverse correspondence.

Distribution of Tung's extraordinary points is very much based upon biological holography. Master Tung emphasized that all the local points could treat diseases of the whole body. Thugh he divided the whole body into 12 therapeutic regions, each of them can be used to treat diseases of the whole body. In his clinical treatment, it was often the patients that decided to select points on either hand or foot. The points of the same therapeutic category are located on both upper and lower limbs. The examples are *Zhiwujin* (11.08), *Shouwujin* (33.08) and *Zuwujin* (77.25), and *Zhisima* (11.07) and *Zusima* (88.17, 18, 19). Moreover, one group of points may also imply the significance of holography. For instance, *Linggu* (22.05) and *Dabai* (22.04) are often selected to warm *yang* and supplement *qi* and their indications almost cover the whole body. Their therapeutic effect is so high that the other points cannot compare. Point *Dabai* (22.040) overlaps *Sanjian* (LI3) that is the point of large intestine meridian, and point *Linggu* (22.05) is located between *Hegu* (LI4) and the junction of the first and second metacarpal bones. Simultaneous selection of the two points covers the location of the *yuan*-source and *shu*-stream points. From the point of view, *Dabai* (22.04) dominates the upper energizer and *Linggu* (22.05) dominates the lower energizer. Besides, the two points are needled deeply, penetrating through all the three energizers transversely and perpendicularly, and thus the therapeutic effect.

Another example is point *Wuhu* (11.27) that has five points distributing from the fingertip to the palm, respectively known as *Wuhuyi* (11.27-1), *Wuhu'er* (11.27-2), *Wuhusan* (11.27-3), *Wuhusi* (11.27-4), and *Wuhuwu* (11.27-5). Master Tung used to select this point to treat swelling of joints. Actually, the location and indication of the points imply holographic significance. *Wuhuyi* is often selected to treat finger pain, palm pain and tenosynovitis. *Wuhusan* is often needled to treat pain of toes. *Wuhu'er* is mainly used to enhance the therapeutic effect of *Wuhuyi* and *Wuhusan*. *Wuhusi* is used to treat pain of the dorsum of foot. *Wuhuwu* is needled to treat heel pain.

Furthermore, some groups of points on the thigh and leg are indicated in disorders of the whole body. For example, *Simashang* (88.18), *Simazhong* (88.17) and *Simaxia* (88.19) are indicated in diseases of the lung system; *Tianhuang* (88.13), *Minghuang* (88.12) and *Qihuang* (88.14) are indicated in liver diseases; *Shenguan* (77.18), *Renhuang* (77.21) and *Dihuang* (77.19) are indicated in disorders of renal system. The meeting point (lowerest point of each part and the upmost point of the connected one) is indicated in diseases of both the corresponding upper and lower. For example, *Linggu* (22.05) can be selected to treat both heel pain and dizziness, and *Quchi* (LI11) can be needled to treat both dizziness and knee pain.

In the point-coupling technique, Master Tung often selected 2 or 3 needles puncturing together in row, and the method implies the significance of correspondence in holography, the points on the thigh in particular, which are often used to treat disorders of internal *zangfu* organs. For example, *Simashang* (88.18), *Simazhong* (88.17) and *Simaxia* (88.19) are indicated in diseases of the lung system; *Tongguan* (88.01), *Tongshan* (88.02) and *Tongtian* (88.03) are indicated in diseases of the heart system; *Minghuang* (88.12), *Renhuang* (88.13) and *Qihuang* (88.14) are indicated in liver diseases; and *Tongshen* (88.09), *Tongwei* (88.10) and *Tongbei* (88.11) are indicated in diseases of the kidney. It can be seen that the upper point is indicated in diseases of the upper, the middle point is indicated in diseases of the middle and the lower point is indicated in diseases of the lower. The therapeutic effect of such integral correspondence is quite prominent.

Now let's see the holographic distribution of the head. It was expounded early in Chapter 49 of *Lingshu* (Spiritual Pivot). It is considered that the tip of the nose is taken as the center (*Taiji*), corresponding to the head and face; the midpoint between the eyebrows corresponds to the lung and the point slightly above it corresponds to the throat; the midpoint between the eyes corresponds to the heart; the midpoint of the nasal spine corresponds to the liver; the tip of the nose corresponds to the spleen; the ala nasi corresponds to the stomach; the lateral side of the point Liver corresponds to the gallbladder; the area below the zygoma and cheek corresponds to the large intestine (directly between the outer canthus, see Illustration 8); the area from the zogyma to the cheek corresponds to the kidney (it levels with the lower border of the nose).

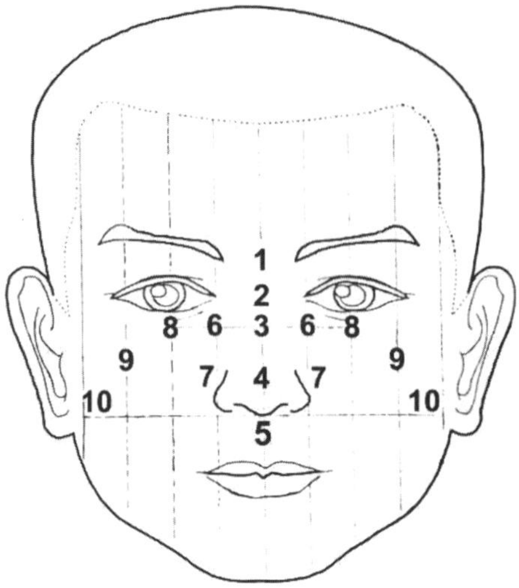

1 Lung
2 Heart
3 Liver
4 Spleen
5 Urinary Bladder and Uterus
6 Gallbladder
7 Stomach
8 Small Intestine
9 Large Intestine
10 Kidney

Illustration 8

According to the holographic correspondence, *Renzhong* (DU26) is often clinically selected to treat pain of the spine and lumbus; *Juliao* (ST3) (corresponding to *Shenshu*, BL23) is often selected to treat diseases of the lumbus; *Majinshui* (which is located below zygoma and corresponds to the kidney and lumbus) is often selected to treat lower back pain and renal stone; *Duiduan* (DU27) is often selected to treated diseases of the urinary system; and *yintang* (Extra) is often selected to treat insomnia with its sedative function, etc.

Each part of the body has both consequent and reverse correspondence, so does the head. As shown in Illustration 9, the area below *Chengjiang* (REN24) corresponds to the throat; mouth corresponds to the heart; *Renzhong* (DU26) corresponds to the esophagus; nose corresponds to the stomach; the area around the eye corresponds to the kidney; forehead corresponds to the intestines; and the top of forehead corresponds to the bladder and uterus.

Clinically, this kind of correspondence could be used in observation and treatment of diseases. Areas 13 and 26 correspond to bronchus; areas 11 and 24 correspond to the lungs, and needling *Shuijin* (1010.20) and *Shuitong* (1010.19) obliquely downward and subcutaneously through zygoma (from the bronchus to the lung) is very effective for cough and asthma; in case of pulmonary tuberculosis, deficiency of *yin* of the lung and heat in the lung, there may appear redness in areas 11 and 24, the areas below zygoma; in case of asthmatic breathing, there may appear bluish color in the areas 13 and 26; the lips correspond to the heart, and pathological changes of the heart often change the color of the lips such as white in case of blood deficiency and purple in case of blood stasis; area 10, the tip of the nose, corresponds to the stomach, and brandy nose suggests damp heat in the stomach; areas 9 and 22, the zygomatic areas, correspond to the liver and spleen, and there may appear brown patches in these areas in case of damp in the liver and spleen or disharmony of the liver and spleen; areas 6 and 19 at the orbit correspond to the kidney, and dark color around the eyes suggests kidney deficiency, and edema of the eyelids suggests nephritis; area 5 corresponds to the traverse colon and lumbus, and needling *Jingming* (BL1) and *Zanzhu* (BL2) can treat lower back pain, and this therapeutic effect is based upon not only the meridian system but also holography.

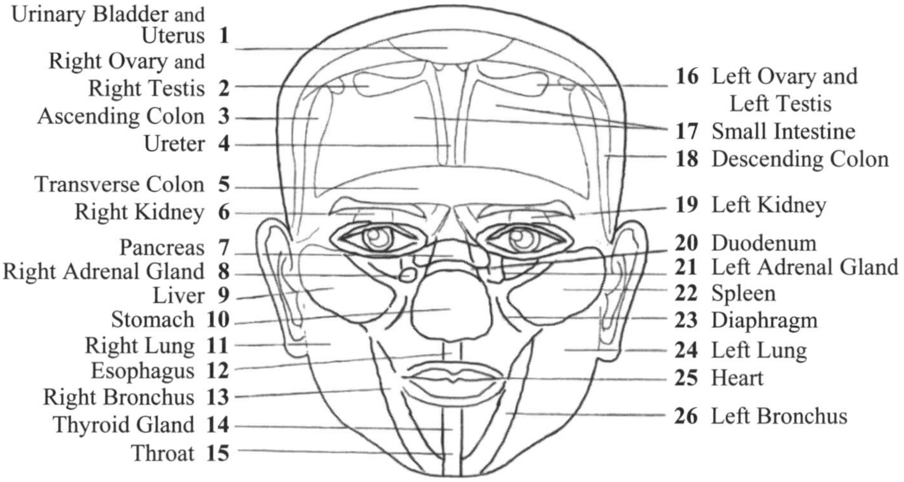

Illustration 9

Chapter Three

Diseases of *Zangfu*

For treating *Zangfu* organ diseases, I want first to introduce some general points. I will try to help you grasp the mechanism and therapeutic methods for various kinds of diseases in this limited period, and meanwhile, grasp the principles of points' selection as well. What will be introduced in this paragraph will give you a general understanding of a disease and its therapeutic methods in the shortest time. If you have profound research on some diseases, you will know more about point applications. Of course the therapeutic effect will be better. The more properties of points you are able to grasp, the deeper understanding of the points you will know, the better therapeutic effect there will be. Considering this, it will take more time to give further explanation. I will try to explain the therapeutic principles in this lecture even though the time is limited.

1. Cardiac Diseases

1) Angina Pectoris

a. *Tongguan* (88.01), *Tongshan* (88.02).
b. It will bring a fairly good therapeutic effect by pricking *Huobao* (55.01) to induce bleeding.
c. It will bring a fairly good therapeutic effect by pricking a place around the cubital crease located at *Quze* (PC 3) and *Chize* (LU 5).
d. *Tianzong* (44.10) and *Dizong* (44.09).
e. *Huozhu* (66.04) and *Huoying* (66.03).

The most commonly used points Master Tung selected for treating cardiac diseases are *Tongguan* (88.01) and *Tongshan* (88.02). The most commonly used point from the fourteen meridians is *Zusanli* (ST 36). The reason is the son could strengthen the mother. Also because the stomach communicates with the pericardium and the *He*-sea points for treating viscera's diseases, thus *Zusanli* (ST 36) could be applied to treat cardiac diseases. It is a very good idea to combine *Neiguan* (PC 6) and *Zusanli* (ST 36) for treating cardiac diseases. *Tongguan* (88.01) and *Tongshan* (88.02) are both points often used by Master Tung, which are both on the stomach meridian and the function of these two points are exerted because of the stomach communicating with the pericardium. *Futu* (ST 32) is between *Tongguan* (88.01) and *Tongshan* (88.02). *Zhen Jiu Da Cheng* (The Great Compendium of Acupuncture and Moxibustion) says *Futu* (ST 32) is the confluence of blood vessel. Therefore, *Futu* (ST 32) is a very good point for regulating cardiac blood circulation. Because the stomach communicates with the pericardium and *Futu* (ST 32) is the confluence of blood vessel, this point could bring a very good therapeutic effect in treating cardiac disease by considering treating the vessel by needling the vessel and treating the heart by needling the vessel.

The place where *Tianzong* (44.10) and *Renzong* (44.08) are locates stout muscle. If the arm rotates forwardly, the hardness could be avoided. These two points are located on the lung meridian. It is easier to insert a needle alongside the blood vessel when the arm is rotated; if not, it will be difficult to insert the needle. In classic books, it recorded that needles were forbidden in this place. According to my opinion, maybe it is because thick needles were used at that time, and therefore susceptible to injuring blood vessels and nerves. This point is close to the artery, therefore, it can regulate blood circulation according to the theory of treating vessels by using vessels. Meanwhile the heart is closely related to blood vessels, thus this point can be applied to treat cardiac diseases, even for bringing back a life.

The chief therapeutic property of *Huoying* (66.03) is to strengthen heart and can be applied for coma. Sometimes when *Renzhong* (DU 26) and *Neiguan* (PC 6) were applied without bringing back consciousness, by stimulating *Huoying* (66.03) consciousness could be brought back, so as *Taichong* (LR 3). *Huozhu* (66.04) can treat paralyses of the heart. Both *Huoying* (66.03) and *Huozhu* (66.04) can treat cardiac diseases. Underneath *Huoying* (66.03) and *Huozhu* (66.04), there is the *chong* meridian. The theory of treating the vessel by stimulating the vessel and treating the heart by stimulating the vessel, and the location of *Huozhu* (66.04) is same as *Taichong* (LR 3 the *Yuan*-source point) and the meridian where *Taichong* (LR 3) bears the same name of Pericardium Meridian of Hand *Jueyin*. Those are the reasons for why *Huozhu* (66.04) has the function of strengthening the heart. Another saying: recent research proves that coronary artery spasm could not only induce angina pectoris but is also one of the reasons for acute myocardial infarction and sudden death. TCM classifies blood vessel as aponeurosis. Chapter 44 of *Su Wen* (Essential Questions) states liver dominates aponeurosis. In Chapters 5, 19 and 3 of the same book, there are records about aponeurosis. Liver dominates aponeurosis which composes tendons, thus in the TCM field, there is a perception of liver dominating aponeurosis. Liver and heart are closely related. Aponeurosis spasm will be induced if liver *qi* is stagnated due to liver *yang* deficiency or emotional disturbance. Hence, heart vessel spasm will occur too. This is one of the reasons why *Huozhu* (66.04) and *Huoying* (66.03) from the liver meridian have the therapeutic effect. Because blood circulation could be regulated by following the theory of treating the vessel by stimulating the vessel, therefore the heart could be treated by following the theory of treating the heart by stimulating the vessel. *Huoying* (66.03) and *Huozhu* (66.04) work better than *Renzhong* (DU 26) in more conditions as first aid. When there is acute coma, and *Renzhong* (DU 26) and *Neiguan* (PC 6) can't bring back consciousness, puncture *Taichong* (LR 3) or *Huoying* (66.03) or *Huozhu* (66.04), the consciousness will be brought back. This is a very good example for the application of five element theory.

Acupuncture clinics could be better helped if extra studying is applied to Chapter 51 of *Su Wen* (Essential Questions) and Chapter 7 of *Ling Shu* (Spiritual Pivot). According to my own study, Master Tung used Chapter 51 and Chapter 7 frequently, though he never said it clearly. After my study to his knowledge, I'd like to summarize his essence and present it to the public. If we know the mechanism, the applications of his points will be improved. Each of Master Tung's points has a profound reason. Not only in South Korea, but also China and USA, Master Tung's points are widely known. At present, plenty of people think that Master Tung's points and points from the fourteen meridians are two separate equal systems. In fact, the theory of Master Tung's points is a very complete system. At the beginning of the lecture, I've already explained it by applying extraordinary connection of *zangfu*, *Yi Jing* (The Book of Changes) and the theory of Open, Close and Pivot. *Tianzong* (44.10) and *Renzong* (44.08) are very good points for strengthening the heart so that they can be used to treat cardiac diseases. *Huoying* (66.03) and *Huozhu* (66.04) also have the function of strengthening heart. The application of all those points is based upon the body parts correspondence.

For treating pectoris angina and myocardial infarction, *Huobao* (55.01) could be applied. The Chinese name of *Huobao* makes people think of pericardium which is *Xinbao* in Chinese. The location of *Huobao* (55.01) is underneath the second toe on the course of stomach meridian which communicates with pericardium meridian through extraordinary connection of *zangfu*. This point is very near the *Jing*-well point, thus it has the function of first aid. The therapeutic effect will be very good if bleeding method is applied. Here I tried to display the explanation and supplement to the function and mechanism of each point. After this lecture, Da Xing Medical Press will publish what is taught in this lecture for your reference. If you can understand the property of each point, it will benefit your clinical practice. We are looking forward to its publication and providing you with a lot of reference.

For acute angina pectoris, our ancestors like to prick the cubital crease to induce bleeding for first aid. I also bleed this place. By inducing more bleeding in this place it could release pain and promote blood circulation. It is a good method to help patients with coronary arterosclerotic heart disease and myocardial infarction by either puncturing or pricking. There are many patients who should have received an operation but didn't because of the acupuncture treatments. Many patients got cardiac diseases in their fifties, but with acupuncture and bleeding treatments, they are still very healthy in their eighties, even in their nineties. We've cured many patients completely who had cardiac diseases. When myocardial infarction or acute pectoris angina occurs, the above mentioned methods could be followed. Usually puncture *Neiguan* (PC 6) and *Zusanli* (ST 36), or *Tongguan* (88.01) and *Tongshan* (88.02). In addition, prick one of the points from two groups to induce some bleeding about once every 10 days: one group includes *Sihuazhong* (77.09) and *Sihuawai* (77.14), another group includes *Chize* (LU 5) and *Quze* (PC 3). With 3 or 4 months' such treatment, patients will feel very good; for severe condition, it may take longer period.

For prevention of hyperlipemia and myocardial infarction, food therapy is advisable and important. The best food is Jew's ear, and garlic would decrease blood lipid. It is better to eat raw garlic. Cut the garlic and eat it after oxidation which brings a better effect. There is no effect if garlic's cooked. Some TCM physicians would like to add 15g or 20g Jew's ear in the prescription for treating coronary cardiac disease which could increase the therapeutic effect. In the herbal prescription, *Gualou* (Fructus Trichosanthis) and *Xiebai* (Bulbus Allii Macrostemi) are used the most. If the pathological condition is severe, *Xue fu Zhu yu Tang* (Decoction for Removing Blood Stasis in the Chest) is a very good formula. *Gua lou Xie bai Tang* (Decoction of Trichosanthes and Allium) works very well for regulating *Qi* circulation and resolving phlegm, but weak in regulating blood circulation. For enhancing blood circulation, *Si Ni San* (Powder for Treating Cold Limbs) and *Danshen* (Radix Salviae Miltiorrhizae) should be added. *Si Ni San* (Powder for Treating Cold Limbs) formula is good at regulating *Qi*. If *Shaoyao* (Paeonia lacti flora Pall) is replaced by *Chishao* (Radix Paeoniae Rubra), the blood circulation could be enhanced. If *Danshen* (Radix Salviae Miltiorrhizae) added, the function of strengthening blood circulation is enhanced. Nowadays more and more people suffer from hyperlipemia and high cholesterol. The basic treatment for those people is to regulate diet, after which the blood lipid will decline. *Danshen* (Radix Salviae Miltiorrhizae), *Shanzha* (Fructus Crataegi), *Chishao* (Radix Paeoniae Rubra), *Juemingzi* (Semen Cassiae) and *Zexie* (Rhizoma Alismatis) and other herbs work very well for decreasing cholesterol. *Chuanxiong* (Rhizoma Chuanxiong) and *Gegen* (Radix Puerariae) added will bring a better effect in decreasing blood lipid. In addition, *Wumei* (Fructus Mume) and *Cuchaihu* (Radix Bupleuri prepared with vinegar) added on the base of this prescription to treat fatty liver.

2) Stomach Distention (distending sensation occurring inferior to heart)

a. *Xinmen* (33.12).
b. *Tongguan* (88.01) and *Tongshan* (88.02) with effect.

Patients suffering with stomach distention sometimes will have difficulty to explain clearly their symptoms. There is a term of inferior to heart recorded in *Shan Han Lun* (Treatise on Injury by Cold) which refers to stomach. For treating common stomach diseases, Master Tung usually prick *Sihuazhong* (77.09) to induce bleeding, then puncture *Tongguan* (88.01) and *Tongshan* (88.02). These points treat stomach distention fairly well. *Neiguan* (PC 6) is also an effective point. If combined with *Zusanli* (ST 36) it also will create a better effect. As well, *Menjin* (66.05) is a good point for stomach distention.

3) Tachycardia

a. *Xinchang* (11.19) with good effect.
b. *Xinmen* (33.12) with good effect.
c. *Tongguan* (88.01) and *Tongtian* (88.03) with effect.
d. *Sihuazhong* (77.09) and *Sihuawai* (77.14), prick to induce bleeding with effect.
e. *Chasan* Points (A.04).
f. Prick ear apex to induce some bleeding with effect.

Same as palpitation, *Xinchang* (11.19) is a commonly used point for tachycardia which is on the middle finger. *Xinchang* (11.19) brings a very good therapeutic effect for treating palpitation, arrhythmia, and abnormal heart beating. *Xinmen* (33.12) is also a good point for palpitation. *Xinchang* (11.19) and *Xinmen* (33.12) are effective points for arrhythmia. For tachycardia, besides *Xinchang* (11.19) and *Xinmen* (33.12), *Chasan* (A.04) is another often used point. *Tongguan* (88.01), *Tongshan* (88.02) and *Tongtian* (88.03) are also good. If pathological condition is severe, prick *Sihuazhong* (77.09) or ear apex to induce bleeding.

Xinchang (11.19) and *Xinmen* (33.12) can also be used for bradycardia. *Tongguan* (88.01), *Tongshan* (88.02) and *Tongtian* (88.03) have the same function as well. *Neiguan* (PC 6) and *Zusanli* (ST 36) are effective too.

4) Cardiac Paralysis

a. *Quling* (33.16) with pricking method to induce bleeding brings a very good effect.
b. *Sihuazhong* (77.09) with bleeding method brings a very good effect.
c. *Huobao* (55.01) with pricking method to induce bleeding brings a fairly good effect.
d. *Huoying* (66.03) and *Huozhu* (66.04) with effect.
e. *Dizong* (44.09) with effect.

The difference between heart paralysis and angina pectoris is the severity of pathological condition. When pathological condition becomes severe, angina pectoris will turn to heart paralysis. It is very clearly recorded in the book of "Points Study" that there are many points which can treat heart paralysis. Among those previously mentioned points: *Tianzong* (44.10), *Renzong* (44.08) and *Dizong* (44.09), *Dizong* (44.09) is the most frequently used one. *Huoying* (66.03) and *Huozhu* (66.04) are also commonly used points for heart paralysis. Both of them have the function of strengthening heart. Pricking method to induce bleeding to *Huobao* (55.01) brings a very good effect. Pricking the area where *Quze* (PC 3) and *Chize* (LU 5) could achieve good effect as well. *Zhongchong* (PC 9) with bleeding technique will bring fairly good effect. When first aid given to wind stroke, prick *Zhongchong* (PC 9) as a key point for rescue, next, prick *Shaoshang* (LU 11) to induce bleeding. As we know that the thumb is correspondent to the head, for treating mental diseases, points on the thumb, for example, *Shaoshang* (LU 11), usually are pricked. Because thumb moves most frequently and closely relates to cerebral neuron, and middle finger is directly related to pericardium, thus, *Jing*-well point of pericardium meridian is pricked. Master Tung usually used *Linggu* (22.05) and *Dabai* (22.04) for treating hemiplegia, *Muhuo* (11.10) on the middle finger is also often used. About *Muhuo* (11.10) will be explained in details when treatment of wind stroke is introduced.

5) Cardiac Pain

a. *Tongguan* (88.01), *Tongshan* (88.02) and *Tongtian* (88.03).
b. *Sihuazhong* (77.09) and *Sihuawai* (77.14) with pricking method to induce bleeding bring fairly good effect.

6) Pain on Both Sides of Heart

a. *Sihuazhong* (77.09) and *Sihuawai* (77.14) with pricking method to induce bleeding will bring a fairly good effect.

Precordial pain and pain on both sides of heart could be treated by puncturing *Tongguan* (88.01), *Tongshan* (88.02) and *Tongtian* (88.03). *Sihuazhong* (77.09) and *Sihuawai* (77.14) with pricking method to induce bleeding will bring a fairly good effect too. *Neiguan* (PC 6) and *Zusanli* (ST 36) also work well. For severe condition, pricking method should be applied.

7) Myocarditis

a. *Xinmen* (33.12).
b. *Tongguan* (88.01), *Tongshan* (88.02) and *Tongtian* (88.03).
c. Prick ear apex.
d. Prick *Sihuazhong* (77.09) and *Sihuawai* (77.14) to induce bleeding.

It is not rare to see myocarditis; especially many youth suffer from myocarditis, manifested in stuffy chest, unsmooth breath, or even arrhythmia. After enquiry, we know that those patients have common cold before myocarditis occurring. Many patients' myocarditis can be considered as after effect of common cold. Heart is injured, though the common cold cured, the after effect remains: stuffy chest or unsmooth breath or arrhythmia. On considering herbal medicine, combined formulas of *Sheng Mai San* and *Zhi Gan Cao Tang* is very good. It is very effective to puncture *Xinmen* (33.12). Combination of *Neiguan* (PC 6) and *Zusanli* (ST 36) is very good too.

2. Liver and Gallbladder Diseases

1) Hepatocirrhosis

a. Prick *Sihuazhong* (77.09) and *Sihuawai* (77.14) to induce bleeding, and then puncture *Minghuang* (88.12), *Qihuang* (88.14), and *Tianhuang* (88.13).
b. Prick *Shangqu* (44.16) to induce bleeding, and then puncture *Ganmen* (33.11) and *Minghuang* (88.12).

2) Hepatitis

a. *Ganmen* (33.11) and *Minghuang* (88.12) bring a fairly good effect for acute and chronic hepatitis. The therapeutic result will be better if *Changmen* (33.10) is combined.

For acute hepatitis, *Ganmen* (33.11) could be punctured first. Combination of *Ganmen* (33.11) and *Changmen* (33.10) is mainly applied. I've treated many patients with hepatitis. Some patients only have herbal treatment without needles; some patients only have acupuncture treatment without medicine; some receive both medication and acupuncture treatments. The best acupuncture treatment is the combination of *Ganmen* (33.11) and *Changmen* (33.10). Among points from the 14 meridians, *Wangu* (SI 4) is the most frequently used point which is *Yuan*-source point of Small Intestine Meridian. TCM considers that small intestine communicates with spleen. Spleen could resolve dampness; small intestine could also remove dampness, as an official separating clear water from the turbid. Both of them are important points for resolving dampness. Because both *Ganmen* (33.11) and *Changmen* (33.10) are located on the Small Intestine Meridian, the underlying reason of application of those two points is same as the one for application of *Wangu* (SI 4) treating jaundice and hepatitis; next, location of *Ganmen* (33.11) is on the middle of arm which is corresponding to Middle Energizer in arm holography, thus it is very good at treating disorders occurring in the Middle Energizer.

When I was in Taiwan, there is a saying among colleagues that a doctor will not be considered as an internal medical doctor if he can't cure liver and kidney diseases properly. Taiwan is surrounded by the sea in a semitropical area. The climate is very humid and hot which is liable to attack liver and kidney. Meanwhile, Chinese don't pay enough attention to food hygiene and there are too many peddlers; in addition, no disposable chopsticks, thus liver diseases were often seen. Nowadays the public sanitary condition is better. Kidney diseases will be induced if food is too salty. On considering ENT diseases, a doctor is not considered as a good doctor if he is incapable of curing rhinitis. There is a tendency that more and more people are suffering from rhinitis. People who drink more cold water can easily accumulate hidden cold fluid. In winter, the external cold may induce the internal cold fluid which may flare and rise upward resulting in nasal diseases. Modernized people like to eat cold, raw food such as ice cream which is available all year around. Also with air conditioning every where, it is very easy to induce rhinitis by the cold air. This indicates an important reason for the occurrence of allergic rhinitis resulting from stimulation by polluted air to respiratory tract. A gynecological doctor is not considered a good doctor if she does not have the ability to cure infertility. In the neuro-department, a neurologist is not considered good if he is not competent in treating spur.

Many patients I have treated with acute hepatitis by using a very good empirical prescription which my students also have applied to cure many patients. Ingredients include *Yinchen* (Herba Artemisiae Scopariae), *Pugongying* (Herba Taraxaci), *Xiaoji* (Herba Cirsii), *Zelan* (Herba Lycopi), *Yujin* (Radix Curcumae), *Dazao* (Fructus Jujubae), *Cheqianzi* (Semen Plantaginis), *Huashi* (Talcum), *Gancao* (Redix Glycyrrhizae), *Danshen* (Radix Salviae Miltiorrhizae) and other herbs. Although not so many herbs are included but extremely good results has been achieved. Many patients were cured by using this prescription. Some patients' GOT and GPT mounts to thousand units, but test results show a drop of 300 or 400 in one week with the help of this prescription. Dosage of the prescription: *Yinchen* (Herba Artemisiae Scopariae) 40g to 50g, *Pugongying* (Herba Taraxaci) 15g to 25g, *Xiaoji* (Herba Cirsii) 15g, *Zelan* (Herba Lycopi) 15g, *Yujin* (Radix Curcumae) 15g, *Dazao* (Fructus Jujubae) 4 pieces, *Cheqianzi* (Semen Plantaginis) 25g, *Huashi* (Talcum) 15g, *Gancao* (Redix Glycyrrhizae) 5g, *Danshen* (Radix Salviae Miltiorrhizae) 15g. After one week use of decoction, the index will drop from one thousand to about 300; at least 500 degree could be dropped. With two weeks treatment, the index will reach 200 or within 100. Most patients' index will drop within 100 with about two weeks' of treatment. About three weeks, it will drop to about 30, which is almost normal. Essentials from the *Jin Gui Yao Lue* (Golden Cabinet) says jaundice will be cured within two to three weeks' treatments if it is appropriate; but if the pathological condition became worse after 10 days' treatments, it will be difficult to cure the disease since the pathogen is predominant but anti pathogen is weak, such as fulminant hepatitis.

Without knowing other puncturing methods, it will take about 3 weeks to cure acute hepatitis completely by applying *Ganmen* (33.11) and *Changmen* (33.10). About acupoints from the fourteen meridians system, for acute hepatitis, *Wangu* (SI 4) and *Zhiyang* (DU 9) mainly applied; for chronic hepatitis, *Ganmen* (33.11) is added; possibly add *Minghuang* (88.12), *Qihuang* (88.14), and *Tianhuang* (88.13). It is fairly difficult to treat hepacirrhosis, try to prick *Sihuazhong* (77.09) and *Sihuawai* (77.14) to induce bleeding, add *Minghuang* (88.12), *Qihuang* (88.14), and *Tianhuang* (88.13) or *Mudou* (66.07) and *Muliu* (66.06).

3) Cholecystitis

a. *Huozhi* (88.15), *Huoquan* (88.16) and *Qihuang* (88.14).
b. *Muzhi* (1010.18).
c. *Qili* (A.01) and *Jiuli* (88.25, 88.26, 88.27).
d. Hand-*Menjin* (66.05).

Cholecystitis can be easily developed nowadays because people are fond of delicious food. The gallbladder colic pain may radiate to the back when acute cholecystitis attacks. Several groups of points could be applied for this symptom. First one includes *Qili* (A.01) and *Jiuli* (88.25, 88.26, 88.27) with point coupling technique and it brings good therapeutic effect for cholecystitis and biliary colic. *Huozhi* (88.15) and *Huoquan* (88.16) on the leg, combining with *Qihuang* (88.14) can also treat cholecystitis. In addition, *Muzhi* (1010.18) on the face is a commonly used point for cholecystitis. Among acupoints from the fourteen meridian system, tenderness may be felt on pressing the point *Dannangxue* (Extra Point) below *Yanglingquan* (GB 34) when cholecystitis attacks, then puncture the tender point. Xiabai (22.07) mentioned previously is also a very good point for cholecystitis and gallbladder colic pain.

For treating cholecystitis, same as Master Tung, I also use *huozhi* (88.15), *Qihuang* (88.14) and *Huoquan* (88.16) or *Muzhi* (1010.18). Meanwhile, I discovered *Qili* (A.01) and *Jiuli* (88.25, 88.26, 88.27) or Hand-*Menjin* (66.05). With regard to herbal formulation, commonly used is *Da Chai hu Tang* (Major Bupleurum Decoction) modification.

4) Cholilithiasis

a. *Muzhi* (1010.18) with special effect.
b. It will bring a better effect if *Xiabai* (22.07) or *Jiuli* (88.25, 88.26, 88.27) is added.

The most commonly used point for pain induced by gallbladder stone is *Muzhi* (1010.18). Other points are also effective, such as *Qili* (A.01), *Jiuli* (88.25, 88.26, 88.27), *Xiabai* (22.07) and *Dannangxue* (Extra). *Da Chai Hu Tang* (Major Bupleurum Decoction) plus *Jinqiancao* (Herba

LySimachiae), *Jineijin* (Endothelium Corneum Gigeriae Galli) and *Yujin* (Radix Curcumae) are also good.

3. Pulmonary Diseases

1) Pulmonary Emphysema (distention and stuffy sensation in the lung area)

a. Pricking *Sihuazhong* (77.09) and *Sihuawai* (77.14) to induce bleeding is effective.

2) Pneumonia

a. *Chongzi* (22.01) and *Chongxian* (22.02).
b. *Dabai* (22.04) with pricking method.
c. *Quling* (33.16) with pricking method.
d. *Tushui* (22.11).

3) Bronchitis (cough)

a. *Shuijin* (1010.20) and *Shuitong* (1010.19) have special effect.

4) Pulmonary Tuberculosis

a. Prick *Sihuazhong* (77.09) and *Sihuawai* (77.14), and then puncture *Sima* (88.17, 88.18, 88.19).

Firstly we will address bronchitis, which takes cough as a chief symptom and can be divided into acute and chronic types. *Shuijin* (1010.20) or *Shuitong* (1010.19) is the best and most often used points for both acute and chronic bronchitis. Generally speaking, *Shuitong* (1010.19) is enough with a technique of oblique insertion upward and subcutaneously. The area where this point is located and the where the needle covers is corresponding to bronchus and the lung according to holography. Upward oblique insertion method is to insert from bronchus to the lung. It is a specially-effective point for treating cough. In addition, *Yangming* Meridians of hand and foot connect with each other at this place. The Large Intestine Meridian of Hand *Yangming* is externally and internally related to the Lung Meridian, thus it can be used to treat lung disorders. Master Tung gave the name of *Shuijin* (1010.20) to this point with a special significance. As we know, the respiration is fulfilled by the cooperation of the lung and kidney. Spleen is the earth which could produce metal. *Jin* means metal, referring to the lung which dominates descending; *Shui* means water, referring to the kidney which dominates reception. If lung fails in descending, it will bring difficult breath; if kidney fails in reception, there will be not enough *Qi*. Respiration is accomplished with a combined effort of the lung in descending and the kidney in reception. The nomination of *Shuijin* (1010.20) is related to respiration. Both *Shuijin* (1010.20) and *Shuitong* (1010.19) can be used for dysfunction of *Qi* activity, including cough, asthma, belching, abdominal distention, profuse urination or unsmooth urination. *Shuitong* (1010.19) could make water metabolism flow smoothly. Regardless of the type of *Qi* disturbance, *Shuijin* (1010.20) or *Shuitong* (1010.19) can help. *Yuji* (LU 10) or *Chize* (LU 5) can be used for cough and asthma.

It will bring a better therapeutic effect for treating cough in the treatment with a puncturing technique following four periods in a day. There are four seasons in a year; four periods in a day. *Huang Di Nei Jing* (Yellow Emperor's Inner Classic) has a statement of puncturing according to four periods in a day. The principle of acupuncture according to four seasons is to puncture *Ying*-spring points in spring, *Shu*-stream points in summer, *He*-sea points in autumn, and *Jing*-well points in winter. According to four periods in a day, it is to puncture *Ying*-spring points in the morning because morning is like spring, *Shu*-stream points at noon because noon is like summer, *He*-sea points in afternoon and evening because they are like autumn, *Jing*-well points at night because night is like winter. In short, puncture *Ying*-spring points in the morning, *Shu*-stream points at noon, *He*-sea points in the evening, and *Jing*-well points at night. But almost there is no one requiring acupuncture treatment at night. Patients are most probable to come before or after noon during day time. For treating cough, *Yuji* (LU 10) is punctured if patients come in morning; if they visit in the afternoon, add *Chize* (LU 5). It is very effective for treating cough and asthmatic breath with *Shuitong* (1010.19) and *Chize* (LU 5). Because *Chize* (LU 5) is the *He*-sea point of lung meridian and *He*-sea points can relieve rebellious *qi*, thus, *Chize* (LU 5) with a very good effect can be used for treating lung rebellious *qi* causing cough. *Chize* (LU 5) is a water point of the lung meridian so that it can be applied for both lung and kidney diseases, which is another reason why *Chize* (LU 5) can achieve a very good effect for cough.

I explained the treatment relationship between cough and the five *shu* points, and *Chize* (LU 5) could be applied for both lung and kidney. Chronic cough may influence lower Energizer resulting in kidney deficiency, on considering this, lung metal and kidney water are both involved. Thus *Chize* (LU 5) as *He*-sea point of lung meridian can be punctured because the *He*-sea points can relieve rebellious *qi*. There is rebellious *qi* in each meridian. Rebellious *qi* in the lung meridian manifests in cough. Rebellious *qi* in the spleen meridian manifests in belching and diarrhea. Rebellious *qi* in the liver meridian is hypertension due to hyperactivity of liver yang. In stomach meridian, rebellious *qi* manifests in vomit. *He*-sea points of each meridian can be applied for their own rebellious *qi*. Regardless in what type of pathological condition, so long as it is rebellious *qi* in the lung meridian, *Shuijin* (1010.20) or *Shuitong* (1010.19) and *Chize* (LU 5) will bring an effect. If patient only has a cough, *Shuijin* (1010.20) or *Shuitong* (1010.19) and *Chize* (LU 5) are more than enough; one more point could be added by puncturing according to four periods in a day. All those have been explained clearly in my books, entitled "*Zhen Jiu Jing Wei* (Strategy of Acupuncture)" and "*Zhen Jiu Wu Shu Xue* (Five Shu Points in Acupuncture)." If points are punctured based on considering time the therapeutic effect will be better and quicker.

For treating intercostal pain, puncture *Yanglingquan* (GB 34) and if time is considered when this point is punctured, the therapeutic effect will be better and quicker. *Yanglingquan* (GB 34) is a *He*-sea point which should be applied in autumn or evening from 3:00 pm to 9:00 pm, then a better effect would occur. Same as treating cough *Yuji* (LU 10) is added in the morning, *Taiyuan* (LU 9) added at noon, *Shaoshang* (LU 11) with pricking method at night, *Chize* (LU 5) better applied at 3:00 pm to 9:00 pm. But if time is not under consideration, *Shuijin* (1010.20) or *Shuitong* (1010.19), combining with *Chize* (LU 5) will suffice.

Acute bronchitis could be treated by the method mentioned above. For chronic bronchitis, patients may have symptoms of kidney deficiency due to coughing for a long time. Patients with chronic bronchitis are more middle aged or older. Symptoms start in late autumn and last until next spring. The kidney should be nourished because of the deficient condition. Both *Shuijin* (1010.20) and *Shuitong* (1010.19) can nourish the kidney. If *Shenguan/Tianhuangfu* (77.18) is added, it will be better. *Shen* means kidney. From the name of this point, we could see that it can nourish kidney. It also nourishes the spleen because the point is located on the spleen meridian. So *Shenguan/Tianhuangfu* (77.18) can nourish both kidney and spleen. Spleen earth produces lung metal. On considering this, *Shenguan/Tianhuangfu* (77.18) brings a very positive effect because it can treat not only earth, but also metal and water.

There are *Ganjiang* (Rhizoma Zingiberis) and *Wuweizi* (Fructus Schisandrae) in *Xiao Qing Long Tang* formula. *Ganjiang* (Rhizoma Zingiberis), with a pungent flavor, has the function of nourishing spleen. *Wuweizi* (Fructus Schisandrae), with an astringent property, it has the function of nourishing kidney. One herb is pungent, the other is astringent; treating both the spleen and kidney, which is also a very important treatment principle for cough. For treating chronic bronchitis, *Shenguan/Tianhuangfu* (77.18) is added which can nourish both kidney and spleen. At the beginning of *Qi* deficiency, it is a very good idea to add *Linggu* (22.05) which has a strong function to nourish *Qi*. Not long ago, I read a book published in mainland China about single point application. It is said in this book that *Hegu* (LI 4) only has reducing function while not reinforcing which I find is a very strange concept. According to my experience, *Linggu* (22.05) has a very strong function of nourishing *Qi* and kidney.

5) Asthmatic Breathing

a. *Shuijin* (1010.20) and *Shuitong* (1010.19) with special effect.
b. *Chongzi* (22.01) and *Chongxian* (22.02) with good effect.
c. *Tushui* (22.11) with special effect.
d. Pricking *Sihuazhong* (77.09) and *Sihuawai* (77.14) achieving special effect.
e. Pricking *Dabai* (22.04) to induce bleeding is effective.
f. Pricking *Quling* (33.16) to induce bleeding achieves good effect.

Asthmatic breath is a very commonly seen disorder. I've treated more than 10 patients with asthmatic breath. Many patients with severe pathological conditions were cured. They are very fortunate. If patients with asthmatic breath don't receive proper treatment, there will be a risk of death. *Shuijin* (1010.20) or *Shuitong* (1010.19) are the main points for treating asthmatic breath. *Chize* (LU 5) is a good point too, especially for chronic ones. When asthma occurs, *Tushui* (22.11) should be punctured which equals to *Yuji* (LU 10), treating earth, metal and water simultaneously. It is a good point to stop asthmatic breathing. For some patients, the asthmatic breathing will be stopped right after this point is punctured.

I'd like to share a real story of mine treating a patient with asthmatic breathing. Seven years ago I was in Taipei. I lived on the eighth floor while my clinic was on the third floor. One night, I went out for dinner, and when I returned, I met my neighbor and his son who was very pale with asthmatic breath. He had great difficulty in breathing. The father asked me whether I could treat this disease or not. I brought them to my clinic on the third floor and gave the son an immediate treatment. I punctured *Yuji* (LU 10) because this point can stop asthmatic breath immediately; if not, *Neiguan* (PC 6) should be added. I punctured *Yuji* (LU 10) bilaterally. The asthmatic breathing stopped immediately, but I still punctured *Neiguan* (PC 6) on one side and left in the needles in there for 30 minutes. One month later, this neighbor came for a visit and presented me with a gift, telling me that his son passed examinations for the best high school. He appreciated my help tremendously. His son had a history of asthma but had not had an attack for many years. The day when he had the attack, he was working very hard for the next day's examination. The asthma attacked him because of the stress and tension in working hard. If I hadn't given him the immediate treatment, he would have been sent to hospital for rescue, thus he could not pass the examination next day successfully. Then I forgot this event, but after three years, the father came with flowers to show his appreciation again and told me that his son passed exams for the best university. If three years ago, he failed to study in the best high school, he would not be allowed to study in the best university then. He was very grateful. *Yuji* (LU 10) which is the middle *Tushui* (22.11) changed the boy's fate. Such university entrance examination is only held once a year. If students failed in this year, it will be more difficult in the next year, that's why they were so grateful.

It is a very good first aid method to help asthmatic breathing by acupuncture. For chronic condition *Yuji* (LU 10) should be punctured first. When there is no attack, puncture *Shuitong* (1010.19) or *Chize* (LU 5) which will achieve a very good effect too. But if the therapeutic effect expected, needs to be improved and obtained quicker, bleed *Chize* (LU 5). This is the best method which could eliminate underlying causes. Pricking *Sihuazhong* (77.09) and *Sihuawai* (77.14) to induce bleeding will produce the same function. Those two groups of points could be applied alternatively. Furthermore, bleeding some points on the back related to the lung meridian can achieve a good result as well. If it is too difficult to prick points on hands or feet due to fright or unskillful technique or failure of holding vein, select points on the back instead; if not enough blood is induced, put cups over those points to draw out more blood. The following points are frequently used: *Dazhui* (DU 14), *Feishu* (BL 13), *Fengmen* (BL 12) and *Gaohuang* (BL 43). In China, there is a physician named Wang Xiu Zhen who brought good effect to patients with asthmatic breath by pricking *Taiyang* (Extra) to induce bleeding. The quantity of bleeding in the point is fairly large. Without acupuncture, but with bleeding method once every two weeks, asthmatic breath would be cured.

Shuitong (1010.19) and *Chize* (LU 5) are very good for treating asthmatic breath with acupuncture technique; if *Yuji* (LU 10) added with bleeding technique once every 10 days, the patient could be cured completely after several months of treatment.

Here is another example of a successful case of treating asthmatic breathing. The patient had been treated for many years and was often sent to the emergency department. He was easily attacked with asthmatic breath. He was recommended to visit me. I applied those commonly used points for him as well: *Shuitong* (1010.19), *Yuji* (LU 10) and *Chize* (LU 5). Sometimes I bled *Chize* (LU 5), sometimes *Sihuazhong* (77.09) and *Sihuawai* (77.14). This patient visited me often in winter when he had attacks.

In the TCM field, there is a principle of treatment which is to treat winter diseases in summer, i.e., it is easy to cure diseases in summer which tend to attack in winter. It is difficult to treat those winter diseases during cold days because the attack is easily induced and aggravated at that time. In winter, the patients had to use western medical inhalers several times a day. Anyway, these patients do not require the inhaler after several treatments and the patient had no recurring attacks again for many years, even in winter.

There were altogether five patients who were sent to the emergency room including the previous mentioned patient. After several years, others died, except him. He was still alive because he relied on TCM treatment. After treatments when he was sure that the disease would not attack him again, he went back to the original western doctor and telling them: you said it is very difficult to cure asthma, but now look at me, I am completely cured. He was eating ice cream when he talked. Of course his eating behavior is improper.

There are many herbs which can cure asthma. *Gejie* (Gekko gecko Linnaeus) is a good medicine for asthmatic breathing. In the thirties of last century, there was a famous physician in Beijing named Shi Jin Mo. In Sichuan province, he was very surprised to see a lot of people pulling or carrying heavy things without shortness of breathe even when they ran, because they had the tail of *Gejie* (Gekko gecko Linnaeus) in their mouth. *Ben Cao Bei Yao* (Essential Preparation of Herbs) has the same saying. Medical function will be improved if *Gejie* (Gekko gecko Linnaeus) prepared into powder or decoction was eaten. Zhu Danxi said *Jiaomu* (Fructus Zanthoxylum bungeanum Maxin) could be applied for asthmatic breathing which achieves a good therapeutic effect. When I treat asthmatic breathing, I differentiate whether it is cold or heat type. According to my experience, the cold type is often seen. Modification of *Xiao Qing Long Tang* formula is most often used.

Treat winter diseases in summer is to treat winter diseases in the hottest period in midsummer which include 30 to 40 days after summer solstice. In those days, *yin Qi* is hidden because of predominant *yang Qi*. That period is the most suitable time to treat diseases of *yin* predominance and *yang* deficiency. The hot weather could help to penetrate the medical function of moxibustion or paste into the root. Points selected include: *Dazhui* (DU14), *Fengmen* (BL 12), *Feishu* (BL 13) and *Gaohuang* (BL 43). Moxibustion could be used first and then herbal paste. Herbal paste consists of *Baijiezi* (Semen Sinapis Albae), *Yanhusuo* (Rhizoma Corydalis), *Gansui* (Radix Kansui, Euphorbia Kansui) and *Xixin* (Manchurian wildginger herb). First, prepare into granulated powder and mix them with *Shexiang* (Musk) or without. Use ginger juice to make the paste, fix the paste on the points with tape until skin becomes red or even blisters induced to enhance the function of expelling cold and resolving phlegm. Remove it after 4 to 6 hours. If the red skin lasted for several days or 2 to 3 weeks, the therapeutic effect would be better. If blisters were induced, put some anti inflammation ointment to avoid infection. Many patients will not suffer from asthma in the coming winter after such treatment. Many patients with chronic bronchitis and asthma will never have such diseases attacking for the rest of their life if they could have continuous treatments for 1 to 3 years. The effective rate is higher than 90%. With the help of herbal paste, many patients' body constitution obviously improved and it reduces the risk of them to catch cold easily, thus this method has the function to strengthen body constitution too.

4. Spleen and Stomach Diseases

1) Stomach Diseases

a. Pricking *Sihuazhong* (77.09) and *Sihuawai* (77.14) to induce bleeding has special effect.
b. Pricking *Sihuashang* (77.08) to induce bleeding has fairly good effect.
c. Pricking *Tongguan* (88.01) and *Tongshan* (88.02) to induce bleeding and then puncturing them has fairly good effect.

2) Stomach Ulceration

a. Pricking *Sihuazhong* (77.09) and *Sihuawai* (77.14) has special effect.
b. Pricking veins from *Jiexi* (ST 41) to *Menjin* (66.05) has good effect.

3) Acute Stomachache

a. Pricking *Sihuashang* (77.08) or *Sihuazhong* (77.09) has special effect, combination of two points brings a better effect.
b. *Tushui* (22.11).

4) Duodenum Ulceration

a. Pricking *Sihuazhong* (77.09) and *Sihuawai* (77.14) has special effect.
b. Pricking veins from *Jiexi* (ST 41) to *Menjin* (66.05) has good effect.

For treating acute stomachache, *Sihuazhong* (77.09) with pricking method could stop the pain immediately. Last year when I was giving a lecture in Los Angles, there was a student who had severe stomachache. It was so severe that even his asthma was induced. If it were simple the stomachache by puncturing *Liangqiu* (ST 34) would stop the pain because *Liangqiu* (ST 34) is the *Xi*-cleft point of stomach meridian. *Xi*-cleft points have the function of checking acute pain related to their own meridian. But after puncturing, though his pain reduced, it still remained. He had stomach problems for long time, so I pricked *Sihuashang* (77.08) to induce some bleeding. As soon as a bit blood oozed out, he felt his stomach felt much better. He had no pain as soon as he was pricked. His asthmatic breath was alleviated too. The next week when he came for the lecture again, he said he had no stomachache and the asthma was much better too and he didn't need to use an inhaler or other medicine after.

Some old acupuncturists retained needles longer for *Neiguan* (PC 6) and *Zusanli* (ST 36) which also could treat chronic stomachache and asthmatic breath. Pricking to induce bleeding is a very effective therapeutic method and obtains a quick result. Mild stomach diseases will be cured by acupuncture treatment. If it is still not completely cured, then prick *Sihuazhong* (77.09) and *Sihuashang* (77.08) to induce bleeding, the pain could be stopped immediately. Besides, *Tushui* (22.11) is also a good point for treating stomachache. When there is cold invasion to stomach, there will be a lot of veins visible around *Tushui* (22.11). The acute stomachache I mentioned here includes ulceration in the duodenum and stomach. According to the differentiation, ulceration in duodenum and stomach can be categorized into both the spleen and stomach deficiency and cold, disharmony between liver and stomach, dampness and heat accumulation in the spleen and stomach, stomach *yin* deficiency and *Qi* retention and blood stagnation. But according to clinical experience, the spleen and stomach are mostly involved. Modification of *Huangqi Jianzhong Tang* (Decoction of Astragalus for Tonifying Middle Energizer) is the most often used formula for ulceration occurring in digestive system.

5) Profuse Stomach Acid

a. *Tianhuang* (77.17) and *Shenguan/Tianhuangfu* (77.18).
b. *Tongtian* (88.03) and *Tongwei* (88.10).

Tianhuang (77.17) and *Shenguan/Tianhuangfu* (77.18) may bring fairly good effect for profuse stomach acid. *Tongtian* (88.03) and *Tongwei* (88.10) are good points too. Acid regurgitation has similar symptoms as those of stomachache, but also has reverse flow of stomach acid. *Tianhuang* (77.17) and *Shenguan/Tianhuangfu* (77.18) are also main points for acid regurgitation which may bring good therapeutic effect. About herbal medicine, a lot of people like to use *Wuzeigu* (cuttlefish bone), *Zhebei* (Bulbus Fritillariae), *Walengzi* (Concha Arcae) and other herbs related to the condition. My own experience is to add *Wumei* (Frucus Mume), *Shanzha* (Fructus Crataegi) which are better than *Wuzeigu* (cuttlefish bone), *Zhebei* (Bulbus Fritillariae) and *Walengzi* (Concha Arcae). Because they have the function to astringe and soothe the liver, both treat the branch and root.

6) Vomit

a. Pricking *Zongshu* (1010.07) has special effect.
b. Pricking *Sihuazhong* (77.09) has fairly good effect.
c. Puncturing *Shuijin* (1010.20) and *Shuitong* (1010.19) has effect.

The most effective method is to prick *Zongshu* (1010.07) to induce bleeding. It is also possible to prick *Fengfu* (DU 16) to induce bleeding. If there is apprehension of using three edged needle and a blood extraction needle, a small needle can be replaced, although the quantity of blood induce is small, the vomit could be stopped too. This method is an application of "correspondence between the front and back."

7) Regurgitation

a. Puncture *Tianhuang* (77.17) and *Shenguan/Tianhuangfu* (77.18).
b. Prick *Zongshu* (1010.07) to induce bleeding.

What's regurgitation? Here is an example. Those people who do not exercise will have unsmooth breath, nausea, and even vomit after over exertion in exercises. That's regurgitation. For this problem, bleed *Zongshu* (1010.07) or *Fengfu* (DU 16) which is 0.2 *cun* above the previous point. These two points also can be bled for treating nausea and vomiting. *Sihuazhong* (77.09) with bleeding technique also works for the symptoms.

Among the 14 meridians, the most effective meridian for vomit is the pericardium meridian. There are many points from the pericardium meridian that can be applied for vomiting. The most effective one is *Jianshi* (PC 5). Vomiting is a kind of *Qi* rebellion and vomiting makes a loud sound. *Jianshi* (PC 5) is *Jing*-River point, pertains to metal which is related to voice and *Qi*. This is because *Jing*-River points should be selected for vocal pathological changes. In addition, because the pericardium communicates with the stomach, points on the pericardium meridian can be applied for vomiting, such as *Daling* (PC 7), *Laogong* (PC 8) and *Neiguan* (PC 6). *Fengfu* (DU16) or *Zongshu* (1010.07) can treat vomiting because of the "correspondence between the front and back" (mouth and occiput).

8) Gastritis

a. *Menjin* (66.05).
b. Prick *Sihuashang* (77.08).
c. *Tongguan* (88.01) and *Tongshan* (88.02).

Gastritis is manifested in stomachache and frequent vomiting. *Menjin* (66.05) is often used for those symptoms. There are various kinds of stomach diseases, such as ulceration in duodenum and the stomach. For treating these conditions, Master Tung always used *Sihuazhong* (77.09) with pricking method to induce bleeding, and then puncture *Tongguan* (88.01) and *Tongshan* (88.02). For treating stomach diseases, Master Tung first used pricking method, and then puncturing method.

9) Poor Appetite

a. *Linggu* (22.05).
b. *Sihuashang* (77.08).
c. *Menjin* (66.05).

It brings good effect by puncturing *Linggu* (22.05) for poor appetite. Other fairly good points include *Zusanli* (ST 36) and *Menjin* (66.05). The location of *Sihuashang* (77.08) is same as *Zusanli* (ST 36). For treating ulceration in the duodenum and stomach, Master Tung often pricked the dorsum of the foot to induce bleeding. Prick *Sihuazhong* (77.09), *Sihuawai* (77.14) and the dorsum of the foot where more veins are present.

10) Splenomegaly

a. Puncture *Mudou* (66.07) and *Muliu* (66.06).
b. Prick *Sanchong* (77.07) to induce bleeding.

Mudou (66.07) and *Muliu* (66.06) are good at treating not only splenomegaly but also hepatocirrhosis. *Sanchong* (77.07) also could be applied for splenomegaly. The locations of *Mudou* (66.07) and *Muliu* (66.06) are between the stomach and the gallbladder meridians. They are especially good at treating diseases due to liver and spleen disharmony. If pathological condition is severe, it is better to prick *Sihuazhong* (77.09) and *Sihuawai* (77.14) to induce bleeding.

5. Kidney and Urinary Bladder Diseases

1) Nephritis

a. Puncturing *Tongshen* (88.09), *Tongwei* (88.10) and *Tongbei* (88.11) may bring fairly good effect.
b. Prick *Shuiyu* (44.17) with three edged needle to induce yellow fluid.

2) Edema

a. Puncture *Tongtian* (88.03) for edema leg.
b. Puncture *Tongshen* (88.09), *Tongwei* (88.10) and *Tongbei* (88.11) for treating edema of the face and the entire body.

Acute nephritis is manifested in edema of the face and body. *Tongshen* (88.09), *Tongwei* (88.10) and *Tongbei* (88.11) can be applied for treating acute nephritis. All those points which are on the spleen meridian have the function to nourish both the spleen and kidney. It is in accordance with the principle of nourishing earth to check water. *Tongshen* (88.09), *Tongwei* (88.10) and *Tongbei* (88.11) are the most commonly used points for edema with a very good effect. Those points also could be used for chronic nephritis. In Master Tung's original book, he said not to use those six points at the same time, but according to my experience, it still brings a good effect if those six points punctured at one time. Of course, it is the best that fewer points could bring a better effect. If only the leg is swollen, which is related to heart, puncturing *Tongguan* (88.01) and *Tongshan* (88.02) brings effect. When I treat leg edema, I often combine *Sihuashang* (77.08) and *Tianhuang* (77.17). Such combination plays an extremely good function that the edema could be removed by the promotion of urination. Among points from the 14 meridians, *Zusanli* (ST 36) and *Yinlingquan* (SP 9) are often used to sooth and promote *Qi* in Foot *Yangming* and *Taiyin* Meridians, in order to strengthen the spleen and stomach *Qi* to maintain a normal water metabolism, and this in accordance with nourishing earth to check water, and thus both the spleen and kidney are treated. According to records in ancient lyrics, *Shuifen* (REN9) is the most frequently used point for edema, thus it is better to treat the diseases related to water if *Shuifen* (REN 9) is added. *Sanyinjiao* (SP 6) and *Fuliu* (KI 7) are also for promoting water metabolism. *Shuigou* (DU 26) could be added if there is edema on the face. Edema in acute nephritis is due to a fight between wind and water. *Yuepi Jia Zhu Tang* (Decoction for Strengthening the Spleen to relieve Edema) or modified *Jingfang Baidu San* (Antiphlogistic Powder of Schizonepeta and Ledebouriella) could be applied for acute nephritis. Modification of Formulas of *Zhen Wu Tang* (Decoction for Strengthening the Spleen-yang) and *Fangji Huangqi Tang* (Tetrandra and Astragalus Decoction) is for chronic nephritis more often due to water overflow because of *yang* deficiency.

3) Renal Calculus

a. Puncture *Majinshui* (1010.13).

Majinshui (1010.13) is punctured for both acute and chronic renal calculus. The therapeutic effect will be better if *Makuaishui* (1010.14) added with point coupling technique. *Xiabai* (22.07) is effective in checking colic pain induced by renal calculus. Puncturing *Majinshui* (1010.14) and *Xiabai* (22.07) alongside bone is very effective for treating renal colic pain, because the place where *Majinshui* (1010. 14) is located is corresponding to the kidney; because it is on the Triple Energizer (*San Jiao*) Meridian and the kidney communicates with the triple energizer, that's why *Xiabai* (22.07) can be applied for kidney diseases. Meanwhile *Xiabai* (22.07) is located on the palm at the level of *Linggu* (22.05) and *Wanshun'er* (22.09). According to holography, they all indicate kidney and lumbar diseases. The therapeutic effect will be better if they are punctured alongside the bone for kidney diseases.

4) Cystolithiasis

a. Puncture *Makuaishui* (1010.14).

5) Urethral Calculus

a. Puncture *Liukuai* (1010.16) and *Qikuai* (1010.17).

6) Dysuria

a. *Tianhuang* (77.17) and *Sihuashang* (77.08).
b. *Huozhu* (66.04) and *Huoying* (66.03).

Symptoms of cystolith are similar to those of cystitis and urethritis, including painful urine, dysuria, and radiation pain toward bladder, perineum and both sides of the thigh, accompanied with pale complexion, nausea, vomiting and cold sweat. Puncturing *Makuaishui* (1010.14) and *Majinshui* (1010.13) is effective. If the symptoms of cystolith include urgent, frequent and painful urination with gravels, puncture *Liukuai* (1010.16) and *Qikuai* (1010.17). Besides, *Xingjian* (LR 2) and *Taichong* (LR 3) can be applied for dysuria, because the liver meridian winds around the external genitalia. The liver meridian is effective for treating painful syndromes in the external genitalia. Because the locations of *Huoying* (66.03) and *Huozhu* (66.04) are near *Xingjian* (LR 2) and *Taichong* (LR 4) and also on the liver meridian, those two points have the therapeutic effect as well. For treating dysuria due to senile prostate gland enlargement, puncturing *Tianhuang* (77.17) – *Yinlingquan* (SP 9) and *Sihuashang* (77.08) – *Zusanli* (ST 36) will bring a best effect. It will be better if *Huozhu* (66.04) (puncture alongside bone) added. *Yinlingquan* (SP 9) is a water point in the spleen meridian which pertains to earth, having the function of nourishing both the spleen and kidney. *Zusanli* (ST 36) is genuine earth on the earth meridian, having a very good function of nourishing *Qi*. Both of them are *He*-Sea points, strong in regulating *Qi*. *Huozhu* (66.04), on the liver meridian, has a soothing function; if this point is punctured alongside the bone, the kidney can be treated. Most of the patients with prostate gland enlargement are result of kidney *Qi* deficiency. Those points are very effective. TCM classifies dysuria into *Lin* Syndrome, which can be varied as five types according to different symptoms: *Qi Lin*, Milky *Lin*, Gravel *Lin*, Blood *Lin* and Heat *Lin*. The first type is *Qi Lin* referring to dysuria due to *Qi* deficiency, such as prostate gland enlargement. The second type is Milky *Lin* manifested in greasy urine which is chyluria. The third type is Gravel *Lin* referring to symptoms due to stones in the urinary system, manifested in sand or gravel within urine. The fourth type is Blood *Lin*, manifested in bloody urine, such as pyelonephritis. The fifth type is Heat *Lin*, referring to cystitis, urethritis or infection in urinary system. It is agreed *Qihai* (REN 6) is the key point for the five *Lin* syndromes in *Xi Hong Fu* (Ode of Xi Hong), *Bai Zheng Fu* (Ode of One Hundred Symptoms) and *Ling Guang Fu* (Ode of Spiritual Brightness). Thus *Qihai* (REN 6) is the best point for dysuria due to various kinds of reasons. *Xingjian* (LR 2) and *Taichong* (LR 3) are also good points for *Lin* syndromes. *Huozhu* (66.04) and

Huoying (66.03) bring good effect for *Lin* syndromes as well. The treatment principle for urinary stones is to resolve dampness and clear heat; the prescription is modified *Zhu Ling Tang* (Umbellate Pore Decoction). Senile patients with stones in the urinary system are more often due to kidney *Qi* deficiency, and can be treated by following the principle of nourishing kidney and *Qi* to promote urination. For such a condition, I always apply modified *Shenqi Wan* (Bolus for Tonifying the Kidney-*qi*) with which I have cured many senile patients suffering from urinary stones. TCM thinks *Niuxi* (Radix Achyranthis Bidentatae) is a key herb for various kinds of *Lin* syndromes. Three Jins, *Jinqiancao* (Herba LySimachiae), *Haijinsha* (Spora Lygodii) and *Jineijin* (Endothelium Corneum Gigeriae Galli), bring the best effect on expelling stones.

6. Large Intestine and Small Intestine Diseases

1) Acute Enteritis

a. Puncturing *Menjin* (66.05) has special effect.
b. Puncturing *Changmen* (33.10).
c. Pricking *Sihuazhong* (77.09) and *Sihuawai* (77.14) has special effect.

Acute enteritis is acute diarrhea. Puncturing *Menjin* (66.05) brings the best effect. The next effective point is *Changmen* (33.10). Besides, *Quchi* (LI 11) is very effective too. Why that *Menjin* (66.05) can be applied for acute diarrhea? It is because *Menjin* (66.05) is on the Stomach Meridian of Foot *Yangming* which communicates with the hand *yangming* meridian, thus it can be applied for diseases of the large intestine, such as diarrhea. *Jin* means metal which refers to lung. Lung and large intestine are internally and externally related, this is another reason. In Master Tung's acupuncture, both *Zuqianjin* (77.24) and *Zuwujin* (77.25) can be applied for diseases in the lung and large intestine, and disorders in the throat system, such as tonsillitis and sore throat. *Shouqianjin* (33.09) and *Shouwujin* (33.08) can regulate the lung to nourish *Qi* and treat sciatic neuralgia because they are related to *jin* which means metal. *Menjin* (66.05) can be applied for both the stomach and large intestine diseases. Location of *Menjin* (66.05) is the same as that of *Xiangu* (ST 43) recorded in ancient classics. Modern location of *Xiangu* (ST 43) is a bit anterior to *Menjin* (66.05). Ancient location of *Xiangu* (ST 43) was slightly posterior and alongside the bone, according to my book *Zhen Jiu Jing Wei* (Strategy of Acupuncture). As a wood point of stomach meridian, *Xiangu* (ST 43) has the function of soothing the liver, regulating *Qi* and strengthening the spleen, regulating and harmonizing the liver and spleen. It brings great effect for painful diarrhea. *Menjin* (66.05) could be applied for both acute and chronic diarrhea; it brings better effect if *Quchi* (LI 11) is added. *Quchi* (LI 11) is *He*-Sea point of the large intestine meridian. *He*-Sea points indicate diarrhea due to *Qi* rebellion. For severe condition, bleeding

Sihuazhong (77.09) and *Sihuawai* (77.14) achieves a very good effect. If bowel movement is urgent but there is no toilet available, pinch *Changmen* (33.10) which could reduce the urgent sensation and then take time to look for a toilet. The formula for acute enteritis is *Gegen Qin Lian Tang* (Decoction of Pueraria, Scutellaria and Coptis) which may achieve good effect.

2) Chronic Enteritis

a. Puncturing *Menjin* (66.05) achieves special effect.
b. *Changmen* (33.10) and *Zuqianjin* (77.24).
c. *Yinlingquan* (SP 9) and *Quchi* (LI 11).

Menjin (66.05) is also effective for chronic enteritis; next point is *Changmen* (33.10) and *Zuqianjin* (77.24). Location of *Zuqianjin* (77.24) is between the stomach and gallbladder meridians, therefore they can treat both wood and earth diseases and regulate the disharmony between wood and earth. Master Tung thought they also could regulate the lung and large intestine on considering the names which contains *Jin*-metal. Because this point locates between wood and earth meridians, it can function on both wood and earth meridians. If the five *shu* points are grasped and applied in this manor, it will bring fairly good effect. Among points from the fourteen meridians, *Yinlingquan* (SP 9) is most often used for chronic diarrhea, if *Quchi* (LI 11) is added, the therapeutic effect will be better. At the beginning of this year, I've treated two patients who suffered from chronic diarrhea. One grandmother started to have diarrhea every morning as soon as she got up, and several times during the day. Such pathological condition lasted for about five months. Thus *Menjin* (66.05) and *Quchi* (LI 11) were selected, plus four days' of decoction, afterward, she was normal again. Altogether, this patient had seven days' of decoction and her chronic diarrhea was cured completely. The formula used for her is the combination of *Sishen Wan* (Pill of Four Miraculous Drugs) and *Lizhong Tang* (Decoction for Regulating the Function of Middle-energizer). Ingredients of *Sishen Wan* (Pill of Four Miraculous Drugs) include: *Wuweizi* (Fructus Schisandrae), *Wuzhuyu* (Fructus Evodiae), *Roudoukou* (Semen Myristicae), *Buguzhi* (Fructus Psoraleae), which are good at treating morning diarrhea due to kidney yang deficiency. This grandmother also had asthma but I didn't add other special medicine for it, because *Lizhong Tang* (Decoction for Regulating the Function of Middle-energizer) is for spleen *yang* deficiency and *Sishen Wan* (Pill of Four Miraculous Drugs) is for kidney *yang* deficiency. Such prescription also works for asthma. The other patient was a beautiful girl from USA about 23 years old. She had diarrhea 4 to 5 times a day for three years. She took a lot of western medicine and was diagnosed as having colitis. I also used *Quchi* (LI 11) and *Menjin* (66.05). I used *Li Zhong Tong* and *Shenling Baizhu San* (Powder of Ginseng, Poria and Bighead Atractylodes) for her.

After decoction, she felt much more comfortable. With a combination of treatments using needles and herbs, she was cured very quickly. Altogether she visited twice and took ten days of decoction, and then her three years of disease was cured. From these two examples, we can see that either needles or herbal decoction brings very good therapeutic effect for chronic diarrhea. The combination of two methods is even better.

3) Lower Abdominal Distention

a. *Wanshunyi* (22.08) and *Wanshun'er* (22.09).
b. *Menjin* (66.05).
c. *Linggu* (22.05).

The reason for lower abdominal distending pain or uncomfortable sensation in lower abdomen is more often due to *Qi* deficiency in large and small intestines and the lower energizer, thus the treatment principle is to nourish kidney. Uncomfortable feeling in the large and small intestines is often related to kidney *Qi*, thus *Wanshunyi* (22.08) and *Wanshun'er* (22.09) could be punctured, because they are on the small intestine meridian which can be applied for treating small intestine and nourishing the kidney as well. If there is distending pain on both the stomach and lower abdomen, puncture *Menjin* (66.05), *Wanshunyi* (22.08) and *Wanshun'er* (22.09). The combination of those points brings a better effect. *Zhen Jiu Da Cheng* (The Great Compendium of Acupuncture and Moxibustion) says puncturing *Neiting* (ST 44), *Zusanli* (ST 36) and *Sanyinjiao* (SP 6) together is very effective for abdominal distention. But I always use *Xiangu* (ST 43) instead of *Neiting* (ST 44). *Menjin*'s (66.05) function is included in that of *Xiangu* (ST 43) and *Jin* is related to *Qi*, therefore, it can nourish *Qi* and very good at treating stomach distention. *Linggu* (22.05), on the large intestine meridian, is also good at treating lower abdominal distention, regulating *Qi* and blood. According to holography of the second metacarpal bone, *Linggu* (22.05) is corresponding to the lower energizer; if it is punctured along bone, it is corresponding to kidney. Puncturing *Gongsun* (SP 4) brings good effect for lower abdominal pain. If the pain didn't stop well after puncturing *Gongsun* (SP 4), we should think that there might be organic changes.

4) Enterorrhagia

a. Prick *Sihuazhong* (77.09) and *Sihuawai* (77.14) to induce bleeding (blood letting), then puncture *Jiemei* (88.04, 88.05, 88.06).

There are two conditions of enterorrhagia: bleeding before and after a bowel movement. For a common condition, prick *Sihuazhong* (77.09) and *Sihuawai* (77.14) to induce bleeding which may bring an effect. For treating bleeding due to hemorrhoids, it brings the most special effect by bleeding *Weizhong* (BL 40). Formula for enterorrhagia is *Huangtu Tang*

(Decoction of Baked Yellow Earth). The most commonly used formula for stomach hemorrhage is *Sanhuang Xiexin Tang* (Decoction of Three Yellow Drugs to clear Heart Fire). Single herb, such as *Baizi* (Radix Angellicae Dahuricae) or *Sanqi* (Radix Notoginseng) powder is also very effective. Prescriptions for enterorrhagia could be divided into two types: *Huangtu Tang* (Decoction of Baked Yellow Earth) for cold type; *Chixiaodou Danggui San* (Phaseolus Seeds and Chinese Angelica Root Powder) with modification for dampness and heat type. If bleeding often occurs, be cautious that cancer might occur in the large intestine.

5) Hemorrhoids

a. Pricking *Weizhong* (BL 40) to induce bleeding or blood letting method brings special effect.
b. Puncturing *Qimen* (33.01), *Qizheng* (33.03) and *Qijiao* (33.02) is effective.

The best effect for bleeding due to hemorrhoids, ensure that *Weizhong* (BL 40) is bled. It is easy to have hemorrhoids with indulgence in eating spicy food, because pungent and spicy food enters into the lung and large intestine. Too much spicy food may injure the large intestine and produce fire. Furthermore, standing for a long time, sitting or staying up late will lead to hemorrhoids. The best method for treating hemorrhoids is create a large quantity of bleeding which is better than pricking to induce some drops of blood. Puncturing *Qimen* (33.01), *Qizheng* (33.03) and *Qijiao* (33.02) brings effect, because those points are on the large intestine meridian. If it is possible to apply bleeding technique, it will be better. For common acupuncturist, *Shangqiu* (SP 5) is most frequently used. In addition, some people may puncture *Erbai* (Extra) which is one *cun* proximal to *Jianshi* (PC 5). All those points are good but not as effective as *Weizhong* (BL 40) with the blood letting technique. Blood letting technique is good for both internal and external hemorrhoids. It is very effective to bleed *Chengshan* (BL 57), that is it brings good effect when veins were pricked at the region from *Weizhong* (BL 40) to *Chengshan* (BL 57). For internal hemorrhoids, bleed the place around *Yinlingquan* (SP 9). Veins around *Lougu* (SP 7) and *Diji* (SP 8) could be bled. In the past, there was printed information that hemorrhoids can be cured without an operation and asking days to leave in Master Tung's business card. At the beginning, I was very curious what kind of special secret remedy he had. After I learned from Master Tung, I know that this secret remedy is blood-letting. Some patients with hemorrhoids may have a second attack after a period of time if they still indulge in taking spicy and pungent food, and then bleeding *Weizhong* (BL 40) still brings the effect.

In January of this year (2003) according to the moon calendar, there was a young man visiting, complaining of severe pain. It was so painful that he couldn't sit straight but deviated. I bled the veins from *Weizhong*

(BL 40) to *Chengshan* (BL 57) and also veins on the medial aspect around *Yinlingquan* (SP 9). Several days later, this young man visited me again with a friend. He was happy at the second visit. He didn't have pain when he sat straight down. For him, I only used the bleeding technique and his pain caused by hemorrhoids was completely cured. Though sometimes hemorrhoids were very severe, it could still be cured by acupuncture without taking medicine. Bleeding technique brings the most special effect. But if herbs could be used simultaneously, it will speed up the process to cure the patients.

For treating hemorrhoids, a Chinese herbal formula that Japanese always use is *Yi Zi Tang* (Decoction for Hemorrhoids). The simple prescription I often use for hemorrhoids include: *Jinyinhua* (Flos Lonicerae) 15g, *Gancao* (Redix Glycyrrhizae) 5g, *Xiakucao* (Spica Prunellae) 15g; for treating hemorrhoids bleeding, *Diyutan* (Carbonic Radix Sanguisorbae) and *Huaihuatan* (Carbonic Flos Sophorae) could stop bleeding. *Huangqin* (Radix Scutellariae) is also good at stopping bleeding. For treating bleeding, usually carbonic herbs are applied. I always apply *Sanhuang Xiexin Tang* (Decoction of Three Yellow Drugs to clear Heart Fire) formula to treat bleeding due to heat invasion. There is *Huangqin* (Radix Scutellariae) in it to stop bleeding. Patients with hemorrhoids could be treated with bleeding technique or using an herbal formula. In addition, there are always blisters around *Yinjiao* (DU 28) in patients with hemorrhoids. So, it is also an effective method to treat hemorrhoids if blisters are pricked. Hemorrhoids can be considered as phlebangioma in the rectum. Bleeding *Weizhong* (BL 40) is a method to promote blood circulation to resolve stagnation. The bladder meridian doesn't reach the rectum, but its divergent meridian reaches the anus. It is suitable to bleed *Weizhong* (BL 40) once a week. Once or twice, treatments may cure a mild condition. Three or four treatments may cure a severe condition.

6) Hernia

a. Prick the area from medial malleolus to *Sanyinjiao* (SP 6) to induce bleeding.
b. Puncture any 2-3 points from *Dajian* (11.01), *Xiaojian* (11.02), *Waijian* (11.04), *Zhongjian* (11.05) and *Fujian* (11.03).

Nowadays there are not so many people suffering from hernia. Hernia is more often due to both *Qi* and blood deficiency and malnutrition. Sometimes it is because of standing for a long time or forceful speaking, such as teachers giving instructions or children's excessive crying. I often use *Bu zhong Yi qi Tang* (Decoction for Reinforcing Middle-energizer and Replenishing *Qi*) plus herbs with function of warming the liver, such as *Xiaohuixiang* (Fructus Foeniculi), *Lizhihe* (Semen Litchi) to warm the liver and plus *Yanhusuo* (Rhizoma Corydalis) and *Wuyao* (Radix

Linderae) to sooth liver *Qi*. Such treatment brought fairly good effect. Many patients were cured.

More than thirty years ago, when I studied in the university, my teacher's son had a hernia. He asked me how to treat him. It was summer when litchi is in abundance. So I told him to eat more litchis, because it was unnecessary to give treatment yet. Litchi can warm the liver to expel cold. If he couldn't be cured by eating litchis, then treatment would be necessary. After summer vocation, I asked the teacher about his son and I was told that his son was cured. For treating hernia, Master Tung always prick veins from the medial malleolus to *Sanyinjiao* (SP 6) to induce bleeding. Regarding acupuncture treatment, select 2-3 points among *Dajian* (11.01), *Xiaojian* (11.02), *Waijian* (11.04), *Zhongjian* (11.05) and *Fujian* (11.03). TCM considers that liver meridian curves around external genitalia, meanwhile the liver dominates tendons. *Dajian* (11.01), *Xiaojian* (11.02), *Waijian* (11.04), *Zhongjian* (11.05) and *Fujian* (11.03) are on the index finger beside the large intestine meridian. Large intestine communicates with liver, so that they can be applied for intestinal hernia. About points from the fourteen meridians, *Dadun* (LR 1) and *Sanyinjiao* (SP 6) can be applied. *Dadun* (LR 1), *Jing*-well point of liver meridian, can open the orifice to expel cold. *Sanyinjiao* (SP 6) can warm the liver and nourish spleen *Qi* to strengthen the ascending function, because hernia is a cold disease and a tendon disease. Liver is related to the tendons, thus the wood point of the wood meridian – *Dadun* (LR 1) can be applied. *Dadun* (LR 1) is not only a *Jing*-well point of the liver meridian but also a wood point on wood meridian with the function of soothing the liver, regulating *Qi*, promoting the meridian and expelling cold. At this point, I'd like to briefly explain the five *shu* points.

The application of the five *shu* points, according to *Nan Jing* (The Classic of Difficulties): *Jing*-well points are indicate in fullness sensation in the gastric region, *Ying*-spring points are indicate of fever; *Shu*-stream points are indicate in heaviness sensation in the body and painful joints; *Jing*-river points are indicate of cough, asthmatic breath, chills and fever; *He*-sea points are indicate of rebellion of *Qi*. Chapter 44 of *Ling Shu* (Spiritual Pivot) says *Jing*-well points apply for mental symptoms; *Ying*-spring points applied when the disease manifested on the complexion; *Shu*-stream points should be punctured when the disease is alleviated and aggravated now and then; when the disease is manifested in abnormal voice and when the collateral is full with stagnated blood, *Jing*-river points should be punctured; for stomach diseases and diseases caused by intemperance of food and drink, *He*-sea points should be punctured. Bleed 12 *Jing*-well points for acute mental disorders. For example: when patients with wind stroke have mental symptoms, it will bring effect if the *Jing*-well point is pricked to induce bleeding. The wind pathogen for wind stroke is related to wood. Flare up of phlegm fire may cause wind stroke, resulting in hemiplegia or coma, *Muhuo* (11.10) could be selected. All *yang* meridians of hand and foot run to the head. Among *yin* meridians, only the pericardium and liver meridians reach the head. Liver meridian reaches the head through throat and inside the brain, thus diseases in the head and mental disorders will be induced if there is hyperactivity of liver *yang* and liver fire. Phlegm, fire and liver wind are the major pathogens for wind stroke. For treating hemiplegia, Master Tung first used *Muhuo* (11.10) because it is on the pericardium meridian which has fairly good effect in treating unconsciousness. Besides, unconsciousness could be induced by phlegm blocking heart and heat due to febrile disease attacking the pericardium; mental disorders could be induced by up flaring of liver fire. *Muhuo* (11.10), on the pericardium meridian, could be applied for pathological condition in the pericardium meridian. On considering this, pathological conditions on the liver meridian could be treated by *Muhuo* (11.10), because they are bearing the same name. Location of *Muhuo* (11.10) is near to *Zhongchong* (PC 9) – *Jing*-well point of pericardium. *Zhongchong* (PC 9) is a key point for mental diseases, derives the reason for the name of *Muhuo* (11.10). This example draws our attention to the application of the theory of five elements. If the theory of five elements could be understood fully, the application of the five *shu* points will be well done.

Application of the five *shu* points is based upon the theory of the five elements. The core of the therapeutic application of the five *shu* points is to search the *Qi* of the same category, i.e., inter-crossing, counteracting, inter-promoting, inter-corresponding, inter-communicating and genuine five elements theory. Both *Nei Jing* (Yellow Emperor's Inner Classic) and *Nan Jing* (The Classic of Difficulties) emphasize on the Therapy of Searching the *Qi* of the same category. For example, *Dadun* (LR 1) is wood point on wood meridian. This is so called genuine five elements. It is the wood point of the wood meridian so it has a very good function of soothing liver. *Jing*-well points could open the orifice to expel cold, thus it is a special point for hernia, and for impotence as well. For treating most of the patients with impotence, *Sanyinjiao* (SP 6) is usually punctured. *Sanyinjiao* (SP 6) is a special point for disorders occurring on the lower abdomen. About *Dadun* (LR 1), liver meridian curves around external genitalia and the liver therefore dominates the front external genitalia. Impotence is very closely related to the liver. It is very easy to have impotence if there is liver *Qi* stagnation or bad mood. The function of the liver in storing blood is very closely related to the erection of the penis. It is very easy for patients with hypertension to have impotence because they are taking western medicine for long term to control blood pressure which could easily inhibit liver *yang*. The best way to treat impotence by acupuncture is the combination of *Dadun* (LR 1) and *Sanyinjiao* (SP 6). But *Sanyinjiao* (SP 6) is more for premature ejaculation. *Dadun* (LR 1) is more for impotence. As a wood point of wood meridian, *Dadun* (LR 1) is good at expansion and shrinking of tendon. If the liver is lacking in storing of blood, it fails in helping the congested penis. *Dadun* (LR 1), as a *Jing*-well point, could help open orifices to expel cold (the tip of penis is one of the orifices), and congest the penis, and reduce pressure in the liver meridian, thus this point is good at treating impotence. While premature ejaculation is due to deconsolidation of the kidney *Qi*, thus *Shenguan/Tianhuangfu* (77.18) and *Sanyinjiao* (SP 6) should be punctured. On considering herbs, *Guizhi* (Ramulus Cinnamomi) plus *Longgu Muli Tang* (Decoction of Os Draconis Fossilia Ossis Mastodi and Concha Ostreae) formula for both impotence and premature ejaculation. After a period of taking the decoction, the effect could be seen and the result is very stable. If premature ejaculation is due over excitement, therapy should be both clearing fire and astringency. *Zhi Bai Dihuang Wan* (Pill of Anemarrhena, Phellodendron and Rehmannia) could be applied to clear fire and *Jinsuo Gujing Wan* (Golden Lock Pill for Keeping the Kidney Essence) to consolidate the kidney. If the patient has impotence and premature ejaculation in the meantime, *Dadun* (LR 1), *Sanyinjiao* (SP 6) and *Shenguan* (77.18) should be punctured together. *Guizhi* (Ramulus Cinnamomi) plus *Longgu Muli Tang* (Decoction of Os Draconis Fossilia Ossis Mastodi and Concha Ostreae) could be prescribed. Though this formula is warm in nature, its therapeutic effect lasts long. At present, some patients are using *Kang Wei Ling* (Anti-impotence Agent), the important ingredient of which are *Danggui* (Radix Angelicae Sinensis) and *Wugong* (Scolopendra). Both of them can invigorate *Yang*.

Zusanli (ST 36) is an earth point on the earth meridian, according to genuine five elements theory. It has the function of strengthening the spleen and nourishing the stomach and brings effect for chronic debility diseases. TCM considers the kidney as the congenital foundation and the spleen and stomach an acquired foundation. Thus, acquired diseases, especially diseases due to weak body constitution should be regulated or treated by applying *Zusanli* (ST 36). The application of the genuine five elements theory in selecting the fire point on the fire meridian, the metal point on the metal meridian, and the water point on the water meridian is the same.

7) Appendicitis

a. Pricking *Sihuazhong* (77.09) and *Sihuawai* (77.14) to induce bleeding brings special effect.
b. *Lanweixue* (Extra) and *Menjin* (66.05) are effective.

For treating appendicitis, a deep insertion is necessary. Retention of the needle should be from 60 minutes to 2 hours with strong stimulation of reducing method. Manipulate needles once every five minutes. I've treated many patients with appendicitis. *Lanweixue* (Extra) is mainly punctured. When symptoms exist due to appendicitis, the tenderness will be discovered on this point. This point is in a place between *Zusanli* (ST 36) and *Shangjuxu* (ST 37) where there is obvious soreness and distention when pressed. Most probably it is about 1 *cun* below *Zusanli* (ST 36). It is better to insert a needle longer than half *cun*. After pricking *Sihuazhong* (77.09) and *Sihuawai* (77.14) to induce bleeding, then, puncture this extra point, thus a better effect will be brought. Adding *Menjin* (66.05) will bring the best effect. Acupuncture treatment brings a fairly good effect for treating simple acute appendicitis. If symptoms are severe and treatment delayed resulting in perforation and necrosis, it is necessary to have surgery.

8) Constipation

a. *Huochuan* (33.04).

Acupuncture is also effective for constipation. *Huochuan* (33.04) which is the same as *Zhigou* (SJ6) could be applied. *Zhigou* (SJ 6) is very effective for treating acute constipation. *Yu Long Fu* (Ode of the Jade Dragon) says *Zhaohai* (KI 6) and *Zhigou* (SJ 6) are for constipation. It is better to combine *Zhigou* (SJ 6) with *Zhaohai* (KI 6), which is a key point among the eight extraordinary meridians, and it has an effect of moistening yin because it is on kidney meridian. Thus it is an effective point for chronic constipation. Chronic constipation is often due to *yin* deficiency or blood deficiency. *Zhaohai* (KI 6) could nourish *yin* to promote fluid and benefit *Qi*. *Zhigou* (SJ 6) can promote *Qi* in Triple Energizer (*San Jiao*), thus it is an effective point for acute constipation. But combining these two points brings a better effect. The combination has a function of nourishing *Qi* and *Yin*. It is a very commonly used combination for constipation. *Za Bing Xue Fa Ge* (Song of Points for Miscellaneous Diseases) says reinforcing *Zhigou* (SJ 6) and reducing *Zusanli* (ST 36) for deficient constipation. If constipation is of the *Qi* deficient type, *Zhigou* (SJ 6) combined with *Zusanli* (ST 36) brings very good effect.

In 1990, when I was lecturing in Detroit of Michigan State, there were 20 TCM and western medical doctors. Almost all of them had a Ph.D. degree. The course lasted for one week. Among them was a sixty year old student. He had a very red face on the fourth day because he didn't have a bowel movement for about three to four days. So I punctured his *Zhigou* (SJ 6) and *Zhaohai* (KI 6) and retained needles for 30 minutes. But 20 minutes later, this student had felt a need to use the toilet. So then the needles were taken out. He went to the toilet and his bowel movement was very smooth. There was another female patient, about 40 or 50 years old, who had chronic constipation, having only a bowel movement once every five or six days. When she visited me, she didn't have stool for four days. I treated her with *Zhigou* (SJ6) and *Zhaohai* (KI 6). Then she had smooth bowel movement everyday in the following two or three days. On the third day, the effect reduced. After three and four more treatments, her bowel movement became normal. It is very easy for this type of patient to have cancer in the large intestine and breasts. For treating them, I always use both acupuncture and herbal medicine which bring a better effect. For chronic constipation, it brings good effect to drink a decoction made of *Fanxieye* (Folium Sennae) 10g or 15g everyday. Some patients drink such a decoction for 10 years without any side effect. In case of senile or female constipation due to blood deficiency, *Ji Chuan Jian* (Decoction for Increasing Fluid in Intestines to Promote Bowel Movement) could be prescribed. The causative factors for constipation are many: very fine food and meat; blood or yin deficiency; or not drinking enough water; or ingesting too much spicy food; or less food taken; or standing too long or sitting or lack of exercise. Thus treatment for constipation should be given according to the body constitution and etiology. It is very good to prevent constipation by promoting peristalsis. *Zhigou* (SJ 6) and *Zhaohai* (KI 6) are the best points for constipation.

Huochuan (33.04) of Master Tung's acupuncture has the same effect as *Zhigou* (SJ6). I am introducing Master Tung's points but other TCM theories and methods are mentioned as well. Master Tung's acupuncture is a part from TCM. And TCM emphasizes on a holistic conception, thus if Master Tung's acupuncture is understood deeper, the application of points of the fourteen meridians will be well done. In fact, the theory of Master Tung's acupuncture could be applied on general treatment. If you understand internal diseases more thoroughly and grasp the application very well of the herbal medicine and acupuncture, the mechanism in point selection could be applied in making herbal prescriptions, so that the prescription will be very well organized. These two methods help and supplement each other if they are very well understood. I always emphasize it when lecturing. I try my best to tell you all about Master Tung's points, effective points from the fourteen meridians and special herbal prescriptions, so that the best therapies could be combined in use. Personally, I think these points and the therapeutic methods are good. Master Tung's points and points from the fourteen meridians should be applied alternatively. The theory for Master Tung's points is the one for fourteen meridians, i.e., if you know more about Master Tung's points, you know more about points from the fourteen meridians. I encourage my students to use the fourteen meridians and Master Tung's points skillfully, and recite *Neijing* (Yellow Emperor's Inner Classic) and other classics and lyrics very fluently, because Master Tung's acupuncture uses a lot of theories from those classics. If you want to exert and advance Master Tung's acupuncture, classic books must be read proficiently.

Application of Holographic Acupuncture Technique for Different Parts of the Body

The applications of holographic acupuncture for different parts of the body include correspondence between different parts of the body and *zangfu* organs. It can be considered as a part of holography and the hardcore thought of Master Tung's acupuncture as well. Those techniques originated from *Huang Di Nei Jing* (Yellow Emperor's Inner Classic). A lot of ancestors' experiences are the same. Up to now, there are odd records about application of such technique, but not holistic and complete. Here, I would like to present a brief statement about Master Tung Jingchang's and my own 40 years' of clinical experience. Acupuncture Techniques of Holography Corresponding to Different Parts of Body is also named as puncturing five body parts technique, i.e.: stimulating bone to treat bone diseases; stimulating tendon to treat tendon diseases; stimulating muscle to treat muscle diseases; stimulating skin to treat skin diseases. Meanwhile, five body parts treating five zang organs' diseases, the theory of which is based on *Huang Di Nei Jing* (Yellow Emperor's Inner Classic). Master Tung used those techniques frequently, and I myself even more. So, now let me explain them one by one:

I. Stimulating Body Parts to Treat Diseases of the Corresponding Body Parts

1. Stimulating bone to treat bone disease

The method for treating bone disease by stimulating bone equals to ancient bone pricking method. Chapter 51 of *Su Wen* (Essential Question) says "when pricking bone, tendons shouldn't be hurt," which has two meanings. One is to insert the needle to reach the bone which equals to *shu*-points-needling recorded in *Huang Di Nei Jing* (Yellow Emperor's Inner Classic). Chapter 7 of *Ling Shu* (Spiritual Pivot) says "*shu*-points-needling means thrusting and lifting the needle perpendicularly to reach the bone to treat bone *Bi* syndrome." Second is to insert needle alongside bone which equals to vertical-needling recorded in *Huang Di Nei Jing* (Yellow Emperor's Inner Classic). Chapter 7 of *Ling Shu* (Spiritual Pivot) says "vertical needling is for bone *Bi* syndrome. After insertion, slightly advance the needle and make the needle tip to approach the bone, then lift and thrust the needle to treat the bone *Bi* syndrome." Among Master Tung's points, there are many to be punctured alongside the bone, and many to be punctured approaching to bone. Master *Zhou Kongsi* in *Qing* dynasty said in his book *Zhou Shi Jing Luo Da Quan* (The Complete Collection of Zhou's Meridians and Collaterals) that the symptoms of those internal diseases moving upward or downward, meridians are involved; if moves are to right or left side, collaterals are involved. Those points, when meridian *Qi* arrives, it accumulates, thus points must be with bone. Recent research discovers a theory of periosteum conduction. Periosteum is full of nerves and blood vessels. When needles reach the bone or stimulate nearby bone, some bone diseases could be cured with a better therapeutic effect, because stimulation is conducted through periosteum. For example, puncturing *Linggu* (22.05) alongside bone to treat sciatic neuralgia brings special effect (it brings a better effect if *Dabai* (22.04) is combined); *Renzhong* (DU 26), *Houxi* (SI 3) and *Shugu* (BL 65) can be applied for bone spur, it brings better effect if *Fengshi* (GB 31) is combined. It brings great effect for spur on the heel if *Linggu* (22.05) is pricked alongside bone. If *Shugu* (BL 65) is added, a better effect will be brought. Puncturing *Quchi* (LI 11) alongside the bone is for inflammation in lateral epicondyle of humerus, also known as tennis elbow. Puncturing *Taichong* (LR 3) alongside bone is for pain in the hand or foot, especially for knee pain.

2. Stimulating tendon to treat tendon diseases

The method for treating tendon disease by stimulating the tendon equals to ancient tendon pricking method. Chapter 51 of *Su Wen* (Essential Question) says "when pricking the tendon, muscle shouldn't be hurt" which has two meanings. One is pricking the tendon, which equals to joint needling recorded in *Huang Di Nei Jing* (Yellow Emperor's Inner Classic). Chapter 7 of *Ling Shu* (Spiritual Pivot) says "joint-needling is to prick around the joints of extremities straightly to treat the tendon *Bi* syndrome." In pricking, it must cause bleeding and it is the pricking therapy corresponding to the liver. Second is to prick alongside tendon which equals to relaxing-needling recorded in *Huang Di Nei Jing* (Yellow Emperor's Inner Classic). Chapter 7 of *Ling Shu* (Spiritual Pivot) says "relaxing needling is to prick straight beside the painful muscle, and manipulate the needle up and down and anteriorly and posteriorly to relax the muscle so as to relieve the muscular ache and spasm." Both needling techniques have good effect for tendon diseases, including spasm, rigidity, convulsion and flaccidity. For example, *Zhenjin* (77.01) is on the Achilles tendon. It brings great therapeutic effect for treating neck rigidity, pain and also lumbar sprain. *Chize* (LU 5) is located beside tendon. If this point is punctured alongside the tendon, the entire body's spasm and convulsion, difficulty in raising the arm up due to frozen shoulder and spasmodic palm can be treated with effect. For treating hemiplegia, this point is also very commonly used. It is the son (water) point of lung (metal), needling this point with reducing method makes it impossible for metal to overact on wood, so that tendons could be relaxed and extended. But application of such therapy is based upon the theory "treating tendon disease by stimulating tendons." Other points, such as *Chengshan* (BL 57) and *Yanglingquan* (GB 34), can be used for tendon diseases, because of the same needling technique and theory.

3. Stimulating vessels to treat vessel diseases

The method for treating vessel diseases by stimulating vessel equals to ancient vessel pricking method. Chapter 51 of *Su Wen* (Essential Question) says "when pricking vessels, skin shouldn't be hurt" which has two meanings. One is to prick the vessel to induce bleeding, i.e., pricking method, including collateral pricking, leopard-spot-needling and repeated-shallow puncture recorded in Chapter 7 of *Ling Shu* (Spiritual Pivot) which says "collateral pricking method is to prick superficial and small veins beneath the skin; leopard-spot-needling is to prick the left, right, front and rear and the collaterals must be hit; the repeated-shallow puncture refers to lifting and thrusting of needle are perpendicular, and the pricking is swift and shallow to treat carbuncle and swelling." The other method is to thrust the needle to reach a big artery without injury and bleeding, i.e., treating blood vessel disease by puncturing alongside the vessel. Such method was not recorded in ancient classic, but a method commonly used by Master Tung, which pertain to pricking methods.

Pricking methods are very commonly used which have special therapeutic effect for difficult diseases and protracted diseases, and are also extremely good for acute severe diseases and febrile diseases. The clinical applications of those methods are many, but it is difficult to display them all here. I'll give some examples which are more than enough to help you to understand the applications in wide range. For example, 12 *Jing*-well points with pricking method can be applied for syncope due to wind stroke, high fever, sore throat and so on. Pricking *Weizhong* (BL 40) could treat headache, pain of the neck, back and lumbar region, sciatica, lumbar sprain, leg pain, hemorrhoids, boil, furuncle, carbuncle, cholera, acute vomit, and so on. Pricking cubital area could treat frozen shoulder, arm pain, asthmatic breath cardiac disease, cholera and so on. Pricking the retro-auricle area could treat ophthalmic diseases, facial paralysis, dermatological diseases, insomnia, hydrosis and so on. Master Tung adapts "reducing collaterals by pricking the distal area." The commonly used clinical applications include pricking back to treat foot and knee pain, pricking the lower back to treat pain on the upper arm. Pricking *Sihuazhong* (77.09) and *Sihuawai* (77.14) located on the leg are good for internal organ diseases. The special unique technique Master Tung applied is treating vessels' disease by puncturing an area near the vessel. The application of such technique is not strange to common people. For example, *Taiyuan* (LU 9), the influential point of the vessel, can be used for various kinds of vessel diseases, which is very familiar to acupuncturists. Master Tung developed and enlarged the application of such technique. For example, *Dizong* (44.09) which is near an artery indicates reviving of life for collapse of *Yang*, cardiac diseases and angio sclerosis; *chong* meridian passes *Huoying* (66.03) and *Huozhu* (66.04), so they are also indicated in blood vessel diseases.

4. Stimulating muscle to treat muscle diseases

The method for treating muscle disease by stimulating muscle equals to ancient muscle pricking method. Chapter 51 of *Su Wen* (Essential Question) says "when pricking muscle, vessel and tendon mustn't be hurt." Muscle pricking method includes superficial-needling, inter-muscular-needling and multi-direction-needling recorded in Chapter 7 of *Ling Shu* (Spiritual Pivot) which also says "superficial-needling is to prick shallowly lateral to the surface of the affected muscle to dispel cold and muscle spasm; inter-muscular-needling is to prick the pace of the low-lying muscular layers; multi-direction-needling is to prick one point in different directions towards left and right, like a chicken claw, on the muscle layer to treat muscle Bi syndrome." Superficial puncture is to prick muscle on the shallow layer with oblique or transverse insertion for cold muscle and muscle spasm. Inter-muscular-needling is to puncture the muscle in a fairly deep layer for muscle pain, numbness or atrophy. Multi-direction-needling is to puncture perpendicularly to a certain depth, then lift the needle to skin layer and then thrust the needle leftward, rightward or anteriorly and posteriorly, like a chicken claw, for treating muscle *Bi* due to wind, cold and dampness invasion. Clinically, it brings quite good therapeutic effect for muscle atrophy by stimulating *Hegu* (LI 4), *Quchi* (LI 11), *Shousanli* (LI 10), *Zusanli* (ST 36) and *Sima* points (88.17, 88.18, 88.19) on the thigh where there are rich muscles. Though there is a saying "when treating *Wei*-flaccid syndrome, only *yangming* channel should be selected," the good therapeutic effect is also due to muscle stimulating for treating muscle disease. Those points are also good for muscle spasm, or peripheral neuritis. *Chengshan* (BL 57) and *Jianzhong* (44.06) locate on the area with rich muscle, and they also bring good therapeutic effect for muscle disease.

5. Stimulating skin to treat skin diseases

The method for treating skin diseases by stimulating skin equals to ancient skin pricking methods. Chapter 51 of *Su Wen* (Essential Question) says "when pricking skin muscle shouldn't be hurt." Skin pricking method includes skin needling and shallow needling recorded in Chapter 7 of *Ling Shu* (Spiritual Pivot) which says "skin needling is for skin *Bi* syndrome; shallow-needling is to insert needle swiftly without injuring muscle, like plucking a piece of fine hair and it can purge the skin energy." Skin needling refers to a shallow insertion, like hair growing superficially on the skin and the technique should be gentle and swift; shallow needing also refers to a shallow insertion, like plucking a piece of hair, which is very similar to skin needling, but a bit deeper. Shallow needling is to prick skin without injuring muscle, equals to plum blossom needling. Skin needling is more for local numbness and some dermatological diseases, similar to plum blossom tapping technique, until skin becomes slightly congested or bleeding. It indicated in abnormal feeling on the skin, neurodermatitis, alopecia areata, hair loss and rosacea. Plum blossom needle could be replaced by a three edged needle exerting scattered-spot-prick. But Chapter 7 of *Ling Shu* (Spiritual Pivot) says "it is not suitable to be applied if the skin is pale." Because the techniques (pricking methods to achieve bleeding) are to treat *yang* and excessive condition is more suitable to be applied for heat in blood if the skin is red. For example, dermatological red skin, erysipelas, multiple boil or herpes zoster can be treated by such methods which should be applied on the local area with skin lesion.

Master Tung's pricking method is different from others. He applied such method for treating dermatological diseases on the area where there are big muscles, which has the meaning of nourishing earth to promote metal and to treat skin by stimulating skin. For example, *Sima* points (88.17, 88.18, 88.19) have extreme good effect for skin diseases because they are on the area where the *yangming* meridian passes which is full of *Qi* and blood, good in regulating *Qi* and blood circulations. But deep insertion is not suitable because it doesn't correspond to skin and hair. Or prick with reducing *ying*-nutrient stage method; i.e., first insert a needle to earth layer, then lift to the man layer with strong stimulation of reducing and then lift to heaven layer to retain needle, which follows what is said in *Nan Jing* (The Classic of Difficulties) "when reducing, take *Qi* from *Ying*-nutrient stage." This technique is especially good at treating skin diseases with skin turning to red. *Quchi* (LI 11) applied for skin diseases should be punctured with such technique according to the same mechanism.

II. Stimulating Body Parts to Treat Corresponding *Zang* Organs

The technique of puncturing five body parts includes not only stimulating body parts to treat corresponding body parts, i.e., stimulating bone to treat bone disease; stimulating tendon to treat tendon disease; stimulating vessel to treat vessel disease; stimulating muscle to treat muscle disease; and stimulating skin to treat skin disease; but also stimulating bone to treat kidney; stimulating tendon to treat liver; stimulating muscle to treat spleen; stimulating vessel to treat heart; and stimulating skin to treat lung. Because kidney dominates bone, liver dominates tendon, spleen dominates muscle, heart dominates vessel, and lung dominates skin. Chapter 7 of *Ling Shu* (Spiritual Pivot) says "shallow needling … purges the skin energy and corresponds to lung; leopard-spot-needling … disperses stagnated blood in channels and corresponds to heart; joint-needling … to treat tendon *Bi* syndrome and must cause bleeding, and corresponds to the liver; multi-direction-needling … pricks muscle to treat muscle *Bi* and corresponds to spleen; *shu*-point-needling … deeply inserted to bone, for treating bone *Bi*, and corresponds to kidney."

Such record explains the correspondence between five body parts and five *zang* organs. The following are some simple examples.

1. Pricking skin corresponds to the lung

Clinically for treating cough, asthmatic breath and other lung diseases, stimulate *Shuijin* (1010.20) or *Shuitong* (1010.19) with subcutaneous needles. For treating sore throat or fever due to lung heat, prick *Shaoshang* (LU 11) and *Shangyang* (LI 1). For treating nasal diseases, prick *Muxue* (11.17) on the index finger.

2. Pricking muscle corresponds to the spleen

Pricking the muscle can be used for the spleen. The places with thick muscle have functions of nourishing and regulating *Qi*. *Hegu* (LI 4) and *Taichong* (LR 3) are on the fingers and toes where the muscles are quite thick, so they have strong function of regulating *Qi*. Though it is because they are *Yuan*-source points, it also is due to muscle correspondence between the muscle and spleen. Puncturing *Simaxue* (88.17, 88.18, 88.19) can treat skin disease and strengthen the spleen to supplement the *Qi*. Master Tung emphasized the theory of the spleen and stomach. For example, *Simaxue* (88.17, 88.18, 88.19) for lung diseases; *Tongguan* (88.01), *Tongshan* (88.02), and *Tongtian* (88.03) for heart diseases; *Tongshen* (88.09), *Tongwei* (88.10) and *Tongbei* (88.11) for kidney; *Tianhuang* (88.13), *Minghuang* (88.12) and *Qihuang* (88.14) for liver; *Fengshi* (GB 31), the key point for stopping pain, all located on thigh where there are big muscles. In fact, application of those points is for strengthening spleen.

3. To treat heart by stimulating vessel

It brings best effect to treat heart diseases by pricking the vessel. I applied cubital area, *Sihuazhong* (77.09) and *Sihuawai* (77.14) near *Tiaokou* (ST 38) and *Fenglong* (ST 40) to treat many severe cardiac diseases with the pricking method to induce bleeding. Pricking *Dizong* (44.09) can revive life, heart tonification, heart diseases and angiosclerosis. Pricking *Huoying* (66.03), *Huozhu* (66.04) and *Taichong* (LR 3) with the artery beating underneath, the heart function could be strengthened for treating cardiac palsy. *Taichong* (LR 3) also has function of heart tonification. I used *Taichong* (LR 3) for coma. First I punctured *Renzhong* (DU 26) and Baihui (DU 20) but failed, while *Taichong* (LR 3) brought immediate effect for some cases.

4. To treat liver by stimulating the tendon

Yanglingquan (GB 34) is the key point for treating tendon diseases and also a chief point for liver and gallbladder. Combining with

Chengshan (BL 57), it has effect on treating foot cramp. This point also brings effect on treating stomach spasm and pain, and dysmenorrhea because those diseases are all related to the liver.

5. Pricking bone corresponds to the kidney

Puncture *Linggu* (22.05) along the bone to treat lumbago, and also to nourish kidney to treat heel pain and various kind of diseases due to kidney deficiency. Puncture *Fuke* (11.24) and *Huanchao* (11.06) along the bone for nourishing kidney to treat kidney diseases, such as infertility. Indications of *Wanshun* (22.08, 22.09) are related to kidney. It brings better therapeutic effect if these points are punctured alongside the bone. Puncture *Sanyinjiao* (SP 6) alongside the bone brings stronger function of kidney tonification.

Some points, through having the corresponding relations with tendon, bone and muscle, could relate to more *zang* organs and indicate more diseases. For example, external epicondyle inflammation, tennis elbow can be treated by puncturing *Shousanli* (LI 10) on the tendon and *Quchi* (LI 11) alongside bone. This is because both liver and kidney are nourished when both tendon and bone are treated. Another example, *Shouqianjin* (33.09), between *Taiyang* and *Shaoyang* meridians, is under the tendon and anterior to bone, thus both tendon and bone could be treated, communicating with the liver and kidney. The indications of this point are related to tendon, bone, liver and kidney. *Yemen* (SJ 2), I most often used, is punctured along the bone until *zhongbai* or known as *zhongzhu* (SJ 3), and *Xiabai* (22.07) where there are more muscles, thus this point communicates with the spleen, liver and kidney, so spleen, liver and kidney diseases can be all treated by needling these points. This point has extensive indications and is very effective. It is one of my ten most frequently used points.

Chapter Four

Other Diseases

1. Diseases of the Anterior and Posterior Genitalia

1) Testitis

a. Prick the area from the inner malleolus to *Sanyinjiao* (SP 6) (bloodletting).
b. *Dajian* (11.01), *Xiaojian* (11.02), *Zhongjian* (11.05) and *Fujian* (11.03).

Hernia has been dealt with as a disease of the anterior and posterior genitalia, and now we are going to discuss testitis. In treating this disease, two or three points can be chosen from *Dajian* (11.01), *Xiaojian* (11.02), *Zhongjian* (11.05), *Waijian* (11.04) and *Fujian* (11.03), using the same manipulations as those used for hernia. Master Tung prefers to prick the area from the inner malleolus to *Sanyinjiao* (SP 6) in the treatment. Acupuncture treatment can also be given at *Dadun* (LR 1) and *Sanyinjiao* (SP 6), the mechanism of which has already been discussed in previous chapters.

2) Frequent Micturition

a. *Shenguan* (77.18) (highly effective).
b. *Haibao* (66.01) and *Mufu* (66.02) (effective).
c. *Makuaishui* (1010.14) (also effective).

The most effective point for frequent micturition is *Shenguan* (77.18), owing to its effect of invigorating the spleen and kidney *qi* and astringency. This point can be used to treat premature ejaculation, albuminuria and diabetes. When I was teaching acupuncture in Taiwan, I started with points from *Shi Si Jing* (The Fourteen Meridians), and *Shenguan* (77.18) from *Dong Shi Qi Xue* (Tung's Extraordinary Points) was taught later. Once, when I was teaching I found that a student had to go to the restroom about every 30 minutes. I asked him to try acupuncture at *Shenguan* (77.18) and his problem was solved in two or three weeks. Urgent and difficult urination with little amount indicates cystitis, which should be accordingly. *Shenguan* (77.18) can be used to treat frequent micturition due to deficiency of kidney *qi*, which causes hyposexuality, and that is why *Shenguan* (77.18) can be used. Besides frequent micturition, *Shenguan* (77.18) can also be used to treat premature ejaculation owing to its effect of astringency. Frequent micturition can also be treated with *Sang Piao Xiao San* (Powder of Oötheca Mantidis) and *Suo Quan Wan* (Pill for Controlling Urination), and premature ejaculation can be treated with *Jin Suo Gu Jing Wan* (Pill for Arresting Premature Ejaculation) and *Zhi Bo Di Huang Wan* (Pill of Rhizoma

Anemarrhenae Asphodeloidis, Cortex Phellodendri and Radix Rehmanniae). Being the gate of the kidney, *Shenguan* (77.18) controls fluid and stores semen, and failure in this function may result in frequent micturition and premature ejaculation, which are effectively treated by this point. Since *Shenguan* (77.18) can improve the storing and astringing functions of the kidney *qi*, it can be used in combination with other points to treat asthma in patients with long-lasting diseases. *Shenguan* (77.18) has the combined effect of both *Shenshu* (BL 23) and *Guanyuan* (REN 4), the former lying in the *yang* location of the body having the effect of warming kidney *yang* and the latter in the *yin* location of the body having the effect of nourishing kidney *yin*. Therefore, *Shenguan* (77.18) is the best point for frequent micturition. Other effective points include *Haibao* (66.01) and *Mufu* (66.02), but since the points are on the toes, they are painful and the patient has to take off the shoes and socks, sometimes making it hard for the doctor to bear the disagreeable smell. *Makuaishui* (1010.14) is also effective, but these points are not as effective as *Shenguan* (77.18) in the treatment of frequent micturition. Besides frequent micturition, *Makuaishui* (1010.14) is also an effective point for cholecystolithiasis. In treating difficulty in micturition, attention should be paid to "mainly bringing down *qi*," by puncturing *Makuaishui* (1010.14) first followed by *Shenguan* (77.18). In treating frequent micturition, one should "focus on ascending *qi*," by puncturing *Shenguan* (77.18) first followed by *Makuaishui* (1010.14). This is the preferable method in spite of the dual regulating effect of acupuncture.

It is important to master the principles in differentiation of syndromes based on the eight principles, whether Tung's extraordinary points or points from Fourteen Regular Meridians are used. A veteran doctor knows how to determine the nature of the disease based on the eight principles: deficiency and cold in long-lasting diseases, and excess and heat in new diseases. For instance, when the needle in inserted into a depth of 1.5 inches, it may go further into a depth of 1.8 inches after some time in patients with cold constitution owing to the needle suction effect in such kind of patients; while the needle may withdraw itself to a depth of 1.3 inches or even less in patients with heat constitution or febrile diseases. By observing these phenomena, it is possible to determine the cold or heat nature of the patients. Administering acupuncture is much the same as administering drugs, since acupuncture can treat and regulate cold and heat syndromes and constitutions and also correspond with drug effects. In treating heat syndromes, shallow insertion of the needle with short duration (without retaining the needle) is given, but treatment can be given twice a day. This is also true with using drugs for the same kind of diseases. Both *Gui Zhi Tang* (Decoction of Ramulus Cinnamomi Cassiae) and *Yin Qiao San* (Powder of Flos Lonicerae and Fructus Forsythiae Suspensae) are mild in their dosage, but they are to be taken several times a day. Being an effective pungent-cool diaphoretic recipe, *Yin Qiao San*

(Powder of Flos Lonicerae and Fructus Forsythiae Suspensae) is the most common recipe to be used at the onset of a febrile disease. Chinese medicine holds that the treatment of the diseases of the upper energizer (shangjiao) is just like a feather (namely, by using drugs light in texture and dosage), the treatment of the diseases of the middle energizer (zhonhjiao) is to bring about a balance, and the treatment of the diseases of the lower energizer (xiajiao) is like a poise (i.e. by using drugs heavy in texture). Since long-lasting diseases affect the lower energizer, pills are used over a long period. Besides, heavy drugs such as *Long Gu* (Os Draconis), *Mu Li* (Concha Ostreae) and *Dai Zhe Shi* (Haematitum) are also used. In treating diseases of the upper energizer, *Jin Yin Hua* (Flos Lonicerae Japonicae) is used with mild dosage, about 10-15 grams. Diseases of the middle energizer are mostly caused by cold-heat incoordination and therefore drugs of both cold and heat nature are used to bring about a balance. As an example, the common recipes for gastrointestinal diseases are *Ban Xia Xie Xin Tang* (Decoction of Rhizoma Pinelliae Ternatae Praeparata for Purging Heart) and *Xiao Chai Hu Tang* (Minor Decoction of Radix Bupleuri), which includes both drugs of cold nature such as *Huang Qin* (Radix Scutellariae Baicalensis) and *Huang Lian* (Rhizoma Coptidis), and drugs of heat nature like *Ban Xia* (Rhizoma Pinelliae Ternatae Praeparata) and *Gan Jiang* (Rhizoma Zingiberis Officinalis). This is also true in acupuncture treatment. In treating diseases of the upper energizer, diseases at the onset or diseases of heat nature, shallow insertion of the needle is used, while in treating diseases of the lower energizer, chronic diseases (when the kidney is affected) and diseases of cold nature, deep insertion is applied. A deep understanding of the eight principles is crucial in using either drugs or acupuncture in the treatment of the disease.

3) Galacturia

a. *Tongshen* (88.09), *Tongwei* (88.10) and *Tongbei* (88.11).
b. *Makuaishui* (1010.14).

Galacturia is among the five types of stranguria, namely, uropsammus, urinary incontinence, galacturia, pollakiuria, and hematuria. Since they have already been dealt with in previous chapters, I'm going to talk only about galacturia here. The common recipe for this disease is *Bi Xie Fen Qing Yin* (Decoction of Rhizoma Dioscoreae Hypoglaucae seu Septemlobae for clarifying Urine), which is normally used at the onset of the disease with damp-heat. In a chronic case, which is often due to failure of *qi* to control fluid, *Bu Zhong Yi Qi Tang* (Decoction for Reinforcing *Qi* in the Middle Energizer) can be used, with *Bai Ji* (Rhizoma Bletillae Striatae) or *She Gan* (Rhizoma Belamcandae Chinensis) added to the prescription to achieve better results. Galacturia is often due to damp-heat or deficiency of *qi* and blood, with excess syndromes seen at the onset and deficiency syndromes found in chronic cases. Both can be treated with *Tongshen* (88.09), *Tongwei* (88.10) and *Tongbei* (88.11) as a group, or with *Makuaishui* (1010.14). *Shenguan* (77.18), *Renhuang* (77.21), *Dihuang* (77.19) are also effective for the disease. Points from the fourteen regular meridians can also be used, such as *Qihai* (REN 6) in the Conception Vessel, an important point for treating the five types of stranguria, and *Taichong* (LR 3).

4) Seminal Emission

a. *Xiasanhuang* (77.18, 19, 21).

Shenguan (77.18) is the best point for the disease. Together with *Renhuang* (77.21) and *Dihuang* (77.19), they form a group of points for regulating and reinforcing the spleen and kidney with the effect of astringency. *Gui Zhi* (Ramulus Cinnamomi Cassiae), *Long Gu* (Os Draconis) and *Mu Li* (Concha Ostreae) also make a good prescription, which I often use to treat infantile enuresis. This prescription is also quite effective even for children ten or eleven years of age with enuresis, and many children recover in a week. If the prescription does not work satisfactorily, *Ma Huang* (Herba Ephedrae) (3 grams) can be added to enable the child to wake up for urination. With Chinese drugs, acupuncture is usually not necessary for children with enuresis, but if acupuncture is used, *Shenguan* (77.18) is normally chosen. The decoction of *Gui Zhi* (Ramulus Cinnamomi Cassiae), *Long Gu* (Os Draconis) and *Mu Li* (Concha Ostreae) is also a common prescription for frequent micturition.

Shenguan (77.18) is an important point for seminal emission. When drugs are used, it is advisable to use the decoction of *Gui Zhi* (Ramulus Cinnamomi Cassiae), *Long Gu* (Os Draconis) and *Mu Li* (Concha Ostreae) for different kinds of seminal emission such as seminal emission without dreams or seminal emission during defecation, so as to reinforce the kidney function.

Regular acupuncture points for seminal emission are *Guanyuan* (REN 4), *Qihai* (REN 6) and *Sanyinjiao* (SP 6). *Guanyuan* (REN 4) is an important point for deficiency syndromes owing to its effect in reinforcing the kidney *qi*. It is said in *Bai Zheng Fu* (a book on a hundred diseases) that "treating turbid urine and seminal emission by puncturing the three yin meridians at *Qihai*." *Qihai* (REN 6) has the functions of reinforcing *qi* and inducing astringency. *Sanyinjiao* (SP 6) can be used to treat the diseases of the spleen, liver and kidney, and is also an important point for the diseases of the urogenital system.

5) Hematuria

a. *Xiasanhuang* (77.18, 19, 21).

Hematuria is often caused by nephropyelitis or urolith rubbing against the urethra wall. To treat stones in the bladder, urethra and kidney, *Majinshui* (1010.13), *Makuaishui* (1010.14), *Liukuai* (1010. 16) and *Qikuai* (1010.17) are used in combination. *Xiasanhuang* (77.18, 19, 21) is effective for nephropyelitis. Two effective recipes for hematuria are *Xiao Ji Yin Zi* (Decoction of Herba Cephalanoploris) and *Zhu Ling Tang* (Decoction of Sclerotium Polypori Umbellati).

6) Urethralgia

a. *Fujian* (11.03) and *Waijian* (11.04).
b. *Makuaishui* (1010.14).
c. *Linggu* (22.05) and *Huozhu* (66.04).
d. *Yunbai* (44.11) and *Libai* (44.12).

Urethralgia is usually caused by cystitis or urethritis, which is known as heat stranguria in Chinese medicine. *Waijian* (11.04), *Fujian* (11.03), *Libai* (44.12) and *Yunbai* (44.11) are all effective points for urethralgia owing to the fact that the corresponding area of *Waijian* (11.04) and *Fujian* (11.03), which lie on the fingers, is the pudendum (direct correspondence of hand and trunk) and the corresponding area of *Libai* (44.12) and *Yunbai* (44.11), which are located on the upper arm, is also the pudendum (adverse correspondence of hand and trunk). Alternatively, *Huoying* (66.03) and *Huozhu* (66.04), or *Linggu* (22.05) and *Huozhu* (66.04) can be used with good results. *Huoying* (66.03) and *Huozhu* (66.04), with *Taichong* (LR 3) in between, are all located in the Liver Meridian, which circles the genitalia and therefore can be used to treat the diseases in this area. *Xingjian* (LR 2) is also effective since it is the spring point of the Liver Meridian and has the effect of purging liver fire, similar to the effect of *Long Dan Xie Gan Tang* (Decoction of Radix Gentianae for Purging Liver Fire). Both *Zhongji* (REN 3), the Front-*Mu* point of urinary bladder and *Qihai* (REN 6), an important point for stranguria, can be used to treat urethralgia. *Ba Zheng San* (Powder for Restoring Health) and *Long Dan Xie Gan Tang* (Decoction of Radix Gentianae for Purging Liver Fire) are also used to treat urethralgia of damp-heat type. I often use *Si Ni San* (Powder for Treating Cold Limbs), which include *Chai Hu* (Radix Bupleuri), *Zhi Shi* (Fructus Immaturus Citri Aurantii), *Shao Yao* (Paeonia lactiflora Pall) and *Gan Cao* (Radix Glycyrrhizae Uralensis). *Jie Geng* (Radix Platycodi Grandiflori) and *Fu Ling* (Sclerotium Poriae Cocos) are added to the prescription since the former can discharge pus and relieve inflammation and the latter can induce diuresis. In a severe case, *Pu Gong Ying* (Herba Taraxaci) can be added. Pregnant women with urethritis should be treated neither with acupuncture nor with Chinese drug recipes such as *Ba Zheng San* (Powder for Restoring Health) and *Long Dan Xie Gan Tang* (Decoction of Radix Gentianae for Purging Liver Fire). I prefer to use *Qing Xin Lian Zi Yin* (Decoction of Semen Nelumbinis Nuciferae for Clearing away Heart Fire), which is also effective for chronic cystitis in pregnant women.

7) Dysuria

a. *Tianhuang* (88.13) and *Sihuashang* (77.08).
b. *Xiasanhuang* (77.18, 19, 21).
c. *Jianzhong* (44.06), *Yunbai* (44.11) and *Xiaqu* (44.15).

Dysuria with varying degrees is caused by prostatomegaly, lithiasis, tumors or neurological bladder dysfunction. *Tianhuang* (88.13) and *Sihuashang* (77.08), or *Yinlingquan* (SP 9) and *Zusanli* (ST 36) can be used to treat the disease. *Jianzhong* (44.06), *Yunbai* (44.11), *Xiaqu* (44.15), and *Xiasanhuang* (77.18, 19, 21) is also effective points. For dysuria caused by abdominal dropsy, *Yinlingquan* (SP 9) and *Zusanli* (ST 36) can be used, the former being water in earth capable of reinforcing the spleen and kidney and the latter being the earth in earth with strong effect of both replenishing the earth to reinforce *qi* and replenishing the earth to control water. The two points are also quite effective for dysuria caused by prostatomegaly. It is said in *Zhi Yao Fu* (Gist of Medicine) that "*Yinlingquan* dredges the water passages." According to *Za Bing Xue Fa Ge* (Rhymes of Needle Manipulation for Miscellaneous Diseases), "dysuria is treated effectively with *Yinlingquan* and *Zusanli. Zhongji* (REN 3), the Frong-*Mu* point of the bladder, can also be used by pressing and releasing the point with the finger to promote the function of urination.

A case report: An old man with prostatomegaly had not passed water for more than ten hours, with flushed and bloated face. I promptly treated him with *Tianhuang* (88.13) and *Sihuashang* (77.08), and soon after the acupuncture treatment, he could urinate freely.

8) Balanitis

a. *Xiasanhuang* (77.18, 19, 21).

Balanitis is generally treated with *Xiasanhuang* (77.18, 19, 21), together with *Zhongji* (REN 3), *Dadun* (LR 1) or *Xingjian* (LR 2). Being the Spring and fire point of the Liver Meridian, *Xingjian* (LR 2) is an important point for cystitis and urethritis. Since *Huoying* (66.03) is close to *Xingjian* (LR 2), this point can also be used. Both *Xingjian* (LR 2) and *Huoying* (66.03) are also effective for glaucoma.

9) Impotence and Premature Ejaculation

a. *Xiasanhuang* (77.18, 19, 21) (together with *Shuijin* (1010.20) and *Shuitong* (1010.19) with better effect).
b. *Dadun* (LR 1) and *Shenguan* (77.18).

Although impotence and premature ejaculation are put in the same category here, they are not the same pathologically. To treat impotence, use *Dadun* (LR 1) and *Sanyinjiao* (SP 6) in combination; to treat premature ejaculation, use *Shenguan* (77.18), *Shuijin* (1010.20) and *Shuitong* (1010.19) together. Both impotence and premature ejaculation can be treated with *Dihuang* (77.19) in combination with *Dadun* (LR 1). To treat impotence, one should treat the liver; to treat premature ejaculation, one should treat the kidney. In treating postcoital protrusion due to hyperactivity of the ministerial fire, I often use *Zhi Bo Di Huang Tang* (Decoction of Rhizoma Anemarrhenae Asphodeloidis, Cortex Phellodendri and Radix Rehmanniae Praeparata) to purge fire. Conversely, in treating impotence due to insufficiency of the ministerial fire, I try to replenish the fire of the gate of life, and in treating premature ejaculation due to inconsolidation of the kidney or hyperfunction of the liver in regulating the flow of *qi* and blood, the kidney is mainly treated prior to the liver. In treating impotence, however, the liver is mainly treated prior to the kidney. Emotional stress also causes impotence and therefore it is often treated by soothing the liver, using *Dadun* (LR 1) and *Sanyinjiao* (SP 6). Premature ejaculation is mainly treated with *Shenguan* (77.18). Impotence and premature ejaculation can be treated together, by using *Dadun* (LR 1) and *Xiasanhuang* (77.18, 19, 21), since *Dadun* (LR 1), the *Jing*-Well point of the liver and the wood point of the Liver Meridian, can soothe the liver and dispel cold and *Shenguan* (77.18) can strengthen the kidney. I have mentioned before that deficiency of *yin* leads to hyperactivity of the ministerial fire, and therefore *Zhi Bo Di Huang Tang* (Decoction of Rhizoma Anemarrhenae Asphodeloidis, Cortex Phellodendri and Radix Rehmanniae Praeparata) can be used to clear away fire, thus strengthening the kidney essence. In treating premature ejaculation, not only *Zhi Bo Di Huang Tang* (Decoction of Rhizoma Anemarrhenae Asphodeloidis, Cortex Phellodendri and Radix Rehmanniae Praeparata) can be used to clear away fire, *Jin Suo Gu Jing Wan* (Pill for Strengthening Kidney) can also be used to strengthen the kidney. Impotence is often a cold syndrome. According to *Jin Kui Yao Lue* (Synopsis of Prescriptions of Golden Chamber), glans coldness is treated with *Gui Zhi* (Ramulus Cinnamomi Cassiae) and *Long Gu Mu Li Tang* (Decoction of Os Draconis and Concha Ostreae), which are also effective for premature ejaculation. To sum up, the common points for this group of diseases are *Dadun* (LR 1) and *Xiasanhuang* (77.18, 19, 21); with impotence treated mainly with *Dadun* (LR 1) and *Xiasanhuang* (77.18, 19,

21), and premature ejaculation treated mainly with *Xiasanhuang* (77.18, 19, 21).

2. Gynecopathy

Fuke (11.24) and *Huanchao* (11.06) in Tung's extraordinary points are the main points frequently used for all kinds of gynecopathy. Other points such as *Jiemeiyi* (88.04), *Jiemei'er* (88.05) and *Jiemeisan* (88.06) are also effective in regulating women's diseases, which Master Tung used to use frequently. Since the points are on the thigh, it causes some inconvenience and therefore I do not use it unless it is necessary, and use *Fuke* (11.24) and *Huanchao* (11.06) instead.

1) Hysteralgia

a. *Menjin* (66.05) (specially good effect).
b. *Fuke* (11.24) (specially good effect).
c. *Huanchao* (11.06) (used as an adjunct point).

Fuke (11.24) used in combination with *Huanchao* (11.06) is quite effective for hysteralgia. I prefer *Menjin* (66.05) and *Chengjiang* (REN 24). *Menjin* (66.05) is connected with the lung and large intestine, with similar effect to *Xiangu* (ST 43) in the Stomach Meridian. Since it is a wood point of the earth meridian, it is related to the liver and can soothe the liver *qi* and regulate the functions of the liver and spleen. Also, since this point is on the *Yangming* Meridian, a meridian full of *qi* and blood, it can regulate *qi* and blood with good effect in treating physiological pains. *Chengjiang* (REN 24) is also an effective point for physiological pains. Being the *Jing*-Well point of the Conception Vessel which reaches the pudendal region, it can remove cold from that region. Besides, it is at the crossing point of *Yangming* Meridians of Hand and Foot, which have the function to regulate *qi* and blood, and therefore *Chengjiang* (REN 24) is effective for hysteralgia, which is mostly caused by disharmony between *qi* and blood, stasis of blood or deficiency and cold of the lower energizer.

2) Oviduct Obstruction

a. *Fuke* (11.24) (specially good effect).
b. *Huanchao* (11.06) (used in combination with *Fuke* with better effect).

Oviduct obstruction is mainly responsible for infertility and is treated effectively by *Fuke* (11.24). Better effect can be achieved if the point is used in combination with *Huanchao* (11.06). *Mufu* (66.02) is also effective, but since the point is on the toe it is painful and causes inconvenience. I have a proved recipe for oviduct obstruction: *Tao Hong Si Wu Tang* (Decoction of Four Drugs Including Semen Persicae and Flos Carthami Tinctorii) plus drugs for regulating *qi*, like *Xiao Hui Xiang*

(Fructus Foeniculi Vulgaris), *Lian Qiao* (Fructus Forsythiae Suspensae) and *Xiang Fu* (Rhizoma Cyperi Rotundi). This recipe is quite effective and some patients became pregnant after just corresponding with me for some time.

3) Hysteromyoma

a. *Huanchao* (11.06), *Jiemeiyi* (88.04), *Jiemei'er* (88.05) and *Jiemeisan* (88.06).
b. Prick the area between *Chongzi* (22.01) and *Chongxian* (22.02) to let out blood.
c. *Fuke* (11.24) (quite effective), *Huanchao* (11.06) (more effective when used in combination with *Fuke*).
d. Prick the area between medial malleolus and *Sanyinjiao* (SP 6) to let out blood.

Fuke (11.24) and *Huanchao* (11.06) are the main point for the disease. Pricking the area between *Chongzi* (22.01) and *Chongxian* (22.02) or between medial malleolus and *Sanyinjiao* (SP 6) alternatively to let out blood is also effective, but may be more painful. Small tumors can be resolved but it is difficult to resolve tumors over six centimeters in diameter. Generally, combination of acupuncture with drugs will produce better effect. The commonly used drugs include *Gui Zhi Fu Ling Wan* (Pill of Ramulus Cinnamomi Cassiae and Sclerotium Poriae Cocos) and drugs for softening and resolving hard masses. Recipes for activating blood circulation and resolving phlegm are frequently used of both tumors and gynecopathy. To resolve phlegm, *Er Chen Tang* (Decoction of Two Old Drugs) which, includes *Ban Xia* (Rhizoma Pinelliae Ternatae Praeparata), *Chen Pi* (Pericarpium Citri Reticulatae), *Fu Ling* (Sclerotium Poriae Cocos) and *Gan Cao* (Radix Glycyrrhizae Uralensis). *Ban Xia* (Rhizoma Pinelliae Ternatae Praeparata) and *Chen Pi* (Pericarpium Citri Reticulatae) are important drugs for resolving phlegm since they can remove dampness and promote the flow of *qi*. *Fu Ling* (Sclerotium Poriae Cocos) can eliminate dampness and prevent the formation of phlegm. The prescriptions for resolving phlegm in *Shang Han Lun* (Treatise on Febrile Diseases) does not include *Chen Pi* (Pericarpium Citri Reticulatae) and *Fu Ling* (Sclerotium Poriae Cocos) often used to resolve phlegm. In *Ling Gui Zhu Gan Tang* (Decoction of Sclerotium Poriae Cocos, Ramulus Cinnamomi Cassiae, Rhizoma Atractylodis Macrocephalae and Radix Glycyrrhizae Uralensis), for example, *Fu Ling* (Sclerotium Poriae Cocos) is used as the main herb for resolving phlegm. Activating blood circulation and resolving phlegm is a good method to treat miscellaneous diseases, and Master Tung Jingchang often treats these with *Sihuawai* (77.14), which is located very close to *Fenglong* (ST 40). *Fenglong* (ST 40) is the collateral point of the Stomach Meridian, and therefore can be used to treat diseases of the spleen and stomach. Also, since "phlegm accumulates at

Fenglong (ST 40)," puncturing this point can treat phlegm disorders. Pricking the point to let out blood can also treat blood stasis, and so this point can treat both phlegm retention and blood stasis. According to the theories of Chinese medicine, both blood stasis and phlegm retention are likely to occur in chronic, intractable, miscellaneous and weird diseases. *Sihuawai* (77.14) can be used as the main point for serious diseases by pricking it to let out blood. As far as herbs for softening and resolving hard masses in the treatment of hysteromyoma are concerned, the commonly used ones are *Xiang Fu* (Rhizoma Cyperi Rotundi), *Xuan Shen* (Radix Scrophulariae Ningpoensis), *Zhe Bei Mu* (Bulbus Fritillariae Thunbergii) and *Mu Li* (Concha Ostreae). In a severe case, *Chuan Shan Jia* (Squama Manitis Pentadactylae), *San Leng* (Rhizoma Sparganii Stoloniferi) and *E Zhu* (Rhizoma Curcumae) can be added to enhance the effect of activating blood circulation. Sometimes, *Gui Zhi Fu Ling Wan* (Pill of Ramulus Cinnamomi Cassiae and Sclerotium Poriae Cocos) is used in combination with *Yi Yi Ren* (Semen Coicis Lachryma-jobi) with good effect. Activating blood circulation to remove blood stasis by acupuncture can be done by pricking the area between medial malleolus and *Sanyinjiao* (SP 6) to let out blood.

4) Leucorrhea with Red and White Discharge

a. *Huanchao* (11.06).
b. *Fuke* (11.24).
c. *Jiemeiyi* (88.04), *Jiemei'er* (88.05), *Jiemeisan* (88.06) and *Mufu* (66.02).
d. *Tongshen* (88.09), *Tongbei* (88.11) and *Tongwei* (88.10).

Fuke (11.24) and *Huanchao* (11.06) are effective for this disease. *Jiemei'er* (88.05), *Jiemeisan* (88.06) and *Mufu* (66.02) are also very effective, but because of their locations, it is not so convenient to use them. *Yunbai* (44.11) and *Libai* (44.12), at the thick muscles of the shoulder, have the effect of invigorating the spleen *qi* and removing dampness, and according to the "adverse correspondence of hand and trunk" their corresponding area is the pudendal part of the body. Therefore they can also be used to treat the disease. Leucorrhea with red and white discharge is often caused by spleen deficiency, severe dampness or failure of *qi* function. When caused by spleen deficiency, *Linggu* (22.05) and *Dabai* (22.04) can be used, and *Yunbai* (44.11) and *Libai* (44.12) are also frequently used. *Linggu* (22.05) and *Dabai* (22.04) can treat leucorrhea by invigorating *qi*. Other points such as *Xiasanhuang* (77.18, 19, 21), *Tongshen* (88.09), *Tongbei* (88.11) and *Tongwei* (88.10) are also effective for leucorrhea owing to the fact that they are all on the Spleen Meridian and can reinforce both the spleen and kidney. However the commonly used points are *Xiasanhuang* (77.18, 19, 21), which include *Shenguan* (77.18), for enhancing the function of *qi*, and *Renhuang* (77.21), for regulating the spleen, liver and kidney, and these make a desirable group of points for leucorrhea with red and white discharge.

The prescription *Wan Dai Decoction* (Decoction for removing mucus) for leucorrhea with red and white discharge is effective. It is the formula of Fu Qing-Zhu's works on women's diseases in Qing dynasty. It has the effect of invigoring the spleen, regulating Qi, and removing dampness and mucus. The yellowish leucorrhea is caused by damp-heat, and *Xingjian* (LR 2) can be used for removing damp-heat of liver and gallbladder. *Mufu* (66.02) is also effective, since it treats the disharmony of liver and spleen and damp-heat of liver and gallbladder. If itching of pudendum caused by leucorrhea with yellow discharge, hip bath can be done with decoction make from *Ku Shen* (Radix Sophorae Flavescentis) (15 grams) and *She Chuang Zi* (Fructus Cnidii Monnieri) (25 grams).

5) Pudendum Swelling

a. *Huanchao* (11.06).
b. *Fuke* (11.24).

Besides *Huanchao* (11.06) and *Fuke* (11.24), *Huozhu* (66.04), *Huoying* (66.03) and *Xingjian* (LR 2) can also be used for this disease. In a severe case, bloodletting can be performed along the area from medial malleolus and *Sanyinjiao* (SP 6). Since the Liver Meridian runs through the lower abdomen and circles the pudendum, and the kidney opens into the Anterior and Posterior Genitalia, diseases of the pudendum is often treated by treating the liver and kidney. Besides, since diseases of the pudendum are often due to damp-heat, treatment is usually given to remove damp-heat.

6) Vaginitis

a. *Yunbai* (44.11) and *Haibao* (66.01).
b. *Fuke* (11.24).
c. *Huozhu* (66.04) and *Huoying* (66.03).

Vaginitis is often accompanied by yellow leucorrhea and can be treated effectively with *Yunbai* (44.11) and *Haibao* (66.01). But the latter is on the toe and is therefore painful. Besides, *Huozhu* (66.04) and *Huoying* (66.03) are also effective for the disease since diseases of the pudendum are mostly due to damp-heat. *Fuke* (11.24) is also effective. If itching of the local area occurs, hip bath can be done with decoction made from *Ku Shen* (Radix Sophorae Flavescentis) (15 grams) and *She Chuang Zi* (Fructus Cnidii Monnieri) (25 grams).

7) Dysmenorrhea

a. *Menjin* (66.05) (specially good effect).
b. *Mufu* (66.02).
c. *Fuke* (11.24) (specially good effect).

Menjin (66.05) is an effective point for dysmenorrhea since it can relieve pain, soothe the liver *qi* and regulate the liver and spleen. *Neiting* (ST 44), which lies just in front of *Menjin* (66.05), is also quite effective. *Fuke* (11.24) is the main point for gynecopathy and is also effective for dysmenorrhea. Generally speaking, *Menjin* (66.05) is used to treat acute painful diseases and *Fuke* (11.24) is for the chronic ones. All the diseases of the uterus can be treated with *Fuke* (11.24).

8) Difficult Labor

a. *Huobao* (55.01).

Huobao (55.01) as a point from Tung's extraordinary points is used for difficult labor. Generally, *Zhiyin* (BL 67) and *Sanyinjiao* (SP 6) from the fourteen regular meridians are used for this disease. Ancient people used to use *Hegu* (LI 4) and *Sanyinjiao* (SP 6) for abortion. *Huobao* (55.01), *Zhiyin* (BL 67) and *Sanyinjiao* (SP 6) used together are quite effective for difficult labor. *Huobao* (55.01) alone is effective but it is better to combine it with *Sanyinjiao* (SP 6).

I met with a case of difficult labor in 1998 when I was giving volunteer treatment in northern Burma. A pregnant woman was having difficult labor after three days of delivery pains and I was asked to help. I used *Huobao* (55.01), *Zhiyin* (BL 67) and *Sanyinjiao* (SP 6) and the position of the fetus returned to the normal position in less than an hour so that the woman finally had a smooth labor.

These points have the effect of relieving the obstruction in the lower energizer and regulating the function of the uterus. They can also be used to treat retention of placenta. As for Chinese herbal medicine, I use *Zhang* Zhongjing's *Tuo Hua Jian* (Decoction for Difficult Labor) with good result. The components of this recipe include *Dang Gui* (Radix Angelicae Sinensis), *Rou Gui* (Cortex Cinnamomi Cassiae), *Chuan Xiong* (Rhizoma Ligustici Chuanxiong), *Niu Xi* (Radix Achyranthis Bidentatae), *Che Qian Zi* (Semen Plantaginis) and *Hong Hua* (Flos Carthami Tinctorii), all of which can be used to treat difficult labor.

9) Long-lasting Infertility

a. *Fuke* (11.24) (specially good effect).
b. *Huanchao* (11.06).
c. Bilateral alternate use of *Fuke* (11.24) and *Huanchao* (11.06) (better effect).

Fuke (11.24) and *Huanchao* (11.06) are most effective for infertility, and not any of the points from the fourteen regular meridians are comparable with these two points. The theories of Chinese medicine state that long-lasting infertility is in most cases accompanied by blood stasis and therefore in treating this disease bloodletting can be performed between medial malleolu and *Sanyinjiao* (SP 6) before *Fuke* (11.24) and *Huanchao* (11.06) are used. The two points can be used alternately, i.e. left *Fuke* (11.24) and right *Huanchao* (11.06) at a time and vice versa. It is preferable to give treatment everyday or every other day, which was the case 30 years ago, with good results. Nowadays people are too busy to receive treatment so frequently and of course it takes longer to see the therapeutic effect, two to three months for young people and four to five months for older women. Generally the younger the patient results in a better the therapeutic effect and vice versa. A 28-year-old woman who has not been pregnant for eight years, for example, is treated more effectively than a 30-year-old newlywed. This shows that it doesn't matter how long you have been married, but age is an important factor. For older patients, the needle should be retained for longer time and the treatment is to be given mainly to activate blood circulation and resolve phlegm, and also to regulate the liver and kidney. Infertility due to oviduct obstruction is best treated with *Fuke* (11.24) and *Huanchao* (11.06). It doesn't matter if a patient who is unaware of her own pregnancy continues to use these two points, since they have dual-regulating effect, being also able to prevent abortion. Both *Fuke* (11.24) and *Huanchao* (11.06) can reinforce the liver and kidney, regulate the flow of *qi*, activate blood circulation and resolve phlegm, and are very good point for women's diseases. *Fuke* (11.24) is on the Lung Meridian and therefore can regulate the flow of *qi*. *Huanchao* (11.06) is on the Triple Energizer Meridian and can regulate the flow of *qi* and resolve phlegm. Through internal organs, *Fuke* (11.24) is connected with the kidney and can reinforce the liver and kidney, and *Huanchao* (11.06) is connected with the bladder, which includes the uterus according to the theories of Chinese medicine. For example, the syndrome of blood retention among the syndromes of *Taiyang fu*-organ in *Shang Han Lun* (Treatise on Febrile Diseases) include blood retention in the uterus, which can be treated with Tao *Hong Cheng Qi Tang* (Decoction of Semen Persicae and Flos Carthami Tinctorii for Purgation). As another example, both *Tao Hong Cheng Qi Tang* (Decoction of Semen Persicae and Flos Carthami Tinctorii for Purgation) and *Gui Zhi Fu Ling Wan* (Pill of Ramulus Cinnamomi Cassiae and Sclerotium Poriae Cocos) commonly used for women's diseases include *Gui Zhi* (Ramulus Cinnamomi Cassiae), which is a drug for *Taiyang* Meridian.

Since there are many different causes of infertility, treatment should be given accordingly. For instance, it is complicated to consider using drugs to promote ovulation if corpus luteal hormone does not solve the problem, but the problem is easily solved by using acupuncture with the points mentioned above. For infertility due to emotional depression and stress, *Xiao Yao San* (Ease Powder) and *Dang Gui Shao Yao Tang* (Decoction of Radix Angelicae Sinensis and Paeonia lactiflora Pall) can be used in combination with *Tu Si Zi* (Semen Cuscutae Chinensis), *Xian Ling Pi* (tip of Radix Angelicae Sinensis) and *Zi Shi Ying* (Amethystum) to reinforce the kidney and warm the uterus. I used this method to treat many patients, mostly due to deficiency of the liver and kidney and accumulation of cold in the uterus. During 30 plus years of clinical practice, I have used *Wen Jing Tang* (Decoction for Warming Uterus) from *Jin Kui Yao Lue* (Synopsis of Prescriptions of Golden Chamber) to treat many patients. Sometimes infertility is caused by oligozoospermia in the male, and male infertility should be treated, using *Liu Er Wu Tang* (Six Two Five Decoction), i.e. *Liu Wei Di Huang Wan* (Pill of Six Drugs Including Radix Rehmanniae), *Er Xian Tang* (Decoction of Rhizoma Curculiginis Orchioidis and Tip of Radix Angelicae Sinensis) and *Wu Zi Yan Zong Wan* (Pill of Five Drugs for Infertility). Generally, after taking these recipes for two months, the patient will have enough sperm for pregnancy.

To treat metrorrhagia, *Sanchayi* (A.02) can be used to invigorate *qi* and induce astringency. Its location corresponds with the extraordinary point *Duanhong*, a common point for metrorrhagia. As for points from the regular fourteen meridians, *Dadun* (LR 1) is the best point and *Yinbai* (SP 1) is also effective. Chinese medicine holds that "the liver stores blood and the spleen controls blood." Metrorrhagia is related to the liver and spleen, and since *Dadun* (LR 1) is the *Jing*-Well point of the Liver Meridian and *Yinbai* (SP 1) is the *Jing*-Well point of the Spleen Meridian, both can be used to treat acute cases. To treat the disease with Chinese drugs, *Jiao Ai Si Wu Tang* (Decoction of Four Main Ingredients Including Colla Corii Asini and Folium Artemisiae Argyi) can be used to arrest bleeding followed by *Dang Gui Shao Yao San* (Powder of Radix Angelicae Sinensis and Paeonia lactiflora Pall) to regulate blood. The reason why powder is used is that decoction may have adverse effect of failure to stop bleeding. To regulate menstruation, just use *Fuke* (11.24) and *Huanchao* (11.06), or use *Dang Gui Shao Yao San* (Powder of Radix Angelicae Sinensis and Paeonia lactiflora Pall). It is important to determine the nature of the menstruation. Premenstrual period is due to heat and *Quchi* (LI 11), *Hegu* (LI 4) and *Sanyinjiao* (SP 6) can be used; delayed menstrual period is often due to cold, and *Linggu* (22.05), *Shenguan* (77.18) and *Sanyinjiao* (SP 6) can be used. Irregular menstrual period is often caused by disorder of liver *qi*, and this is treated with *Hegu* (LI 4), *Taichong* (LR 3) and *Sanyinjiao* (SP 6). For heat syndromes, use *Dan Zhi Xiao Yao San* (Powder of Cortex Moutan Radicis and Fructus Gardeniae Jasminoidis); for cold syndromes, use herbs for warming and invigorating purposes.

3. APOPLEXY

1) Apoplexy (coma)

a. Prick the twelve *Jing*-Well points (bloodletting).
b. *Renzhong* (DU26), *Neiguan* (PC 6), *Yongquan* (KI 1) and *Taichong* (LR 3).
c. *Zhenghui* (1010.01), *Qianhui* (1010.05), *Houhui* (1010.06) and *Linggu* (22.05).

At the acute phase of apoplexy, coma may occur, which can be treated with either acupuncture or Chinese drugs, with good results. It is commonly known that apoplexy with coma can be treated by pricking the twelve *Jing*-Well points to let out blood. According to *Shang Han Lun* (Treatise on Febrile Diseases), "coma occurs when *yin* and *yang* fail to connect with each other." The *Jing*-Well points are the starting or terminating points of the meridians, and pricking these points may "connect *yin* and *yang*." According to *Nei Jing* (Yellow Emperor's Inner Classic), "to treat diseases of the *zang*-organ, use the *Jing*-Well points." It follows that the *Jing*-Well points are especially effective for an acute case of apoplexy. Sometimes it is inconvenient to use the points on the foot, and points on the hand are more often used. The points on the foot can be used selectively, e.g. Dadun (LR 1), *Yinbao* (LR 9) and *Lidui* (ST 45) used first, followed by other points such as *Baihui* (DU 20), *Renzhong* (DU 26), *Neiguan* (PC 6) and *Taichong* (LR 3).

Over the past 30 years, I have treated many patients with apoplexy, including those with coma or hemiplegia. In 1980, I treated a patient named Ruan, who was in coma with dysuria and high B.U.N. level. I performed bloodletting at all the *Jing*-Well points on the hand and *Dadun* (LR 1), *Yinbao* (LR 9) and *Lidui* (ST 45) on the foot. Then, I give an acupuncture treatment at *Baihui* (DU 20), *Neiguan* (PC 6) and *Yongquan* (KI 1). I didn't use *Renzhong* (DU 26) because the patient was wearing an oxygen hood tent. After that, I tube fed the patient with *An Gong Niu Huang Wan* (Pill of Calculus Bovis for Resurrection). Soon afterwards the patient could pass water freely and B.U.N. level went down greatly. I continued to use *An Gong Niu Huang Wan* (Pill of Calculus Bovis for Resurrection) and he regained consciousness on the third day.

Another case involved a woman named Wan, who was in coma for over fifty days caused by angioma rupture due to brain vein malformation. I also treated her with bloodletting at the *Jing*-Well points and prescriptions for activating blood circulation and resolving phlegm. *An Gong Niu Huang Wan* (Pill of Calculus Bovis for Resurrection) was not used since this prescription works well soon after coma occurs and the patient had been in coma for two or three months. Instead, I used *Er Chen Tang* (Decoction of Two Old Drugs) to resolve phlegm and *San Qi Fen*

(Powder of Radix Notoginseng) to activate blood circulation. Later I also used *Gua Lou* (Fructus Trichosanthis) to resolve phlegm and *Da Huang* (Radix et Rhizoma Rhei) to relax the bowels and promote blood circulation. I also used *Ting Li Zi* (Semen Lepidii seu Descurainiae) and *Long Dan Cao* (Radix Gentianae), and these two drugs played a very important part in curing the disease. According to *Shang Han Lun* (Treatise on Febrile Diseases), *Ting Li Da Zao Tang* (Decoction of Semen Lepidii seu Descurainiae and Fructus Zizyphi Jujubae) can be used to treat hydrothorax, suggesting that *Ting Li Zi* (Semen Lepidii seu Descurainiae) is a good herb for fluid retention in the upper part of the body. *Long Dan Cao* (Radix Gentianae) can purge the liver fire, and the two herbs used together are very effective for brain edema with brain hypertension in coma patients. Finally the patient regained consciousness after the ninth day of coma.

In fact, the patient became partially conscious in the course of the treatment. After coma was completely gone, I tried to treat hemiplegia as the sequela of the disease, and the patient gradually fully recovered. In a word, herbs for activating blood circulation and resolve phlegm can cure many unusual diseases.

2) Hemiplegia

a. *Linggu* (22.05) and *Dabai* (22.04) (especially effective).
b. *Jiuli* (88.25, 88.26, 88.27) with point-coupling technique (especially effective).
c. bilateral *Chongzi* (22.01) and *Chongxian* (22.02) (very effective).
d. *Shenguan* (77.18).
e. *Zhenghui* (1010.01) and *Houhui* (1010.06).
f. *Wuling* (DT.04) (bloodletting).

Hemiplegia responds well to Chinese medicine, especially acupuncture, which is far more effective than western medicine. The first point to use is *Muhuo* (11.10), which should be used only several times and should not be used any longer. We use *Muhuo* (11.10) because apoplexy is closely related to the liver wind and phlegm fire, and is sometimes caused by the falling off of the heart thrombus. Also, all the *yang* meridians reach the head and the Pericardium and Liver Meridians among the *yin* meridians also reach the head. Acupuncture at *Muhuo* (11.10), therefore, corresponds with the liver (wood) and the pericardium (fire). Besides, this point is adjacent to the *Jing*-Well point of the Pericardium Meridian, just between the *Jing*-Well (wood) point and the *Ying*-Spring point (fire), and that is why it is called *Muhuo* (wood-fire) in Chinese. Since *Jing*-Well points can treat mental diseases, it is very effective for apoplexy. According to Master Tung's experience, *Muhuo* (11.10) should not be used too many times and the needling time should not be long. For apoplexy with hemiplegia, the first treatment with this point is about seven to eight minutes, and then *Linggu* (22.05), *Dabai* (22.04) and preferably *Qili* (A.01) and *Jiuli* (88.25, 88.26, 88.27) with point-coupling technique can be used. *Linggu* (22.05) and *Dabai* (22.04) are mainly used to treat weakness and spasm of the lower limbs, and of the upper limbs as well. They are the most effective points for hemiplegia. For weakness and spasm of the upper limbs, *Qili* (A.01) and *Jiuli* (88.25, 88.26, 88.27) are also effective. The needling time of *Muhuo* (11.10) should be five to six minutes during the second and third sessions of treatment, four to five minutes during the fourth and fifth sessions and three to four minutes during the sixth and seventh sessions. Severe cases can be treated by bloodletting at *Wuling* (DT.04) at the back every week or every 15 days.

Early treatment is very important. The following conditions can certainly be cured. The first is early treatment given within three months after the onset of apoplexy, certainly with good effect. Very good effect can also be obtained as long as the patient receives treatment within six months after the onset. The second is related to the age. Good effect can be obtained for patients under 60 years of age, and apoplexy patients are mostly between 50 to 60 years old. There are also many patients about 60 to 70 years of age, and the earlier the treatment, the better the effect. As a rule, the effect of treatment for the first attack is the best; the effect is less satisfactory for the second attack, and even worse for the third attack. Generally speaking, acupuncture treatment for apoplexy should be given mainly on the unaffected side of the body, but for chronic cases (two or three years), the affected side should also be punctured to achieve better effect. During the first attack, many patients have paralysis only on one side, but during the second attack, both sides are affected. Physiotherapy is given to some patients but the effect is not so satisfactory. Chinese medicine, especially acupuncture, is absolutely superior to western medicine in this area. It is still possible to cure apoplexy lasting for two or three years, but the treatment takes longer time and Chinese herbs should be used in conjunction with acupuncture. Therefore, getting treatment earlier is the better.

Linggu (22.05) and *Dabai* (22.04) are very effective for hemiplegia, more effective than *Quchi* (LI 11), *Yanglingquan* (GB 34), *Xuanzhong* (GB 39) and *Taichong* (LR 3). In fact, *Linggu* (22.05) and *Dabai* are a group of “wood-fire points,” similar to *Muhuo* (11.10). *Dabai* (22.04), a wood point according to the theory of the five elements, is close to *Sanjian* (LI 3) of the Large Intestine Meridian, and *Linggu* (22.05), a fire point, is close to *Yangxi* (LI 5). The two points used together with point-coupling technique can treat both wood and fire. *Muhuo* (11.10) on the middle finger connects with the Foot *Jueyin* Meridian (Liver Meridian) through the Hand *Jueyin* Meridian (Pericardium Meridian), and therefore can be used to treat liver wind. *Linggu* (22.05) and *Dabai* (22.04) on the Large Intestine Meridian connect with the large intestine through the liver and therefore can also be used to treat liver wind. Besides, *Dabai* (22.04) is related to the lung, and since the large intestine and the lung are internally and externally related to each other, points on the Large Intestine Meridian can also be used to treat lung diseases or invigorate *qi*. *Linggu* (22.05) should be inserted just against the bone, which corresponds with the kidney, and can be used to reinforce the kidney *qi*. Thus, *Linggu* (22.05) and *Dabai* (22.04) are a group of points very effective for apoplexy since they can be used to reinforce the spleen, liver, kidney, *qi* and blood. Generally speaking, doctors would like to use *Bu Yang Huan Wu Tang* (Decoction for Invigorating *Yang* for Recuperation) to treat apoplexy, but I prefer to use *Zhen Wu Tang* (Decoction for Strengthening Spleen *Yang*) as well to enhance the effect. The former is effective in invigorating *qi* and activating blood circulation, while the latter can warm the kidney yang and invigorate both the liver and kidney. These two recipes are important ones for hemiplegia. Kidney deficiency, a common cause of hemiplegia, can be dealt with by using *Shenguan* (77.18) in the lower limbs or *Shuitong* (1010.19) and *Shuijin* (1010.20) on the face to enhance the effect of invigorating the kidney. Besides, *Jiuli* (88.25, 88.26, 88.27), *Qili* (A.01), *Zhenghui* (1010.01) and *Houhui* (1010.06) with point-coupling technique are all the points Master Tung frequently used to treat the disease. Several groups of points can be selected and used alternately, but *Linggu* (22.05) and *Dabai* (22.04) are certainly the most important and most commonly used points.

3) Apoplexy with Aphasia

a. *Zhenghui* (1010.01) and *Houhui* (1010.06).
b. Prick to let out blood.

To treat apoplexy with aphasia, *Zhenghui* (1010.01) should be punctured first and then *Houhui* (1010.06), followed by *Shangqiu* (SP 5), the *Jing*-River point of the Spleen Meridian, which connects with the root of the tongue. It is stated in *Nei Jing* (Yellow Emperor's Inner Classic) that "*Jing*-River points can be used to treat disorders of the voice." Pricking *Zongshu* (1010.07), *Fengfu* (DU16) and *Yamen* (DU 15) to let out blood is also quite effective. This method also works for apoplexy with dysphagia, or supranuclear paralysis. The best recipe for the disease is *Di Huang Yin Zi* (Decoction of Radix Rehmanniae), which can be used in combination with bloodletting at *Fengfu* (DU 16) and *Yamen* (DU 15). The ingredients of *Di Huang Yin Zi* (Decoction of Radix Rehmanniae) include *Ba Ji Tian* (Radix Morindae Officinalis) and *Rou Gui* (Cortex Cinnamomi Cassiae) for warming *yang* and *Di Huang* (Radix Rehmanniae) for nourishing *yin*. Most cases are due to *yang* deficiency and are treated with *Bu Yang Huan Wu Tang* (Decoction for Invigorating

Yang for Recuperation) and *Zhen Wu Tang* (Decoction for Strengthening Spleen *Yang*) used in combination, while those with *yin* deficiency are treated more effectively with *Di Huang Yin Zi* (Decoction of Radix Rehmanniae). *Zongshu* (1010.07), which is between *Fengfu* (DU 16) and *Yamen* (DU15), *Fengfu* (DU 16) and *Yamen* (DU 15) are the most frequently used points for apoplexy with aphasia.

4) Limb Tremor (Parkinson's syndrome)

a. *Shenguan* (77.18), *Fuliu* (KI 7) and *Minghuang* (88.12).
b. *Minghuang* (88.12), *Qihuang* (88.14) and *Shenguan* (77.18).
c. *Zhenghui* (1010.01), *Qianhui* (1010.05) and *Muzhi* (1010.18).

Limb tremor, including Parkinson's syndrome, is in most cases due to *yin* deficiency, and a minority of cases is due to "deficiency of *yang* and stirring of wind." Acupuncture is quite effective for this kind of diseases of the neurological system, but it takes relatively longer time to treat those due to deficiency of *yin* and stirring of wind with acupuncture. Chinese medicine believes that limb tremor is related to the liver and kidney. In *Bing Ji Shi Jiu Tiao* (Pathogenesis No. 19) from *Nei Jing* (Yellow Emperor's Inner Classic), it is said that "the various kinds of trembling and dizziness due to wind are related to the liver" and "the various kinds of trembling and dizziness due to cold is related to the kidney." Since most patients with Parkinson's syndrome are due to wind and deficiency of *yin* of the liver kidney, treatment should be given to treat both the liver and kidney. In using acupuncture, the main principle is "two liver points and one kidney point" or "two kidney points and one liver point." *Shenguan* (77.18) and *Fuliu* (KI 7) are points for reinforcing the kidney; *Minghuang* (88.12) and *Qihuang* (88.14) are points for the liver. In treatment, two kidney points, *Shenguan* (77.18) and *Fuliu* (KI 7) or *Taixi* (KI 3), and one liver point, *Minghuang* (88.12) or *Qihuang* (88.14) or *Taichong* (LR 3), are used at one time, and at another time, two liver points, *Minghuang* (88.12) and *Qihuang* (88.14) or *Taichong* (LR 3), and one kidney point, *Shenguan* (77.18) or *Fuliu* (KI 7) or *Taixi* (KI 3) are used. This method used alternately is quite effective. Besides, *Zhenghui* (1010.01) and *Houhui* (1010.06) can be used to enhance the sedative effect, and can also be added to treat senile asthenia and dispel wind. These Tung's extraordinary points can be used together with the points from the fourteen regular meridians, with good effect. Thus, *Hegu* (LI 4) and *Taichong* (LR 3) can be used together with *Sanyinjiao* (SP 6). In scalp acupuncture, Tung's extraordinary points can be used together with these points at the tremor control area, and Tung's extraordinary points can be used alternately. For *yang* deficiency with stirring of mild wind accompanied by aversion to cold, *Zhen Wu Tang* (Decoction for Strengthening Spleen *Yang*) can be used with modification; for *yin* deficiency with stirring of wind, *Tian Ma* (Rhizoma Gastrodiae Elatae), *Gou Teng* (Ramulus

Uncariae cum Uncis) and *Ling Yang Jiao* (Cornu Saigae Tataricae) can be used in combination. Besides, drugs from shells such as *Mu Li* (Concha Ostreae), *Gui Ban* (Plastrum Testudinis), *Bie Jia* (Carapax Trionycis), *Shi Jue Ming* (Concha Haliotidis) and *Zhen Zhu Mu* (Concha Margaritifera Usta) can also be used. These drugs have sedative effect and can be used to "control mobility with tranquility." Other drugs such as *Quan Xie* (Buthus Martensi), *Wu Gong* (Scolopendra Subspinipes), *Jiang Can* (Bombyx Batryticatus) and *Di Long* (Pheretima) can be used to "control mobility with mobility." In addition, *Mu Gua* (Fructus Chaenomelis), *Shao Yao* (Paeonia lactiflora Pall), *Gan Cao* (Radix Glycyrrhizae Uralensis) and other related herbs can be used to suppress liver wind. At the late stage of the treatment, drugs for reinforcing the kidney *yin*, like *Di Huang* (Radix Rehmanniae) and *He Shou Wu* (Radix Polygoni Multiflori), and drugs for nourishing blood and dispel wind, like *Dang Gui* (Radix Angelicae Sinensis) and *Dan Shen* (Radix Salviae Miltiorrhizae) can be used.

The most commonly used recipes for the disease are *Ding Zhen Wan* (Pill for Easing Tremor), *San Jia Fu Mai Tang* (Decoction of Three Shell Drugs) and *Da Ding Feng Zhu* (Great Pearl for Wind Syndrome), the first being a recipe from *Zheng Zhi Zhun Sheng* (Standards of Diagnosis and Treatment), and the second and the third being recipes from *Wen Bing Tiao Bian* (Treatise on Differentiation and Treatment of Epidemic Febrile Diseases). *San Jia Fu Mai Tang* (Decoction of Three Shell Drugs) is in fact *Zhi Gan Cao Tang* (Decoction of Radix Glycyrrhizae Uralensis Praeparata) plus the three shell drugs, i.e. *Mu Li* (Concha Ostreae), *Gui Ban* (Plastrum Testudinis) and *Bie Jia* (Carapax Trionycis), with astringing and tranquilizing effect.

5) Apoplexy with Hand Convulsion

a. *Chongzi* (22.01) and *Chongxian* (22.02) on the opposite side.
b. Bloodletting at *Quling* (33.16).

Chongzi (22.01) and *Chongxian* (22.02) on the opposite side can be used to treat this disease. In a severe case, *Chize* (LU 5) on the affected side can be used, either by bloodletting or needling with reducing method. Bloodletting is more effective and puncturing *Chize* (LU 5) follows the principle of "treating tendon with tendon," since this point is just next to the great tendon. *Chize* (LU 5) is also the water point or the son point of the metal meridian and therefore can be used to reduce the metal, making it unable to control wood, and as a result the wood or rather the tendon is at ease. This method is also effective for frozen shoulder. Needling *Chize* (LU 5) with reducing method can soothe the liver and bloodletting at the point can activating blood circulation to remove blood stasis, both being good methods for this disease. The disease is very difficult to treat in those whose shoulders drop down two or three finger breadth.

4. Miscellaneous Diseases

1) Hypertension

a. *Wuling* (DT.04) [1.5 inches lateral to the line from the fourth to the seventh thoracic vertebrae, *Jueyinshu* (BL 14) and *Geshu* (BL 17) on the Bladder Meridian], bloodletting along the line between *Huoyun* (DT.IV) and *Tuxie* (DT.X).
b. Bloodletting at *Weizhong* (BL 40) just on the blue vein.
c. Bloodletting at *Sihuazhong* (77.09) and *Sihuawai* (77.14).
d. *Zhongbai* (22.06).
e. Bloodletting at the tip of the ear.
f. Bloodletting at *Taiyang*.
g. *Huoju* (66.11) and *Huoying* (66.03).

The Medical Society of the United States has recently re-formulated a new standard for hypertension. The normal blood pressure is between 80 systolic pressure and 120 diastolic pressures. Those with a blood pressure range of between 80-90 systolic pressure and 120-135 diastolic pressure are considered to have “pre-hypertension,” the former standard for which was between 90 systolic pressure and 140 diastolic pressure.

Hypertension responds well to bloodletting therapy. *Zhongbai* (22.06), *Xiabai* (22.07), *Huoju* (66.11) and *Huoying* (66.03) are all very effective for the disease. When bloodletting is given, the common points include *Sihuazhong* (77.09), *Sihuawai* (77.14), *Weizhong* (BL 40), *Wuling* (DT.04), *Quchi* (LI 11) and *Xingjian* (LR 2). *Huoju* (66.11) is close to *Gongsun* (SP 4) and is also effective for hypertension. Part of its Chinese meaning is chrysanthemum, which has the effect of lowering blood pressure. Diastolic pressure in most cases involves the heart and systolic pressure, the kidney. Most hypotension patients have kidney diseases with edema or uremia. On the other hand, heart diseases are mostly accompanied by hypertension (high diastolic pressure). Renal hypertension can be treated with acupuncture at *Shenguan* (77.18), *Yinlingquan* (SP 9) and *Taixi* (KI 3), which are also effective for edema and albuminuria. For those with high diastolic pressure, the heart blood vessels are affected and should be treated. This is related to long-lasting emotional tension and the etiology may include incoordination between *yin* and *yang* in the liver and kidney, or by accumulation of phlegm-dampness. In treatment, *Huoju* (66.11) and *Huosan* (66.10), or *Quchi* (LI 11), *Neiguan* (PC 6) and *Zusanli* (ST 36) can be used. For hypertension without kidney diseases, *Quchi* (LI 11), *Yanglingquan* (GB 34) and *Taichong* (LR 3) can be used with very good effect. For those with kidney disease accompanied by edema, points for the kidney should be added. The common syndromes of hypertension include hyperactivity of liver *yang* and deficiency of *yin* in the liver and kidney. Besides, deficiency of kidney *yang* may arise as a result of damage to *yin*. Recipes for hypotension include *Liu Wei Di Huang Tang* (Decoction of Six Herbs Including Radix Rehmanniae) and *Zhen Wu Tang* (Decoction for Strengthening Spleen *Yang*), which are also effective for parenchymatous kidney diseases. Alternatively, *Fang Ji Huang Qi Tang* (Decoction of Radix Stephaniae Tetrandrae and Radix Astragali seu Hedysari) and *Liu Wei Di Huang Tang* (Decoction of Six Drugs Including Radix Rehmanniae) can be used in combination. Ordinary hypertension can be treated with *Tian Ma Gou Teng Tang* (Decoction of Rhizoma Gastrodiae Elatae and Ramulus Uncariae cum Uncis), and also with the Chinese drugs like *Ju Hua* (Flos Chrysanthemi Morifolii), *Gou Teng* (Ramulus Uncariae cum Uncis), *Shi Jue Ming* (Concha Haliotidis), *Huang Qin* (Radix Scutellariae Baicalensis), *Du Zhong* (Cortex Eucommiae), *Sang Ji Sheng* (Ramulus Loranthi) and *Ze Xie* (Rhizoma Alismatis Orientalitis). It is comparatively easier to treat a hypertension at the onset than a chronic one. Some hypertension is secondary to brain traumatic injury, brain tumor or diseases of the endocrine system, and therefore should be treated accordingly.

2) Jaundice

a. *Shangsanhuang* (88.12, 13, 14).

Jaundice appears when the liver and gallbladder are diseased. For chronic hepatitis with jaundice, *Shangsanhuang* (88.12, 13, 14) can be used; for acute hepatitis the best points are *Ganmen* (33.11) and *Changmen* (33.10). *Wangu* (GB 12), the *Yuan*-Source point of the small intestine which is capable of distinguishing between the clear and the turbid, is also effective. *Ganmen* (33.11) is on the Small Intestine Meridian and also on the middle portion of the forearm corresponding with the liver, and therefore it is also effective for liver diseases. According to ancient medical books, "*Wangu* (GB 12) can treat jaundice" and "*Zhiyang* (DU 9), which is just below the seventh thoracic vertebra, has the effect of activating yang and removing dampness and is an important point for treating jaundice."

3) Diabetes

a. *Xiasanhuang* (77.18, 19, 21) (with medially perpendicular insertion of the needle), together with *Tongshen* (88.09) if great thirst occurs.

The commonest method of Chinese medicine to treat diabetes is to "invigorate *qi* and nourish *yin*," or rather, invigorating *qi* of the spleen and lung and nourishing the kidney *yin*. Diabetes is likely to occur when both the spleen and the kidney are deficient and most diabetes patients have deficiency of the spleen and the kidney. Thirst is a symptom of kidney deficiency. *Shenguan* (77.18) and *Tianhuang* (77.17) are quite effective for the disease. According to *Jing Xue Pian* (On Meridians and Points),

Tianhuang (77.17) is the main point for diabetes. When *Tianhuang* (77.17), which is the water point of the Spleen Meridian and coincides with *Yinlingquan* (SP 9) of the Spleen Meridian, is used together with *Shenguan* (77.18) (point-coupling technique) they can "reinforce both the spleen and kidney." *Xiasanhuang* (77.18, 19, 21) are also very effective and *Tongshen* (88.09) can be added if thirst occurs. *Chengjiang* (REN 24) and *Yangchi* (SJ4) from the fourteen regular meridians are also effective. *Chengjiang* (REN 24) is the *Jing*-Well point of the Conception Vessel and can invigorate *yin*; it is also at the crossing point of the *Yangming* Meridians of Hand and Foot, and so it can regulate the flow of *qi* and blood; through the crossing point of the Stomach and Large Intestine Meridians it is internally and externally related to the lung and the spleen, and therefore it can invigorate the two organs, reinforce *qi* and nourish *yin*. Since it is a point that can reinforce both *qi* and *yin*, it is a good point for diabetes. As for *Yangchi* (SJ4) of the Triple Energizer (*San Jiao*) Meridian, Japanese has said, "In systemic treatment, *Yangchi* (SJ 4) and *Zhongwan* (REN 12) are absolutely indispensable, and stimulating *Yangchi* (SJ 4) has the effect of regulating the functions of the internal organs. According to *Yi Zong Jin Jian* (The Golden Mirror of Medicine), *Yangchi* (SJ 4) is the main point for diabetes since it can regulate the *qi* of the triple energizer. *Yangchi* (SJ 4) is a *Yuan*-Source point and an earth point, and since a *Yuan*-Source point correspond with *qi* stored between the kidneys, it can regulate *qi* and reinforce the kidney. *Yangchi* (SJ 4) is the point that the Japanese use most frequently, and since it is connected with the triple energizer through the kidney, it can reinforce the kidney. Also, since it is an earth point, it can reinforce both the spleen and the kidney. It is generally believed that in treating diabetes, one should reinforce the spleen and nourish *yin* and herbs for warming *yang* is seldom used. This is also the case with acupuncture, as "the principles used in pharmacotherapy also apply to acupuncture. Chinese drug recipes for the disease include *Mai Wei Di Huang Tang* (Decoction of Radix Ophiopogonis, Fructus Schisandrae Chinensis and Radix Rehmanniae), which is effective for nourishing *yin*, but not so effective for invigorating the spleen *qi*. Therefore, *Huang Qi* (Radix Astragali seu Hedysari) and *Dang Shen* (Radix Codonopsis Pilosulae) should be added. In addition, other herbs can also be added, like *Zhi Mu* (Rhizoma Anemarrhenae Asphodeloidis), *Xuan Shen* (Radix Scrophulariae Ningpoensis) and *Tian Hua Fen* (Radix Trichosanthis Kirilowii) for clearing away fire, *Dan Shen* (Radix Salviae Miltiorrhizae) for activating blood circulation, and *Cang Zhu* (Rhizoma Atractylodis) for invigorating the spleen. Thus these twelve or thirteen kinds of drugs form a very good recipe for diabetes. As long as insulin is not used in the treatment, Chinese medicine treatment is very effective for diabetes even if the blood sugar level is three to four hundred. The therapeutic effect is achieved very quickly for those with the blood sugar level of one to two hundred. Some patients whose blood sugar level is three to four hundred have the normal blood sugar level after receiving treatment for several months. When diabetes is accompanied by hypertension, apoplexy is likely to occur. In such a case, *Bai Hu Jia Ren Shen Tang* (White Tiger Decoction with Radix Ginseng) and *Ge Geng Qin Lian Tang* (Radix Puerariae, Radix Scutellariae Baicalensis and Rhizoma Coptidis) can be used in combination, the former for diabetes and the latter for hypertension. The two recipes used together are quite effective.

It is sometimes said that both cancer and diabetes are incurable. However, some cancer and diabetes patients can live to eighty or ninety. Diet control is very important for diabetes patients, and besides a balanced diet, exercise is also very important. Acupuncture and herbs are effective for diabetes, but if no due attention is paid to diet and exercise, recurrence may follow, making it difficult to cure the disease.

4) Limb Edema

a. *Xiasanhuang* (77.18, 19, 21) and *Tongtian* (88.03).

Limb edema here refers to edema caused by nephritis. Whether an acute or a chronic case, *Tongshen* (88.09) and *Tongwei* (88.10) or *Xiasanhuang* (77.18, 19, 21) can be used. For simple leg edema, *Tongtian* (88.03), or *Tianhuang* and (77.17) *Sihuashang* (77.08), or *Zusanli* (ST 36) and *Yinlingquan* (SP 9) can be used. To treat acute nephritis, *Yue Bi Jia Zhu Tang* (Decoction for Relieving Edema with Rhizoma Atractylodis Macrocephalae) plus *Bai Mao Gen* (Rhizoma Imperatae Cylindricae) can be used to promote dispersing function of the lung and invigorate the spleen; to treat chronic nephritis, *Zhen Wu Tang* (Decoction for Strengthening Spleen *Yang*) can be used with modification to treat the spleen and stomach, and *Gui Shao Zhi Mu Tang* (Decoction of Ramulus Cinnamomi Cassiae, Paeonia lactiflora Pall and Rhizoma Anemarrhenae Asphodeloidis) can also be used in combination.

5) Urticaria

a. Bloodletting along the line between *Tianhuang* (77.17) and *Renhuang* (77.21), and at *Menjin* (66.05), followed by acupuncture at *Sima* (88.17, 88.18, 88.19) and *Jiuli* (88.25, 88.26, 88.27).
b. Bloodletting at ear back (especially effective) followed by acupuncture at *Sima* (88.17, 88.18, 88.19) and *Jiuli* (88.25, 88.26, 88.27).

The simplest method to treat this disease is to prick the back of the ear and tip to let out blood, and then use acupuncture at *Sima* (88.17, 88.18, 88.19) or *Jiuli* (88.25, 88.26, 88.27). *Quchi* (LI 11) and *Xuehai* (SP 10) from the fourteen regular meridians are also effective. In needling these two points, one should use the method of reducing the *ying* system, i.e. "to acquire *qi* from the *ying* system in reducing method," a method similar to the cool-producing method at the withdrawal of the needle in order to cool heat in the blood. As an example, if the needle is to be retained for 30 minutes, then the needle should be withdrawn one third of its depth ten minutes after the insertion, and then it is withdrawn another one third after another ten minutes and finally it is completely withdrawn at the end of the 30 minutes. This method can also be used when *Quchi* (LI 11) or *Xuehai* (SP 10) are used alone, but normally the combination of the two points produced a better effect. Even a better effect can be achieved if *Sanyinjiao* (SP 6) is also used. *Quchi* (LI 11) is the *He*-Sea point of the *Yangming* Meridian of Hand, which is full of *qi* and blood, and therefore this point is effective in regulating the flow of *qi* and blood. Also, there is thick muscle at the location of this point and therefore acupuncture at this point can invigorate the spleen *qi*. Since the large intestine and the lung are internally and externally related, *Quchi* (LI 11) is an important point for skin diseases. *Xuehai* (SP 10) and *Sanyinjiao* (SP 6) are used mainly to regulate the blood system, and "to treat wind one must treat blood, and free flow of blood leads to relief of wind." Urticaria appearing on the upper part of the body can be treated with *Jianzhong* (44.06), and on the lower part, *Jiuli* (88.25, 88.26, 88.27) or *Fengshi* (GB 31). As for herbs, *Xiao Feng San* (Powder for Dispelling Wind) and *Yin Qiao Liang Xue Tang* (Decoction of Flos Lonicerae and Fructus Forsythiae Suspensae for Cooling Blood) can be used for acute cases; *Dang Gui Yin Zi* (Decoction of Radix Angelicae Sinensis) can be used for chronic cases.

6) Insomnia

a. *Xiasanhuang* (77.18, 19, 21) and *Zhengjing* (1010.08) (extremely effective).
b. *Dabai* (22.04) and *Jiuli* (88.25, 88.26, 88.27) (very effective).
c. Bloodletting at the ear tip (specifically effective).

Acupuncture is very effective for insomnia. According to my experience, acupuncture treatment can achieve immediate effect. *Dabai* (22.04) and *Jiuli* (88.25, 88.26, 88.27) are very effective. *Jiangu*, which is between *Dabai* (22.04) and *Hegu* (LI 4), or between *Sanjian* (LI 3) and *Hegu* (LI 4), is also effective for insomnia. We all know that *Dabai* (22.04) is very effective for diseases of the upper energizer, *Hegu* (LI 4) is very effective for diseases of the middle energizer, and *Linggu* (22.05) is very effective for diseases of the lower energizer (such as sciatica). Insomnia with vexation and stuffy chest can be treated with *Jianggu* with very good effect. According to holographic correspondence, *Jianggu* corresponds with the heart and chest area, and therefore it is very effective for insomnia. The effect is more satisfactory if *Fengshi* (GB 31) is also used. In most cases, the therapeutic effect is achieved only after the patient receives treatment once.

Twenty years ago I used to treat insomnia with what I call *Siguan*, i.e. *Hegu* (LI 4) and *Taichong* (LR 3), later with *Jianggu* and *Taichong* (LR 3), and recently with *Jianggu* and *Xingjian* (LR 2). *Jianggu* is anterior to *Hegu* (LI 4) and *Xingjian* (LR 2) is anterior to *Taichong* (LR 3). Therefore I call this combination of *Hegu* (LI 4) and *Xingjian* (LR 2) *Siguan*. Anterior *Siguan* refers to *Xingjian* (LR 2) and *Jianggu*; the middle *Siguan* refers to *Hegu* (LI 4) and *Taichong*. *Siguan* has tranquilizing and antispasmodic effect and is effective for insomnia and also other diseases such as tremor of the hand and foot and Parkinson's syndrome. The posterior *Siguan*, i.e. *Linggu* (22.05) and *Huozhu* (66.04), is often used to treat diseases of the tendons and bones of the hand and foot and general joint pains, owing to the fact that the insertion of the needle at both points is just against the bones. Since they are related to wood, they are also effective for tendon problems and soreness of the whole body. *Huozhu* (66.04) is a point on the Liver Meridian (pertaining to wood) and can be used to treat tendon problems; it is near *Taichong* (LR 3) and is an earth point, and so it can be used to treat diseases of the spleen and muscle; it is near the bone and can treat the kidney. Therefore, this point can be used to treat the spleen, liver and kidney. *Linggu* (22.05) is connected to the large intestine through the Large Intestine Meridian and the liver, and can be used to treat the liver; since the needle is inserted against the bone at this point, it can treat diseases of the tendons and bones. *Linggu* (22.05) and *Huozhu* (66.04) used together can treat general joint pains and pains of the knee and elbow.

I often use *Jianggu* and *Xingjian* (LR 2) to treat insomnia, sometimes also with *Fengshi* (GB 31), with good effect. Some people think that it is difficult to treat *yin* deficiency with acupuncture, but acupuncture is quite effective for insomnia due to *yin* deficiency. Parkinson's syndrome is also due to *yin* deficiency, but it can be treated with acupuncture, and of course it takes longer. The reason why *Siguan* can treat many neurological diseases lies in the fact that *Hegu* (LI 4) is the *Yuan*-Source point of the Large Intestine Meridian (a *yang* meridian) and *Taichong* (LR 3) is the *Yuan*-Source point of the Liver Meridian (a *yin* meridian). Thus, one in the upper part and one in the lower part; one on the hand and one on the foot; one is a *zang* organ and one is a *fu* organ; and one pertains to *yin* and one pertains to *yang*. The combination of the two points has the joint effect of connecting the upper part and the lower part and connecting *yin* and *yang*, and so both *yin* and *yang* can be treated. Being both the *Yuan*-Source point, the primordial *qi* of which are connected with the triple energizer, they can effectively regulate the functional activities of *qi*. Also, since the Large Intestine Meridian can regulate *qi* and blood and the Liver Meridian can regulate blood and soothe the liver, these two points are the frequently used ones for regulating *qi* and blood and soothing liver *qi*. Neurologically speaking, the hand is an organ for work and the foot is one for exercise. They have multiple functions and thus have close connections with the brain, especially the thumb and the big toe. Therefore the responses at the hand and foot are very strong. Since *Hegu* (LI 4) and *Taichong* (LR 3) are *Yuan*-Source points closest to the big toe, they are most effective. Because of the strong functions of the big toe, *Dadun* (LR 1) and *Yinbai* (SP 1) on the big toe are also very important *Jing*-Well points.

Acupuncture treatment is very effective for chronic insomnia patient, who can sleep only two or three hours even if they take sleeping pills. Insomnia in young people is often due to stagnation of liver *qi* turning into fire, causing them to have difficulty falling asleep. This can be treated with *Si Ni San* (Powder for Treating Cold Limbs) or *Dan Zhi Xiao Yao San* (Powder of Cortex Moutan Radicis and Fructus Gardeniae Jasminoidis) to soothe the liver, and *Gan Mai Da Zao Tang* (Decoction of Radix Glycyrrhizae Uralensis, Fructus Tritici Aestivi Levis and Fructus Zizyphi Jujubae) for tranquilization. Insomnia in the elderly is often caused by deficiency of *yin* of the liver and kidney, causing them to wake up early. This should be treated by regulating the liver and kidney with *Qi Ju Di Huang Tang* (Decoction of Fructus Lycii, Flos Chrysanthemi Morifolii and Radix Rehmanniae). Acupuncture is still very effective for patients with a history of chronic insomnia for over ten or even twenty years, and they can also be treated with Chinese herbs such as *Xue Fu Zhu Yu Tang* (Decoction for Removing Blood Stasis in the Chest), which is also effective for insomnia with blood stasis. According to my experience, *Ban Xia* (Rhizoma Pinelliae Ternatae Praeparata) and *Xia Ku Cao* (Spica Prunellae Vulgaris) added to the recipe may have a better effect for all kinds of insomnia.

Jiuli (88.25, 88.26, 88.27), or *Fengshi* (GB 31), is also a very effective point. *Jiuli* (88.25, 88.26, 88.27) has very strong tranquilizing and analgesic effect and is very effective for diseases of the neurological diseases. *Jiuli* (88.25, 88.26, 88.27), or *Fengshi* (GB 31), is on the Gallbladder Meridian connected with the gallbladder through the heart, and it can be used to treat hyperactivity of the heart fire and disturbance of the heart by phlegm-heat. Through the internally and externally related liver and gallbladder, it can also be used to treat insomnia due to hyperactivity of the liver fire. *Yuan Hu Suo* (Rhizoma Corydalis) has analgesic and tranquilizing effect and can be added together with *Suan Zao Ren* (Semen Ziziphi Spinosae) to recipes to treat insomnia. Chinese medicine holds that long-lasting diseases are always accompanied by blood stasis, and this can be treated very effectively with *Xue Fu Zhu Yu Tang* (Decoction for Removing Blood Stasis in the Chest), or by pricking *Wuling* (DT.04) to let out blood. In recent years I have found that bloodletting at the ear tip alone is very effective for insomnia. We all know that the kidney opens into the ear, and, according to *Su Wen* (Plain Questions), "the heart opens into the ear." Thus, both the kidney and the heart open into the ear. Besides, the *Shaoyang* Meridian runs around and then into the ear. That's why bloodletting at the ear tip is so effective. It has the effect of activating blood circulation to remove blood stasis, tranquilizing the mind, dispelling wind and coordinating the heart and kidney.

7) High Fever

a. *Dabai* (22.04) (extremely effective).
b. Bloodletting at *Wuling* (DT.04) on the back.

Extremely good effect can be achieved by pricking the blue vein at *Dabai* (22.04). Bloodletting at *Wuling* (DT.04) is also effective. Good effect can also be achieved by performing bloodletting at *Shaoshang* (LU 11), *Zhongshang* and *Laoshang* or at the ear tip. Points from the fourteen regular meridians include *Dazhui* (DU14) and *Quchi* (LI 11), which can be used alone or in combination, with the former more effective than the latter.

8) Alcoholic Intoxication

a. Bloodletting at *Erhuan* (99.01), combined with *Suliao* (DU25) with better effect.
b. *Huobao* (55.01).

Alcoholic intoxication can be treated by performing bloodletting around *Erhuan* (99.01), followed by acupuncture at *Suliao* (DU 25) to achieve a better effect. Even a better effect can be achieved by bloodletting at the ear tip, because both the heart and kidney open into and ear and *Shaoyang* Meridian runs around and into the ear, making it possible to coordinate the heart and kidney, calm the mind and dispel wind. *Huobao* (55.01) is also effective by tonifying the heart and regulating the stomach. Chinese medicine believes that alcoholic intoxication is due to water toxins; and *Wu Ling San* (Powder of Five Drugs Including Sclerotium Poriae Cocos) with good effect.

9) Epilepsy

a. *Shenguan* (77.18) and *Shangliu* (55.06).
b. *Wanshunyi* (22.08) and *Wanshun'er* (22.09).
c. *Jinqianshang* (88.24) and *Jinqianxia* (88.23).
d. Bloodletting at *Jinji* and *Jinling* which is 1.5 inches lateral to the third thoracic vertebra [*Feishu* (BL 13) and *Jueyinshu* (BL 14)] with very good effect.

In the past, epilepsy was mostly due to hereditary factors, but nowadays many cases are caused by traumatic injuries. The best method is to perform bloodletting on the back or to reinforce the kidney. Since the disease is related to the brain nerve, *Shenguan* (77.18), *Shangliu* (55.06) and *Xiasanhuang* (77.18, 19, 21). Ancient people had it that *Shenmai*

(BL 62) could be used for an epilepsy attack during the day and *Zhaohai* (KI 6), for an epilepsy attack at night. The former comes from the *Yangqiao* Meridian and the latter from the *Yinqiao* Meridian; the former is on the Bladder Meridian and the latter, the Kidney Meridian. So they are both related to the kidney. *Jinqianshang* (88.24) and *Jinqianxia* (88.23), which are below *Fengshi* (GB 31), can also be used to dispel wind and resolve phlegm, since epilepsy is often due to incoordination between the *zang* and *fu* organs, causing stirring or wind and hyperactivity of fire and ascending of the phlegm *qi* to obstruct the upper orifices. *Wanshunyi* (22.08) and *Wanshun'er* (22.09) can also be used to treat the disease. According to *Tong Xuan Zhi Yao Fu* (Ode of the Essentials of Understanding), "epilepsy can be treated with *Houxi* (SI 3)." *Houxi* (SI 3) is just between *Wanshunyi* (22.08) and *Wanshun'er*, and is an important point that Master Tung used to treat kidney diseases. A better method is to prick *Jinji* and *Jinling*, which is 1.5 *cun* lateral to the third thoracic vertebra, to let out blood. Besides, bloodletting can also be performed at *Dazhui* (DU 14), or the middle line (Governor Vessel) at the back at *Wuling* (DT.04) and along the lines 0.5 and 3 inches (Bladder Meridian) lateral to the middle line, since epilepsy is related to the brain and the Governor Vessel. Both the Governor Vessel and Bladder Meridian enter into the brain. It is very important to reinforce the kidney in treating this disease, since treating the kidney means treating the brain. *Shenguan* (77.18), *Shangliu* (55.06), *Wanshunyi* (22.08) and *Wanshun'er* (22.09) can tonify the brain, and *Wanshunyi* (22.08) and *Wanshun'er* (22.09) are also connected with the Governor Vessel (DU). Therefore, these points are all frequently used to treat epilepsy. Besides, Chinese medicine holds that "the heart is in charge of mental activity." *Jiuwei* (REN 15) [punctured perpendicularly towards *Juque* (REN 14)], *Xinshu* (BL 15), *Neiguan* (PC 6), *Hegu* (LI 4), *Taichong* (LR 3) and *Yongquan* (KI 1) from the fourteen regular meridians are also effective for the disease, since these points have something to do with the kidney and liver and with tranquilization. The common recipes include *Chai Hu Jia Long Gu Mu Li Tang* (Decoction of Radix Bupleuri, Os Draconis and Concha Ostreae) or *Chai Hu Gui Zhi Tang* (Decoction of Radix Bupleuri and Ramulus Cinnamomi Cassiae) with *Shao Yao* (Paeonia lactiflora Pall) added to the recipes. Herbs for activating blood circulation can also be added if blood stasis is present.

10) Coma

a. For unconsciousness: *Huoying* (66.03), *Zhenghui* (1010.01), *Qianhui* (1010.05), and *Wuling* (DT.04) with bloodletting.
b. *Huoying* (66.03) and *Huozhu* (66.04).
c. Prick the twelve *Jing*-Well points (bloodletting).

Apoplexy with coma has already been dealt with, with several case reports. I just want to make some supplementary remarks here. In recent years I have treated quite a few coma patients, mainly with *Huoying* (66.03), *Huozhu* (66.04) and also with *Taichong* (LR 3), with quite a good effect. Many doctors would like to use *Renzhong* (DU 26) and *Neiguan* (PC 6), without knowing that the three points mentioned above are also very effective. It often happened that after acupuncture at *Renzhong* (DU 26) and *Neiguan* (PC 6) were given, the patient still did not regain consciousness until one of the three points was then used. This is because that underneath these points there is the *Taichong* Meridian, which, when stimulated, can treat the heart. These points are also on the Liver Meridian of Foot-*Jueyin*, which communicates with the Hand-*Jueyin* Meridian and therefore it is possible to tonify the heart. The Liver Meridian of Foot-*Jueyin* runs from the interior of the brain to the head, and the needling effect at *Taichong* (LR 3) or *Huozhu* (66.04) can penetrate to *Yongquan* (KI 1) to enhance the effect of first aid and bring back consciousness. In a severe case, bloodletting should be given at the twelve *Jing*-Well points. *Shang Han Lun* (Treatise on Febrile Diseases) tells us that "coma occurs when the twelve meridians fail to communicate with each other." The twelve *Jing*-Well points are at the starting or terminating points of the meridians and have the functions of connecting *yin* and *yang* and relieving cold limbs. The first point for bloodletting is *Zhongchong* (PC 9) and then *Shaoshang* (LU 11), because *Zhongchong* (PC 9) is the *Jing*-Well point of the Pericardium Meridian of Hand-*Jueyin* and is an important point for tonifying the heart and also a wood point of the fire meridian. The *Jing*-Well points can treat acute mental diseases and *Zhongchong* (PC 9) can treat mental diseases related to wood and fire, i.e. liver wind and phlegm fire. *Shaoshang* (LU 11) can regulate the flow of *qi* and resolve phlegm. Besides, it is on the thumb and is therefore most closely related to the brain neurologically and holographically.

11) Fainting During Acupuncture

a. *Shoujie* (22.10) punctured towards *Xiabai* (22.07) (especially effective).
b. *Jie* (88.28).

Shoujie (22.10) is in fact the *Ying*-Spring point of the Heart Meridian. According to *Nei Jing* (Yellow Emperor's Inner Classic), "*Ying*-Spring points can be used for diseases with changed facial complexion." During fainting, the facial complexion always changes, and *Shoujie* (22.10), or the *Ying*-Spring point of the Heart Meridian *Shaofu* (HT 8) which can tonify the heart can be used to effectively deal with the problem. *Jie* (88.28) is one *cun* below *Liangqiu* (ST 34), the *Xi*-Cleft point of the Stomach Meridian, and both points are at the area where *qi* and blood converge. *Jie* (88.28) is even nearer to the knee and so is richer in *qi* and blood. Besides, since it is on the *Yangming* Meridian, which is full of *qi* and blood, it has a stronger effect of regulating *qi* and blood and can therefore be used to treat fainting during an acupuncture treatment.

12) *Qi* and Blood Disorder

a. *Jie* (88.28).

Qi and blood disorder occurs as a result of improper ways of practicing *qigong*, or improper ways of acupuncture by using too many needles, or from traumatic injuries. *Jie* (88.28) is quite effective for all these cases, and also for pains and numbness that occur after acupuncture treatment. The mechanism for this is already explained in the previous section "Fainting during Acupuncture."

13) Common Cold

a. *Sanchasan* (A.04).
b. *Mu* (11.17).
c. Bloodletting at *Wuling* (DT.04) to alleviate fever.
d. *Cesanli* (77.22) for nasal obstruction (very effective), *Menjin* (66.05) and *Mu* (11.17) (also effective).

Acupuncture is very effective for treating common cold. *Sanchasan* (A.04) can be first used and *Mu* (11.17) can also be used. For common cold with headache, *Sanchasan* (A.04) and *Dabai* (22.04) can be used together; for cold with sore throat, this point and *Tushuizhong* (22.11) can be used in combination; for running nose and nasal obstruction, *Sanchasan* (A.04) and *Mu* (11.17) can be used. The most important point is *Sanchasan* (A.04). Thc combination of this point and *Dabai* (22.04) has been mentioned before and also in books about the five *Shu* points. The mechanism of the points in treating common cold lies in "*Ying*-Spring points and *Shu*-Stream points that control the superficial meridians." The *Ying*-Spring points pertains to water in *yang* meridians and to fire in *yin* meridians, and can control cold and heat, which is just the features of exterior syndromes. *Shu*-Stream points pertain to wood and controls wind and tendon, and to earth and controls dampness and muscles. And wind, cold, dampness and heat are the features of exterior syndromes and diseases of the meridians. *Sanchasan* (A.04) is close to *Yemen* (SJ 2), the *Ying*-Spring Point of the Triple Energizer (San Jiao) Meridian, and can be used to improve immunity, and since the insertion of this point is just against the bone, it can be used to treat pains of bones and tendons due to wind and cold. *Dabai* (22.04) is close to *Sanjian* (LI 3), the *Shu*-Stream point of the Large Intestine Meridian and is related to the lung, so it can be used to treat common cold. *Tushuizhong* (22.11) is at *Yuji* (LU 10), the *Ying*-Stream point of the Lung Meridian, and is very effective for common cold with sore throat and asthma.

According to *Di Er Zhang Gu Quan Xi Lun* (Holography of Second Metacarpal Bone), *Dabai* (22.04) corresponds with the upper energizer (Upper Jiao) and is therefore effective for diseases of that area, and the combination of *Sanchasan* (A.04) and *Dabai* (22.04) is very good for common cold. For nasal obstruction, *Mu* (11.17), *Cesanli* (77.22) and *Menjin* (66.05) are very effective.

14) Aphonia

a. *Shiyin* (88.32).
b. Bloodletting at *Zongshu* (1010.07).

Shiyin (88.32), meaning aphonia in Chinese, is at the bending part of the knee joint. It is punctured just along the skin to penetrate from the Spleen Meridian to the Kidney Meridian, and both meridians reach the throat. Holographically it also corresponds with the throat. Voice is also related to the lung and puncturing the point along the skin enables it to communicate with the lung. That's why the point is effective for aphonia. Bloodletting at *Zongshu* (1010.07) at the back of the neck, or *Yamen* (DU 15), is also effective. This follows the principle of using both front and back points and using back points to treat diseases of the front. The common recipe is *Mai Men Dong Tang* (Decoction of Radix Ophiopogonis), and *Feng Huang Yi* (Membrana Follicularis Ovi) can also be used together.

Many points from the fourteen regular meridians can also be used to treat aphonia. It is said in *Nei Jing* (Yellow Emperor's Inner Classic) that "diseases of the voice can be treated with points of the corresponding meridians." Since the Spleen Meridian reaches the tongue and the heart opens into the tongue, both *Shangqiu* (SP 5) and *Lingdao* (HT 4) can be used to treat aphonia. Sudden loss of voice is mostly related to the heart and can be treated with *Lingdao* (HT 4) and *Tongli* (HT 5) from the Heart Meridian. *Yamen* (DU 15) is also an important point for aphonia owing to the fact that it is a point of the Governor Vessel related to the mental activity and it is at the neck corresponding with the throat.

15) Cholera with Convulsion

a. Bloodletting at *Sihuazhong* (77.09) and *Sihuawai* (77.14) and needling *Boqiu* (77.04).

The TCM concept of cholera include what the western medicine calls cholera and acute enterogastritis. The first step in treating the disease is to perform bloodletting at *Weizhong* (BL 40) and *Chize* (LU 5), or at *Sihuazhong* (77.09) and *Sihuawai* (77.14). If cramp of the foot occurs, *Chengshan* (BL 57) can also be used. Both acute cholera and acute enterogastritis are accompanied by vomiting and diarrhea, which should be treated according to different symptoms. For acute enterogastritis with both vomiting and diarrhea, the contemporary recipe is *Huo Xiang Zheng Qi San* (Powder of Herba Agastachis for Restoring Health), and the classic recipe is *Ge Geng Qin Lian Tang* (Radix Puerariae, Radix Scutellariae Baicalensis and Rhizoma Coptidis).

16) Adipoma

a. *Minghuang* (88.12) (specifically effective).
b. *Waisanguan* (77.27).
c. Bloodletting at *Sihuawai* (77.14).

Adipoma cases have increased recently. Modern life with ample nutritional supply causes accumulation of fat, and adipoma is likely to occur especially in the parts of the body where there is lots of fat, such as the thighs, shoulders, arms, abdomen, chest, back, hips and even the face. *Minghuang* (88.12) is a very effective point for adipoma, since it is on the thigh where there is much fat so that it is possible to "treat the flesh with the flesh," and it is also on the Liver Meridian and liver is related to the fat secretion. *Waisanguan* (77.27) and bloodletting at *Sihuazhong* (77.09) and *Sihuawai* (77.14) are also effective methods. *Sihuazhong* (77.09) can regulate the spleen and stomach and remove dampness and phlegm. *Sihuawai* (77.14) is just beside *Fenglong* (ST 40), which is "influential point of phlegm" and bloodletting at this point is effective for phlegm retention. Chinese herbs for invigorating *qi*, activating blood circulation and resolving phlegm are also frequently used. *Ying Wei Fan Hun Tang* (Decoction for Restoring Functions of *Ying* and *Wei* System) can be taken over a long period with good effect. *Liu Jun Zhi Tang* (Decoction of Six Ingredients) and *Xiao Yao San* (Ease Powder) used in combination, with the addition of *Bai Jie Zi* (Semen Sinapis Albae) and *Zhe Bei Mu* (Bulbus Fritillariae Thunbergii) are also effective for adipoma. Messenger drugs can also be used to enhance the effect.

17) Phlebangioma

a. Prick the veins above and below the tumor.

Long time standing in work is likely to cause phlebangioma, the best method for which is to perform bloodletting on the veins above and below the tumor. Since this may cause bleeding, it is not advisable to prick thick veins and the bloodletting should be performed several times before the disease is cured. After bloodletting, acupuncture can be given at *Taiyuan* (LU 9) (one of the eight influential points for blood vessel), *Taichong* (LR 3) and *Neiguan* (PC 6), which are related to the blood vessel. Traditional Chinese medicine believes that diseases of the lower energizer, like phlebangioma, are mostly due to damp-heat, and phlebangioma is due to both damp-heat and blood stasis, which should both be treated. Chinese herbal recipes for the disease include *Gui Zhi Fu Ling Tang* (Decoction of Ramulus Cinnamomi Cassiae and Sclerotium Poriae Cocos) for activating blood circulation to remove blood stasis, the effect of which can be enhanced by adding *Fang Ji* (Radix Stephaniae Tetrandrae) and *Huang Qi* (Radix Astragali seu Hedysari) to regulate *qi* and remove dampness, *Fang Ji Huang Qi Tang* (Decoction of Radix Stephaniae Tetrandrae and Radix Astragali seu Hedysari) and *Si Miao San* (Decoction of Four Wonderful Drugs).

18) Angiosclerosis

a. Bloodletting at *Weizhong* (BL 40).
b. Bloodletting at *Sihuazhong* (77.09) and *Sihuawai* (77.14) (specifically effective).
c. Peck needling at *Wuling* (DT.04) (1.3 and 3 inches lateral to the 4th and 7th thoracic vertebrae) (specifically effective).

Angiosclerosis is often due to high levels of blood lipid or triglyceride, which can be treated effectively by performing bloodletting at *Sihuazhong* (77.09) and *Sihuawai* (77.14), or by giving acupuncture at *Zhigou* (SJ 6) and *Fenglong* (ST 40). The disease is often due to phlegm or blood stasis and bloodletting at *Sihuazhong* (77.09) and *Sihuawai* (77.14) can effectively activate blood circulation and resolve phlegm. *Fenglong* (ST 40) is effective since it is "influential point of phlegm" and Chinese medicine considers fat accumulation to be related to phlegm. *Zhigou* (SJ 6) can regulate *qi* activity, relax the bowels and reduce blood lipid. Bloodletting at *Wuling* (DT.04) on the back promotes blood circulation of the body and relieves hardening of the blood vessels.

19) Leucopenia

a. *Qihuang* (88.14) and *Ganmen* (33.11).
b. *Mudou* (66.07) and *Muliu* (66.06).

20) Erythropenia (aplastic anemia)

a. *Ganmen* (33.11).
b. *Shangsanhuang* (88.12, 13, 14).
c. *Mudou* (66.07) and *Muliu* (66.06).

21) Hyperleucocytosis

a. *Sanhuang* (88.12, 13, 14) (specifically effective).
b. *Mudou* (66.07) and *Muliu* (66.06).
c. *Xiasanhuang* (77.18, 19, 21).

The main method of treatment for blood disorders such as hyperleucocytosis or erythrocytosis is to apply acupuncture at *Shangsanhuang* (88.12, 13, 14), which means that both the spleen and the liver are treated, the former controlling blood and the latter storing blood. *Mudou* (66.07), *Muliu* (66.06) and *Sanzhong* (77.07) can also be used alternately and are also quite effective. *Xiasanhuang* (77.18, 19, 21) can "tonify both the spleen and the kidney," which has been mentioned frequently in recent medical reports about the treatment of blood disorders. *Shangsanhuang* (88.12, 13, 14), *Mudou* (66.07) and *Muliu* (66.06) are used to tonify the liver and spleen and when *Xiasanhuang* (77.18, 19, 21) are also used, the spleen, liver and kidney are all tonified, and desirable results will be obtained. In using Chinese herbal recipes, *Jin Kui Yao Lue* (Synopsis of Prescriptions of Golden Chamber) provides us with *Huang Qi Jian Zhong Tang* (Decoction of Radix Astragali seu Hedysari for Tonifying Middle Energizer) and *Liu Wei Di Huang Tang* (Decoction of Six Herbs Including Radix Rehmanniae) for tonifying both the spleen and kidney, and the two recipes are often used together. *Han Lian Cao* (Herba Ecliptae Prostratae) and *Xian He Cao* (Herba Agrimoniae Pilosae) can also be used to blood deficiency and bleeding. *Huang Qi Jian Zhong Tang* (Decoction of Radix Astragali seu Hedysari for Tonifying Middle Energizer) can invigorate the spleen, and this recipe can be used together with *Gui Zhi Tang* (Decoction of Ramulus Cinnamomi Cassiae) to regulate the *Ying* and *Wei* systems and invigorate the spleen and stomach. When fever and bleeding occur, *Xi Jiao Di Huang Tang* (Decoction of Cornu Rhinocerotis and Radix Rehmanniae) can be used for patients with acute hyperleucocytosis, and *Huang Qi Jian Zhong Tang* (Decoction of Radix Astragali seu Hedysari for Tonifying Middle Energizer) and *Liu Wei Di Huang Tang* (Decoction of Six Drugs Including Radix Rehmanniae) can be used for patients with chronic hyperleucocytosis.

22) Odontoprisis

a. *Sihuazhong* (77.09) (specifically effective).
b. *Fuchang* (77.12).
c. Bloodletting at ear tip.

Traditional Chinese medicine believes that restless sleep, such as sleepwalking, often occurs in those with stomach upset or heat in the gallbladder. This is often treated with *Wen Dan Tang* (Decoction for Warming Gallbladder). For the stomach problem, drugs for "regulating the functions of the stomach and resolving phlegm" should be used. I myself prefer to use *Ban Xia Xie Xin Tang* (Decoction of Rhizoma Pinelliae Ternatae Praeparata for Purging Heart), a famous recipe recorded in *Shang Han Lun* (Treatise on Febrile Diseases), with good effect for sleepwalking and also for odontoprisis. Also, since people who indulge in drinking are likely to have damp-heat in the stomach and therefore have odontoprisis, *Huang Qin* (Radix Scutellariae Baicalensis) and *Huang Lian* (Rhizoma Coptidis) in *Ban Xia Xie Xin Tang* (Decoction of Rhizoma Pinelliae Ternatae Praeparata for Purging Heart) can purge the heart fire and clear away heat in the stomach. Acupuncture treatment can be given by using *Sihuaxia* (77.11) and *Fuchang* (77.12), which are both on the Stomach

Meridian and can regulate the spleen and stomach. Bloodletting can be performed for a mild case.

23) Fatigue

a. *Sanchasan* (A.04) (relieve fatigue).
b. *Biyi* (1010.22) (prevent fatigue).

Biyi (1010.22) is very effective in relieving fatigue, since this point can refresh the mind. This point can also be used to treat loin and back soreness and pains, and also sciatica. *Sanchasan* (A.04) is also quite effective. However, since it is on the hand it is not as convenient as *Biyi* (1010.22) is. When the point is punctured, one has to stop working.

Sanchasan (A.04) has its own advantages since it can also be used to treat shoulder pain, loin pain, headache, common cold, and thigh pain.

24) Skin Sensitiveness

a. *Sima* (88.17, 88.18, 88.19) (specifically effective).
b. Bloodletting at ear tip or ear back (specifically effective).

25) Psoriasis

a. *Sima* (88.17, 88.18, 88.19) (specifically effective).
b. Bloodletting at ear back (specifically effective).

All kinds of skin diseases, especially psoriasis, can be treated with *Sima* (88.17, 88.18, 88.19), together with bloodletting behind the ear. Master Tung is very good at treating psoriasis, and even on his business card it is claimed that he can treat the disease effectively. The point that he likes to use is *Sima* (88.17, 88.18, 88.19). Giving acupuncture treatment at *Sima* (88.17, 88.18, 88.19) everyday and bloodletting at the tip of the ear once a week or bloodletting at *Feishu* (BL13) and *Jueyinshu* (BL 14) is a very effective method for psoriasis. Points from the fourteen regular meridian that are effective for psoriasis include *Quchi* (LI 11), *Xuehai* (SP 10) and *Sanyinjiao* (SP 6).

26) Acne

a. *Sima* (88.17, 88.18, 88.19) (specifically effective).
b. Bloodletting at ear back (specifically effective).
c. Bloodletting at the back (specifically effective).

Acne responds well to acupuncture treatment, which is given by using *Sima* (88.17, 88.18, 88.19) and then *Yingxiang* (LI 20), a point where the Hand-*Yangming* Meridian and the Foot-*Yangming* Meridian meet. Since the face is where the *Yangming* Meridians pass, acupuncture at *Yingxiang* (LI 20) has the effect of inducing the needling effect of other points to this area. Another method is to prick the blue veins at the back of the ear to let out several drops of blood. Points from the fourteen regular meridians include *Quchi* (LI 11), *Xuehai* (SP 10), *Sanyinjiao* (SP 6) and *Yingxiang* (LI 20), combined with bloodletting at the tip of the ear.

To treat acne with Chinese herbs, *Pi Pa Qing Fei Yin* (Decoction of Folium Eriobotryae Japonicae for Clearing away Heat from Lung) from *Yi Zong Jin Jian Wai Ke Xin Fa* (The Golden Mirror of Medicine: External Treatment) is the best recipe. There are also other recipes, which I am not going to mention here. The patients with acne should pay attention to the following points: 1. eat less sweet food; 2. eat less greasy food; 3. eat less pungent food; 4. have free-flowing bowel movement; 5. ensure good sleep and don't stay up late; 6. avoid exposure to the sun excessively; 7. eat plenty of fruits and vegetables; and 8. wash the face frequently.

17. Question: How to treat ectopic dermatitis?

Answer: Ectopic dermatitis, also known as specific dermatitis, affects more and more children. This disease is related to heredity. For example, if one of the parents has skin or breathing sensitivities, their children will have a 30% chance to develop the diseases; if both parents have the problems, the chances for their children to develop the disease will increase to 80%. In Taiwan and Los Angeles there are quite a few cases of ectopic dermatitis. I think this is also true with South Korea. Most people have the disease during their childhood, age two or three years or older, and recover in their teen years. This disease should be treated as early as possible.

Ectopic dermatitis didn't occur so frequently in the past, because of the simple diet and eating habits. Nowadays, owing to the development of means of transportation and the use of refrigerators, people can eat complex diets, mostly frozen food, coming from different places and different seasons. Some people are allergic to milk, or develop ectopic dermatitis because of wearing certain sweaters, owning pets, or exposed to air pollution. This disease is characterized by alternate attack of skin eczema and diseases of the respiratory system, which may change into chronic bronchitis or asthma if not properly treated.

Ectopic dermatitis was called "*Si Wan Feng*" (meaning: eczema at four bending parts) in the medical book *Wai Ke Zheng Zong* (Orthodox Manual of External Diseases) in 1665, late *Ming* Dynasty. This is because the disease is likely to occur in the transverse crease of the elbows and knees. Chinese medicine believes that this disease is due to wind, dryness, dampness and stasis. "Wind" refers to the sudden attack of the disease with itchiness, "dampness" indicates purulent discharge, "dryness" suggests desquamation and peeling of the skin, and "stasis" means blood stasis in chronic cases, with discolouration of the skin or thickened hard skin. According to my experience, the best recipe is *Yin Qiao Shu Feng*

Tang (Decoction of Flos Lonicerae and Fructus Forsythiae Suspensae for Dispelling Wind) developed by me, which can be used to treat many skin diseases. The components of the recipe are *Yin Hua* (Flos Lonicerae), *Lian Qiao* (Fructus Forsythiae Suspensae), *Chi Shao* (Radix Paeoniae Rubra), *Sheng Di Huang* (Radix Rehmanniae Glutinosae), *Mu Dan Pi* (Cortex Moutan Radicis), *Gan Cao* (Radix Glycyrrhizae Uralensis), *Huang Qin* (Radix Scutellariae Baicalensis), *Cang Er Zi* (Fructus Xanthii Sibirici) and *Chan Tui* (Periostracum Cicadae). The dosage for each herb is 15 grams, except for *Gan Cao* (Radix Glycyrrhizae Uralensis) (7.5 grams). Of course the dosage for small children should be reduced to 5-10 grams. For itching, *Di Fu Zi* (Fructus Kochiae Scopariae) and *Bai Xian Pi* (Cortex Dictamni Dasycarpi Radicis) can be added. This recipe is also called *Yin Qiao Liang Xue Tang* (Decoction of Flos Lonicerae and Fructus Forsythiae Suspensae for Cooling Blood) and is also effective for psoriasis and neurodermatitis. When it is used to treat acne, *Pi Pa Ye* (Folium Eriobotryae Japonicae) and *Sang Bai Pi* (Cortex Mori Albae Radicis) can be added.

Jin Yin Hua (Flos Lonicerae Japonicae) and *Lian Qiao* (Fructus Forsythiae Suspensae), which is often used to treat skin diseases, can regulate the *Ying* and *Wei* systems. Most skin diseases are due to blood heat, manifested by local redness, for which *Chi Shao* (Radix Paeoniae Rubra), *Mu Dan Pi* (Cortex Moutan Radicis) and *Sheng Di Huang* (Radix Rehmanniae Glutinosae) can be used to cool blood. *Huang Qin* (Radix Scutellariae Baicalensis), which can clear away heat in the lung, *Pi Pa Ye* (Folium Eriobotryae Japonicae) and *Sang Bai Pi* (Cortex Mori Albae Radicis) are also effective for skin diseases. Acupuncture treatment can be given by pricking the back of the ear and tip to let out blood and the treatment will last for two or three months before the disease is cured. I have already cured almost a hundred cases. For severe cases, the paste made from *Di Yu* (Radix Sanguisorbae Officinalis) and *Hu Zhang* (Radix et Rhizoma Polygoni Cuspidati) can be used. The Japanese would like to use recipes to treat ectopic dermatitis, with *Xiao Chai Hu Tang* (Minor Decoction of Radix Bupleuri) during attack, *Xiao Feng San* (Powder for Dispelling Wind) as the main recipe for treatment, and *Liu Wei Di Huang Wan* (Pill of Six Herbs Including Radix Rehmanniae) and *Xiao Feng San* (Powder for Dispelling Wind) used in combination during remission stage. *Xiao Feng San* (Powder for Dispelling Wind) is a very good recipe for most skin diseases, the effect of which can be enhanced by adding *Cang Er Zi* (Fructus Xanthii Sibirici) and *Chan Tui* (Periostracum Cicadae). *Jing Jie* (Herba Schizonepetae Tenuifoliae) and *Fang Feng* (Radix Ledebouriellae Divaricatae) are very effective for patients susceptible to common cold and can be added for this kind of patients, including children. Bloodletting at the back of the ear and tip can also be used to enhance the effect. For older children, acupuncture can be given at *Sima* (88.17, 88.18, 88.19).

Method of Selecting Five *Shu* Points of the Same Five-Element Nature

The correspondence between Five *Shu* Points to the climate and other natural phenomena of different seasons and to *zang-fu* organs has given rise to the "method of selecting points of the same five-element nature." This principle is often applied to the acupuncture practice, but its mechanism is not known to some doctors. This method is also of great importance in the application of the Five *Shu* Points and further study is necessary. The method is also called "Method of Inter-Respondence (*Jiao Ying Liao Fa*)," and can be considered as one form of holographic correspondence and is divided into the following five types: inter-promotion, inter-restriction, genuine five elements, inter-relation and inter-connection.

I. Inter-promotion

This method is developed from the inter-promotion relation among the five elements. For instance, *Taiyuan* (LU 9) is the earth (*Shu*-Stream) point of the metal (lung) and therefore can be used to supplement the earth to generate metal to treat lung *qi* deficiency; *Shangqiu* (SP 5), the metal point of the earth, can also be used to reinforce *qi* to treat diseases due to deficiency of *qi* in the middle energizer; *Xiaxi* (GB 43), the water point of wood (Gall Bladder Meridian), can be used to treat deficiency of the liver due to failure of the water to nourish the wood; the mother point *Fuliu* (KI 7) for reinforcing the Kidney Meridian can be used to treat various diseases due to kidney deficiency, bony spur, long-lasting lumbago and lumbar sprain; *Chize* (LU 5), the son point of the Lung Meridian (metal meridian), can be used with reducing method to decrease the metal in restricting wood and is quite effective for disturbance in the locomotor system such as frozen shoulder and hemiplegia. No more examples are given here, since this is similar to the mother-son reinforcing-reducing method.

II. Inter-restriction

This method is developed from the inter-restriction relation among the five elements. For instance, *Erjian* (LI 2), the water point of the Large Intestine Meridian, is very effective for diseases of this meridian due to heat or fire such as toothache, and *Neiting* (ST 44) is also effective for toothache for the same reason; *Yemen* (SJ 2), the water point of the Triple Energizer (*San Jiao*) Meridian, is effective for diseases of the meridian due to heat or fire, especially diseases of the senses and throat caused by accumulation of heat in the upper and middle energizer. *Bai Zheng Fu* (Ode of One Hundred Patterns) mentions that *Yemen* is effective in sore throat. The author has been exerting it to clinical practice and receiving outstanding result every time. These points are the *Ying*-Spring points of the *Yang* Meridians and pertain to water. Since "*Ying*-Spring points master body heat," they are used to purge fire, which is known to everyone. *Chize* (LU 5), the water (*He*-Sea) point of the Lung Meridian, can be used to treat diseases of the meridian due to fire, and is therefore the specific point for sore throat and tonsillitis; *Quze* (PC 3), the water point of the fire meridian, can be used to restrict fire and is therefore effective for diseases due to water deficiency and heat excess, especially those diseases in which adverse ascending of the heart fire is to be checked such as canker sore, eye redness, etc.

The inter-restriction relation mentioned above also applies to the other four elements. For example, since *Zuqiaoyin* (GB 44) is the metal point of the wood (Gall Bladder) meridian, it can be used to check wood that counteracts on metal in the treatment of diseases due to *qi* deficiency and stagnation with liver dysfunction; *Zhongfeng* (LR 4), the metal point of the Liver Meridian, is considered to be able to treat difficulty in walking in some ancient medical rhymes (Song More Precious than Jade, Song of Jade Dragon, and Ode of Jade Dragon), because metal can restrict wood, if metal lessens in restricting wood, so that wood is at ease; *Quchi* (LI 11), the earth point of the metal (Large Intestine Meridian), and since metal can restrict wood and coursing earth can harmonize wood, this point is often used to treat hyperactivity of the liver yang; *Shaoshang* (LU 11), the wood point of the metal (Lung Meridian), can also be used to treat wood hyperactivity. Both *Quchi* (LI 11) and *Shaoshang* (LU 11) are very effective for hypertension. Those are the applications of "Energy of the same nature seeks one another (*Tung Qi Xiang Qiu*). More examples could be given, and readers can also refer to *Zhen Jiu Jing Xue Xue* (Channels and Acupuncture Points) written by the author.

III. Genuine Five Elements

Genuine five elements refer to genuine metal in metal, genuine earth in earth, genuine fire in fire, and so on. That is to select the point with the same five-element nature as that of the meridian. The indications of these points are simple and limited compared with the points utilizing other four types of the method of the same five-element nature, but their effect is doubled and they are much more effective for the diseases of the corresponding meridian.

For example, *Jingqu* (LU 8), the genuine metal point of the metal (Lung Meridian), is frequently used to treat common cold, asthma and cough with marked effect, especially pediatric acute bronchitis; *Zusanli* (ST 36), the genuine earth of the earth meridian, has strong effect in regulating the spleen and stomach; *Taibai* (SP 3), the earth point of the earth meridian, is effective for diseases of the digestive system such as constipation, indigestion, abdominal pain and vomiting, and is also used to treat general fatigue; *Yanggu* (SI 5), the fire point of the fire meridian, is often used for antipyretic purposes by Honma, a renowned Japanese acupuncturist; *Laogong* (PC 8), also a fire point of the fire (Pericardium Meridian), has excellent effect of purging fire, clearing away heart fire and chest fire and causing fire to descend, and therefore is often used to treat canker sore in children (The Golden Mirror) and heart stuffiness (Ode of Jade Dragon) effectively; *Yingu* (KI 10), the genuine water point of the water (Kidney Meridian), has strong diuretic effect and is used to treat diseases due to kidney deficiency (the Golden Mirror, Song of Supreme Unity); both *Qiuxu* (GB 40) and *Zulinqi* (GB 41) are the wood points of the wood meridian (Gall Bladder Meridian) and therefore the former is used to treat muscle spasm (since wood dominates tendons) and chest and hypochondriac diseases (the location of wood diseases) and the latter is an important point for eye diseases (since wood opens into the eye); *Dadun* (LR 1), also a wood point of the wood (Liver Meridian), is extremely effective for impotence, and hernia since these diseases are diseases of the tendons, and the Liver Meridian circles around the genitalia. Because Liver stores blood, *Dadun* (LR 1) is also very effective in metrorrhagia.

IV. Inter-relation

This is the main and most widely used method in the method of selecting points of the same five-element nature, the principle of which is to fully utilize the close relation between the five elements and visceral manifestation in clinical practice. To apply this method, first choose the corresponding meridian in accordance to the main diseases, and then selects the corresponding five-element point according to the secondary diseases.

For example, *Taiyuan* (LU 9), the earth (*Shu*-Stream) point of the Lung Meridian, is effective for exogenous diseases with body heaviness and arthralgia or vomiting and diarrhea (all diseases of the earth); *Xiangu* (ST 43), the wood point of the earth meridian, is often used to treat diseases due to incoordination between the wood and earth (liver and spleen), especially diarrhea with abdominal pain, headache, migraine and dysmenorrhea; *Dadu* (SP 2), the fire point of the Spleen (earth) Meridian, can be used to treat cold limbs (since the spleen controls the limbs and fire promotes increase of body temperature); *Yinlingquan* (SP 9), the water point of the earth meridian, has strong effect of supplementing earth to control water and is therefore used to induce diuresis in the treatment of dampness, edema, and water swelling and fullness; *Lingdao* (HT 4), the metal point of the Heart Meridian, can be used to treat sudden loss of voice and aphonia (since the heart dominates the mind and metal corresponds to voice); *Shaohai* (HT 3), the water point of the fire (Heart Meridian), is effective for mental diseases due to kidney deficiency; *Shenmen* (HT 7), the earth point of the Heart Meridian, is often used to treat dysfunction of the spleen and stomach due to nervous disorders; *Houxi* (SI 3) is the wood point of the *Taiyang* Meridian, and since wood controls the tendons it can be used to treat diseases along the *Taiyang* Meridian that are related to tendon, such as stiff neck, waist and legs; *Wangu* (SI 4), also pertaining to wood, has similar effect as *Houxi* (SI 3), and is often used as a main point to treat jaundice, since it is the *Yuan*-Source (wood) point of the Small Intestine Meridian and Small Intestine is the officer of separation of clear and turbid.; *Shugu* (BL 65) is the wood point of water meridian, and since wood controls tendons, it is used to treat tendon rigidity along the meridian, especially stiff neck and lumbar sprain (and that is also the reason the *Shu*-Stream points can be used to treat body heaviness and arthralgia), and is used to treat vertex pain with good effect because this point has the effect of supplementing water and nourishing wood and also due to the channel pathway; *Yongquan* (KI 1), the wood point of the water (Kidney Meridian), can also be used to treat vertex pain (or *Jueyin* headache) with the same mechanism, and is used as an important point for epilepsy and wind syndromes since wood dominates wind and the *Jing*-Well point has strong tranquilizing effect.

Kunlun (BL 60), the *Jing*-River (fire) point of the water (Bladder Meridian), is an important point for redness and swelling of the leg and foot (redness and swelling pertain to fire) (according to the Ode and Song of Jade Dragon, and Ode of Essentials of Understanding), and is also used to treat toothache due to ascending of fire (the Golden Mirror)and diarrhea before dawn due to decline of vital gate-fire (deficiency of fire of water) since it is the fire point of water; *Rangu* (same pronunciation to the two words meaning "burning grains") (KI 2), also a fire point of the water (Kidney Meridian), has better effect than *Kunlun* (BL 60) in treating diseases due to decline of vital gate-fire and is also effective for febrile diseases of the Kidney Meridian; *Taixi* (KI 3), the earth point of the Kidney Meridian, is effective for kidney diseases with symptoms of the spleen and stomach such as vomiting and diarrhea or diarrhea before dawn, and is also a frequently used point for deficiency of *yang* in the spleen and kidney, since it is the *Jing*-River (earth) point of water (Kidney Meridian). *Daling* (PC 7), the earth point of the fire (Pericardium Meridian), can be used to treat diseases due to deficiency heat of the Spleen and Stomach Meridians and diseases due to heart fire such as foul breath. (The Ode and Song of Jade Dragon and Song More Precious than Jade).

Yanglingquan (GB 34) is the earth point of the wood (Gall Bladder Meridian) and the tendon point among the eight influential points. Since earth dominates muscles and four limbs, this point can be used to treat diseases of both the tendons and muscles such as dysfunction of the muscles and tendons and locomotor diseases, and is used as a main point for hemiplegia. Since it is also the earth point of the wood meridian, it is effective for incoordination between the liver and spleen.

Taichong (LR 3), also the earth point of the wood, is an important point for regulating the liver and spleen and can be used in the similar way as *Yanglingquan* (GB 34). *Xingjian* (LR 2), the fire point of the wood (Liver Meridian), can reduce the fire caused by liver depression and hence is used as an important point for coursing and rectifying the liver *qi*.

Ququan (LR 8), the water point of the Liver Meridian, is effective for diseases at the genitalia (where the Liver Meridian passes) and diseases related to the kidney water, such as urethritis, strangury (Lin syndrome), edema of the scrotum, etc.

In addition, *Jianshi* (PC 5) (the metal and *Jing*-River point of the Pericardium Meridian) can be used to treat aphonia (Ode of One Hundred Patterns), and *Zhiyin* (BL 67) (the metal and *Jing*-Well point of the Bladder Meridian) can be used to treat aphonia and pruritus (Ode of One Hundred Patterns). Both points are related to metal. *Yinbai* (SP 1), the wood (*Jing*-Well) point of the earth (Spleen Meridian), is responsible for controlling and storing blood, and is therefore effective for metrorrhagia. *Sanjian* (LI 3), the wood point of the Large Intestine Meridian, is used to treat diarrhea with shoulder and hypochondriac pain. Master Tung preferred to use *Erjian* (LI 2) to treat lumbago, since this point is the water point of metal (Large Intestine Meridian) and water is related to the kidney, which also bears the relation of "energy of the same nature seek one another (*Tung Qi Xiang Qiu*)." Those kinds of examples are too many to cxpound piccc by piccc.

It follows from the above explanation that the five shu points are in fact holographic points of the meridians, and their five-element nature reflects the conditions of the five *zang*-organs and hence can be used to treat diseases of the five *zang*-organs.

V. Inter-connection

This is a method in which two five-element points are used in combination. For instance, *Chize* (LU 5) is the water point of the metal (Lung Meridian) and *Fuliu* (KI 7) is the metal point of the water (Kidney Meridian). The two points used together have the effect of connecting metal with water to treat diseases of the lung failing in depurative descending and kidney failing in receiving and accepting with good effect. The author often combines these two points to treat chronic bronchitis and bronchial asthma effectively. Similarly, *Shaohai* (HT 3) is the water point of the fire (Heart Meridian) and *Rangu* (same pronunciation as another two words meaning "burning grains") (KI 2) is the fire point of the water (Kidney Meridian). The two points can be used in combination to treat diseases due to incoordination or disharmony between the heart and kidney (discordance between fire and water), such as symptoms often seen in neurasthenia like heart vexation with insomnia, dream-disturbed sleep with seminal emission, palpitation with poor memory, vertigo, tinnitus, dry mouth and throat, aching loin and knees, tidal fever with spontaneous sweating, etc. Deficiency of both the heart and spleen can be treated with the earth point of the fire meridian and the fire point of the earth meridian in combination; deficiency of both the lung and spleen can be treated with the metal point of the earth meridian and the earth point of the metal meridian in combination; incoordination between the liver and spleen can be treated with the earth point of the wood meridian and the wood point of the earth meridian in combination; deficiency of *yin* of the liver and kidney can be treated with the water point of the wood meridian and the wood point of the water meridian in combination; deficiency of *yang* of the spleen and kidney can be treated with *Taixi* (KI 3), the earth point of the water meridian and *Yinlingquan* (SP 9), the water point of the earth meridian. This method can be applied to other conditions in a similar way, and no more examples are to be given here.

Summary

The method of selecting points of the same five-element nature is flexible and highly effective, with a wide application. Though it is divided into five different sub-methods here, they are not separate but can be used in combination to achieve better effect. Besides, each point is not restricted to one of the five methods. For instance, *Chize* (LU 5), the water point of the metal meridian, is used to treat diseases due to heat and fire of its meridian such as tonsillitis and sore throat. Since metal and water are of the same source and the *He*-sea water points correspond to Kidney water, it can also be used to treat frequent urination, and since metal restricts wood, water nourishes wood and wood controls tendons, it is also an important point for regulating tendons. By needling this point with *Fuliu* (KI 7), the metal point of water, so that metal and water are inter-connected, it can be used to treat chronic diseases of the trachea. This is only one example of the multiple use of one particular point. Other points can be used in a similar way and are not to be discussed here.

The best art of acupuncture treatment lies in the multiple use of one point rather than multiple points for one particular disease. The flexible application of the method of selecting points of the same five-element category will go far towards the accomplishment of this pursuit.

Appendix 1

Application of Bloodletting Therapy

Introduction

Master Tung's bloodletting therapy and the points have been widely adopted by most clinicians, including myself. The main points for bloodletting and their indications have been mentioned before in this book. This appendix is intended to provide the readers with an overall understanding of the bloodletting method and to facilitate further investigation and application.

Bloodletting therapy is an essential procedure in the practice of traditional Chinese medicine, with extremely wide application and surprising therapeutic effects. Bloodletting therapy has been recorded in the medical literature since at least 200 B.C.; however, no one has engaged in a systematic study and documentation of its theory and practice. I have followed Master Tung for many years and have often seen him using the three-edged needle with miraculous effect, e.g. speedy recovery of long-lasting serious diseases and instant relief of great pains. Bloodletting therapy can be used to treat any diseases and the effect is even better than the filiform needle. Master Tung can be considered to be the most significant master who is accomplished in bloodletting therapeutics, he achieved such wonderful effect. I have also found method practical and valuable in the experience of treating over three hundred thousand patients. Many intractable and serious diseases have been cured with this method. In 1988 I went to Anhui to meet the bloodletting expert Wang Xiuzhen, who had distinctive features in bloodletting techniques worthy of further study.

Bloodletting therapy played an important role in the ancient medical practice in China; and according to records on the formation of flint needle and nine forms of needles, has the longest history of medical treatment. As a method, bloodletting refers to the use of a sharp instrument (usually a three-edged needle) to prick certain parts of the patient's body surface: this releases blood in order to treat disease.

The application and importance of bloodletting therapy is mentioned in *Ling Shu* (Spiritual Pivot Chapter 3) which states, "To treat chronic diseases, prick to let out blood." The *Jia Yi Jing* (A-B Classic of Acupuncture and Moxibustion Chapters 1-14) also discusses bloodletting, "To treat diseases, prick the blood vessels which are everywhere in the body, some as thin as a needle and some as thick as tendon."

Bloodletting can be performed on big veins, venules and peripheral capillaries. Venules and peripheral capillaries only appear when disease occurs. They present as red or white streaks or as hemangiomas anywhere on the body surface or hidden beneath the skin. The large veins are prominent and purple or blue in color, and are commonly referred to as "blue veins." They often appear at *weizhong* (BL 40), *chize* (LU 5), and the lateral sides of the four limbs, in the scapular region or on the abdominal wall.

Master Tung's use of bloodletting therapy is not restricted by ancient medical books. In addition to the common parts of the body such as the cubital fossa, popliteal fossa, lateral sides of the forehead, hypoglossis, twelve *Jing*-Well points, *shixuan* (Extra 24) and the back of the ear, he uses bloodletting in almost everywhere, such as the arm, the leg, the ankle, the back of the foot and the acromion. He also prefers to use bloodletting on the back as a flexible method for treating all forms of disease.

Master Tung used bloodletting to treat a wide variety of diseases. For example, he used *weizhong* (BL 40) for sciatica, lumbago, stiff neck, lower limb rheumatism and hemorrhoids. He used *chize* (LU 5) for stuffy chest, asthma and frozen shoulder. *Zusanli* (ST 36) was used for gastropathy and enterogastritis while *taiyang* (EX-HN5) was used for migraine, dizziness and conjunctivitis. Special points such as *sanjin* (DT.07) was used for knee pain, *jinlin* (DT.09) for thigh pain, *jingzhi* (DT.08) for leg pain, *shuangfeng* (DT.05) for numbness of the hand and foot, *sanjiang* (DT.15) for gynecopathy, and *zongshu* (1010.07) was used for conditions such as high fever and vomiting in children. This method addressed pathologies in the following areas of care, internal medicine, external medicine, gynecology, pediatrics and traumatology.

The most prominent feature of Master Tung's bloodletting therapy is the emphasis on distal point selection; this conforms to the ancient orthodox method of "reducing distal points." On the contrary, in our experience, local points (Ahshi points) are less satisfactory.

I have studied Tung's methods of bloodletting intensively, here are some further examples of his work: he used *taiyang* (EX-HN5) to dispel wind and activate blood circulation, he pricked the ear tip to clear heat and activate blood, and pricked the back (where *yang* is) to warm yang and activate blood circulation; he used *weizhong* (BL 40) to remove dampness and activate blood; he used *sihuazhong* (77.09) and *sihuawai* (77.14) which are near *fenglong* (ST 40) for resolving phlegm and activating blood, and he used the twelve *Jing*-Well points for inducing resuscitation and activating blood circulation. His methods are flexible and effective.

1. Common Locations and Indications for Bloodletting Therapy

The most important and common method of bloodletting is to prick the vein. The common locations for bloodletting therapy are as follows.

1) Cubital fossa
This common location has been used since ancient times; it is close to *chize* (LU 5) and *quze* (PC 3). This form of bloodletting is performed on the prominent blue vein.
Indications: Diseases of the respiratory organs and the heart (specifically effective for angina pectoris), cholera, sunstroke, upper limb rheumatic neuralgia, frozen shoulder and hemiplegia.

2) Popliteal fossa
This is a common area for bloodletting with good effect, where *weizhong* (BL 40) is.
Indications: Enteritis, hemorrhoid, lumbago, stiff neck, lower limb rheumatic neuralgia, sciatica, bony spur of the lumbar vertebrae, hemiplegia, cervicospondylopathy, hypertension, apoplectoid stroke, encephalitis sequela, sequela of poliomyelitis in children, thromboangiitis obliterans, rubella, sunstroke, furuncles and sores, retention of urine.

3) Lower arm, where *shousanli* (LI 10) is.
Indications: Facial pustule, carbuncle, conjunctivitis, toothache, eczema, urticaria.

4) Lower leg
   a. *Yangming*
   This area is where one finds *zusanli* (ST 36), *tiaokou* (ST 38) and *sihuazhong* (77.09). Bloodletting should be conducted on the blue vein.
   Indications: Gastritis, enterogastritis, chronic gastropathy, chest pain and stuffiness, chronic trachitis, erysipelas and multiple radiculitis.

   b. *Shaoyang*
   This area is between *yanglingquan* (GB 34) and *yangfu* (GB 38), it is called *sihuawai* (77.14). Bloodletting should be conducted on the blue vein.
   Indications: Acute enterogastritis, pleurisy, heart diseases, chest distention, chronic bronchitis, asthma, sciatica, shoulder pain, migraine, and hypertension.

c. *Taiyang*

This area is where *chengshan* (BL 57) is, and bloodletting should be given on the blue vein.

Indications: Hemorrhoid, backache and phlebangioma.

d. *Taiying*

This area is near *yinlingquan* (SP 9).

Indications: Internal and external hemorrhoid, dysmenorrhea, infertility, urinary tract infection, acute lymphangitis.

5) External malleolus

This area is where *qiuxu* (GB 40) and *kunlun* (BL 60) are.

Indications: Podarthritis, lumbago, sciatica.

6) Internal malleolus

This area is where *Zhongfeng* (LR 4) and *Zhaohai* (KI 6) are.

Indications: Otitis media, hernia, infertility.

7) Dorsum pedis

a. *Yangming*

This area is near *jiexi* (S41).

Indications: Gastric ulcer, duodenal ulcer, erysipelas, peripheral neuritis, thromboarteritis obliterans, lymphedema.

b. *Shaoyang*

This area is where *zulinqi* (GB 41), *xiaxi* (GB 43) and *diwuhui* (GB42) are.

Indications: Toothache, migraine along *shaoyang* channel, sciatica.

8) Parafrontals

This area is where *hanyan* (GB 4) is, and is often referred to as the temple.

Indications: Headache, dizziness, conjunctivitis, hemorrhage of the ocular fundus, apoplexy, asthma and pathological changes of the esophagus.

9) Hypoglossis

This area is where *Jinjing*, *Yuye* (Extra 9) is, i.e. the subglossal blue vein.

Indications: Laryngitis, speech disorder, apoplexy, shock and cardioplegia, serious cold.

2. Other Common Locations for Bloodletting Therapy

Besides the aforementioned locations, other common locations for bloodletting therapy include the posterior ear, the twelve *Jing*-Well points, *shixuan* (Extra 24), the back, the acromion and the face. Since it is difficult to find blue veins and there are no large veins in these areas, bloodletting is accomplished by pricking the point to let out little blood.

1) The twelve *Jing*-Well points.
   Indications: Apoplexy, acute inflammation, cardioplegia, fever.
2) *Shixuan* (Extra 24), at the tip of the ten fingers.
   Indications: Apoplexy and cardioplegia.
3) The ear back or ear tip, with thin veins for bloodletting.
   Indications: Headache, trigeminal neuralgia, conjunctivitis, ceratitis, skin diseases, arthritis of the temple and chin, insomnia, palpitation, and hidrosis.
4) The face, including the cheek, the zygomatic region, the tip of the nose and the nasal ala.
   Indications: Facial paralysis, rhinitis, headache, and trigeminal neuralgia.
5) The oral cavity, the oral mucosa.
   Indications: Facial paralysis.
6) The palm margin, from *houxi* (SI 3) to *wangu* (GB 12).
   Indications: Rubella and asthma.
7) The side of sole, at *rangu* (KI 2).
   Indications: Cerebral concussion.
8) The acromion, around *jianyu* (LI 15).
   Indications: Kidney diseases (when yellowish discharge appears), pain of the wrist and the back of the hand (when dark blood appears), congealed shoulders, frozen shoulders, urticaria, mastitis, etc.
9) The back, including all back-*shu* points.
   Indications: Diseases of *zang-fu* organs and the related Channels.
10) *Qishing* (DT.03), including *zongshu* (1010.07), 0.8 inch into the hairline and the area 1 inch below it.
    Indications: Vomiting, common cold with headache, fever in children, various wind syndromes in children, apoplexy with aphasia and dysphagia.
    ※Remarks: *Qishing* (DT.03) (translation from Chinese: seven star) refers to seven points, including *zongshu* (1010.07), which coincides with *fengfu* (DU16), and *fenshu* (DT.03-II), which coincides with *yamen* (DU 15). The two points are to be used in bloodletting, not all the seven points.

11) *Wuling* (DT.04).

This includes five lines of points. The first runs from *jiangkou* (DT.04-II) at the second vertebra from *dazhui* (DU 14) down *to tuke* (DT.04-XI), below the tenth thoracic vertebra, with one point below each vertebra, altogether ten points. The eight points in between are *houqu*, *huoyun*, *huochang*, *huoming*, *huoxiao*, *huomen, tuyue*, and *tuxie* (DT.04III-X). The second line (two bilateral lines) is four finger breadth from *jiangkou*, running from *jinbei* (XXIII) downwards, with each two points one inch apart, altogether 8 points. The other points are *jindou*, *jinji*, *jinling*, *huojin*, *mudong*, *mudu* and *mumei* (XXIV-XXX). The third line (two bilateral lines) are four finger breadth lateral to the second line, again with each two points one inch apart, altogether seven points, namely, *jinzhi*, *jinjing*, *jinshen*, *muyuan*, *mutai*, *muju*, and *musong* (XXXVII-XLIII).

Indications: Hypertension, severe cold, high fever, chills, sudden dizziness, headache, paralysis of hand and foot caused by hypertension, hemiplegia, various kinds of cholera, vomiting, lumbago due to angiosclerosis and acute gastralgia.

12) *Shuangfeng* (DT.05).

This is in fact two bilateral lines of points going from *huofeng* (XLIV), which is 1.5 inches lateral to the point between the second and the third vertebrae from *dazhui* (DU 14), with each two points one inch apart, altogether fourteen points on the two bilateral lines. The other points are *huozhu*, *huomiao*, *huochao*, *huochong*, *huohua* and *huomi* (XLV-L).

Indications: Pains and numbness of the hand and foot and angiosclerosis of the hand and foot.

13) *Jiuhuo* (DT.06), including *huofeng*, *huozhu*, *huomiao* (XLIV-XLVI), *jintang* (XXII two inches above *jindou*), *jinbei* (XXIII), *jindou* (XXIV), *jinji* (XXV), *jinzhi* (XXXVII) and *jinjing* (XXXVIII).

Indications: Housha.

※Remarks: These points are arranged in three lines. The first line starts from *huofeng*, which is half inch lateral to the second vertebra, altogether three points, with each two points one inch apart; the second line starts from *jintang*, which is three inches lateral to *dazhui* (DU 14), altogether four points, with each two points one inch apart; the third line starts from *jinzhi*, which is six inches lateral to the second vertebra, and ends at *jinjing*, which in one inch below. There are altogether 9 points, thus the name "*jiuhou*" (Chinese meaning: nine monkeys).

14) *Sanjin* (DT.07), including *jindou* (XXIV), *jinji* (XXV) and *jinling* (XXVI).
Indications: Knee pain.
※**Remarks**: These three points are three inches lateral to the third, fourth and fifth vertebrae respectively, which coincide with *pohu* (BL 42), *gaohuang* (BL 43) and *shentang* (BL 44) of the Bladder Channel. Pricking the points to let out little blood and knee pain is relieved instantly. Even long-lasting serious diseases can be cured in this way.

15) *Jingzhi* (DT.08), including *jinjing* (XXXVIII) and *jinzhi* (XXVII).
Indications: Distention and pains of the leg.
※**Remarks**: These two points are six inches lateral to the second and third vertebrae respectively. They are very effective for distention and pains of the leg.

16) *Jinlin* (DT.09), including *jinshen* (XXXIX), *muyuan* (XL) and *mutai* (XLI).
Indications: Sciatica due to angiosclerosis.
※**Remarks**: These three points are six inches lateral to the fourth, fifth and sixth vertebrae respectively, just below *jingzhi*. They are effective for sciatica and neuralgia of the thigh.

17) *Dingzhu* (DT.10), including eleven points: *jingji*, *jinling*, *huojin*, *mudong*, *mudu*, *mumei* (XXV-XXX), *jinshen*, *muyuan*, *mutai*, *muju* and *musong* (XXXIX-XLIII) (twenty-two points bilaterally).
※**Remarks**: These points are arranged in two lines. The six points in the first line are three inches lateral to the fourth to the ninth vertebrae respectively; the five point in the second line are six inches lateral to the fourth to the eighth vertebrae.

18) *Houxin* (DT.11), including three lines of points: the first line starting from *Huoyun* (IV), going down through *huochang*, *huoming*, *huoxiao*, *huomen* and ending at *tuyue* (six points V-IX); the second line, 1.5 inches lateral to the spinal column, including four points: *huomiao*, *huochao* and *huochong*, *huohua* (eight points bilaterally XLVI-XLIX); the third line, 3 inches lateral to the spinal column, including three points: *jinji*, *jinling* and *huojin* (six points bilaterally XXV-XXVII).
Indications: Wool-like fruncles, furuncle, heart failure, gastropathy, acute cardioplegia, invasion of wind-cold, severe cold, apoplexy and various kinds of cholera.

19) *Sanjiang* (DT.15), involves two lines of points: the first line starting from the point just below the thirteenth vertebra, going down through *shuifen*, *shuike*, *shuiguan*, *liuzong*, *fengchao* and ending at *zhuchao* (XII-XVIII), altogether seven points, with each point at each intervertebral space successively; the second line, four finger breadth lateral to the fourteenth vertebra, including six points: *liuyuan*, *liuman*, *liudao*, *huachao*, *huanchao* and *hechao* (twelve points bilaterally XXXI-XXXVI).
    Indications: Amenorrhea, metritis, enteritis, loin sprain, chest pain, acute enteritis.

20) *Shuanghe* (DT.16), including *liuyuan*, *liuman*, *liudao*, *huachao*, *huanchao* and *hechao*, below the fourteenth vertebra (twelve points bilaterally XXXI-XXXVI).
    Indications: Pain of the arm, shoulder and back.

21) *Chongxiao* (DT.17), includes the three points: *Miaochao* (XIX) below the twentieth vertebra, *shangdui* (XX) below the twenty-first vertebra and *shanggao* (XXI) which is one *cun* below *shangdui*.
    Indications: Distention and pain of the cerebellar, distention of the middle of os nuchale.

22) *Hou'ejiu* (VT.01), including nine points, one at the laryngeal prominence, one 1 inch above the laryngeal prominence, one 1.5 inches below it, and the rest six 1.5 inches lateral (to the right and to the left) to the first three points.
    Indications: Throat moth, throat pain, thyroiditis, throat itching, obstruction of the throat by sputum (dyspnea resembling asthma).

23) *Shi'erhou* (VT.02), including twelve points, six points on the line 1.3 inches below the clavicle bilaterally, and another six points on the line 1.5 below the clavicle bilaterally.
    Indications: Scarlet fever, asthma due to angiosclerosis, hepatic cholera (typhoid, severe cold, cholera).

24) *Jinwu* (VT.03), including five points starting from *jingan* (VT.03-1), which is at the depression at the semilunar portion at the top of the sternum, going down through *jinyin*, *jinyang*, *jinzhuan* and ending at *jinjiao* (VT.03-2-5).
    Indications: Hepatic cholera, indigestion (abdominal distention), hypochondriac pain, trachea obstruction, various kinds of chorera.
    ※**Remarks**: *Jingan*, *jinyin*, *jinyang*, and *jinzhuan* and *Jinjiao* (VT.03-1-5) coincide with *tiantu* (REN 22), *xuanji* (REN 21), *huagai* (REN 20), *zigong* (REN 19) and *yutang* (REN 18) of the REN Vessel.

25) *Weimaoqi* (VT.04), includes seven points, one at the depression of the seventh costosternal juncture, the other two are 1 inch and 2 inches below it, and the other four are 1.5 inches lateral to the middle line.

Indications: Wool-like furuncle, gastropathy, various kinds of cholera, palpitation, gastric hemorrhage.

※**Remarks**: If we change the location from "1.5 inches lateral to the middle line" to "2 inches lateral to the middle line," it will be easier to locate the points. In this way, the seven points coincide with *jiuwei* (REN 15), *juque* (REN 14), *shangwan* (REN 13) of the REN Vessel, bilateral *burong* (ST 19) and *chengman* (ST 20) of the Stomach Channel. Of course, bloodletting can be performed one the line 1.5 inches apart.

26) *Fuchao'ershisan* (VT.05), includes twenty-three points, two points above the umbilicus and five points below the umbilicus; two bilateral points one inch lateral to the umbilicus, each having one point above and two points below (eight points bilaterally); two bilateral points two inch lateral to the umbilicus, each having one point above and two points below (eight points bilaterally). All the points are 1 inch apart.

Indications: Enteritis, metritis, nephritis, nephralgia and umbilical pain.

※**Remarks**: Generally, not all the twenty-three points are used, but only the four points around the umbilicus. More points can be used in severe cases.

Besides the common locations for bloodletting mentioned above, there are more locations in the empirical recipes spread among people for bloodletting. The further development of the techniques of bloodletting therapy calls for our joint efforts.

3. Bloodletting Therapy for Common Diseases

Both mainstream practitioners and the historical literature acknowledge that bloodletting therapy can be used to treat a great variety of diseases with speedy effect. It is unfortunate that very few contemporary medical texts discuss this therapy in depth. The following is a summary of bloodletting therapy used in the treatment of common diseases, based on various medical texts and my understanding of Master Tung's experience in bloodletting therapy.

1) Diseases of the head
   a. Vertex pain: *shangxing* (DU 23) and *baihui* (DU 20).
   b. Distention and pain of the occiput or metencephalon: a) *chongxiao* (DT.17); b) *weizhong* (BL 40).
   c. Migraine: a) *sihuawai* (77.14); b) *taiyang* (EX-HN5).

   d. Frontal pain: a) *sifuyi* (1010.11), *sifu'er* (1010.10) and *shangli* (1010.09); b) *sihuazhong* (77.09).
   e. Sudden dizziness: *wuling* (DT.04); dizziness due to hypertension: a) *wuling* (DT.04), b) the ear back.
   f. Common cold with headache: a) *sanshang*; b) *qishing* (DT.03).
   g. Angioneurotic headache: *taiyang* (EX-HN5).

2) Diseases of the eye
   a. Keratitis: a) *taiyang* (EX-HN5); b) *ganshu* (BL 18); c) *wuling* (DT.04) [liver, gall bladder, *xinshu* (BL 15)]; d) ear back.
   b. Distention and pain of the orbit: a) *shaoshang* (LU 11); b) *taiyang* (EX-HN5).
   c. Conjunctivitis: a) *taiyang* (EX-HN5); b) *zanzhu* (BL 2); c) *shaoshang* (LU 11).
   d. Hordeolum: a) ear back; b) *quchi* (LI 11); c) tip of middle toe.
   e. Pterygium: a) *shaoze* (SI 1); b) *zhiyin* (BL 67).

3) Diseases of the ear
   a. Subaural adenitis: a) *shaoshang* (LU 11); b) ear tip; c) *zulinqi* (GB 41), *xiaxi* (GB 43), *diwuhui* (GB42).
   b. Earache: *sihuawai* (77.14).
   c. Otitis media (suppurative): around the ankle.

4) Diseases of the mouth
   a. Sores of the mouth and tongue: a) ear tip; b) *jinjin* (Extra 9), *yuye* (Extra 9); c) the blue vein between *yinlingquan* (SP 9) and *xuehai* (SP 10).
   b. Swelling of the mouth, tongue and throat: *sanzhong* (77.07), *shaoshang* (LU 11).
   c. Sores of the mouth and lips: a) the blue vein between *yinlingquan* (SP 9) and *xuehai* (SP 10); b) *shangchun* (77.15), *xiachun* (77.16).

5) Diseases of the tooth
   Toothache: The area between external malleolus and *zulinqi* (GB 41), *xiaxi* (GB 43), *diwuhui* (GB42).

6) Diseases of the nose
   a. Epistaxis: a) *shaoshang* (LU 11); b) *ganshu* (BL 18).
   b. Acne rosacea: a) *pishu* (BL 20); b) *weishu* (BL 21); c) from the nose tip to *zhengben* (1010.12) (seven-star needle).
   c. Allergic rhinitis: *zhengben* (1010.12).

7) Diseases of the throat
   General treatment: a) First prick *shaoshang* (LU 11) and *shangyang* (LI 1), and then treat the diseases according to different conditions. b) First prick

the ear tip or ear back, and then treat the diseases according to different conditions.

a. Tonsillitis: a) *shaoshang* (LU 11) and *shangyang* (LI 1); b) *sanzhong* (77.07).
b. Laryngitis: a) *shaoshang* (LU 11), *shangyang* (LI 1) and *hegu* (LI 4); b) *sanzhong* (77.07).
c. Pharyngeal swelling with dysphagia: a) *shaoshang* (LU 11), *shangyang* (LI 1) and *hegu* (LI 4); b) *sanzhong* (77.07); c) *guanchong* (SJ 1).
d. Laryngeal pain: a) pricking the area between *yinlingquan* (SP 9) and *xuehai* (SP10); b) *yamen* (DU 15); c) *hou'ejiu* (VT.01).
e. Throat moth: *shaoshang* (LU 11).
f. Aphasia: *zongshu* (1010.07).
g. Obstruction of the throat by sputum: *hou'ejiu* (VT.01).

8) Asthma

a. *Wuling* (DT.04) on the back [including *geshu* (BL 17), *feishu* (BL 13), *xinshu* (BL 15), etc.]; b) *taiyang* (EX-HN5), *chize* (LU 5); c) *sihuawai* (77.14); d) pricking the blue vein from *houxi* (SI 3) and *wangu* (GB 12).

9) Diseases of the neck

a. Goiter: a) *sanzhong* (77.07); b) auricular vein; c) *hou'ejiu* (VT.01).
b. Pain of the middle line of the os nuchale: a) *chongxiao* (DT.17); b) *weizhong* (BL 40).

10) Diseases of the upper limbs

General treatment: First prick the cubital fossa and then treat the diseases according to different conditions.

a. Wrist pain: a) *sihuazhong* (77.09), *sihuafu* (77.10); b) *zulinqi* (GB 41), *xiaxi* (GB 43), *diwuhui* (GB42), c) *shuiyu* (44.17).
b. Shoulder pain: *sihuawai* (77.14).
c. Finger numbness: a) *houxin* (DT.11); b) *shuangfeng* (DT.05).
d. Redness and swelling of the back of the hand and finger pain: *sihuazhong* (77.09), *shuangfeng* (DT.05).
e. Hand pain and numbness, angiosclerosis of hand and foot: a) *shuangfeng* (DT.05); b) *sihuawai* (77.14); c) *shuiyu* (44.17).
f. Arm pain: a) *shuanghe* (DT.16); b) *sihuawai* (77.14); c) *shuiyu* (44.17).
g. Shoulder and arm pain: a) *shuanghe* (DT.16); b) *sihuawai* (77.14).
h. Ganglionic cyst: Applying chicken-claw pricking at the local area to let out mucus and blood.

11) Diseases of the lower limbs
   General treatment: First prick *weizhong* (BL 40) and then treat the diseases according to different conditions.
   a. Soreness of the legs: *jinlin* (DT.09), *jinzhi* (DT.08-XXVII).
   b. Sciatica: a) pain of the *taiyang* Channel – *weizhong* (BL 40) or *jinlin* (DT.09); b) pain of the *shaoyang* Channel – *sihuawai* (77.14) or *jinlin* (DT.09).
   c. Knee pain: *sanjin* (DT.07).
   d. Leg pain and distention: *jingzhi* (DT.08).
   e. Swelling and pain of the ankle: *weizhong* (BL 40), *yanglingquan* (GB 34).
   f. Heel pain: *weizhong* (BL 40).
   g. Foot numbness and pain: a) *shuangfeng* (DT.05); b) *yinbai* (LR 9).
   h. Toe spasm: Center of the external malleolus.
   i. Hong Kong foot with yellow discharge: a) pricking the blue vein from the center of the external malleolus to *zulinqi* (GB 41); b) *zhiwu* (11.26).
   j. Numbness and pain of the four limbs: *Jing*-Well points.

12) Diseases of the chest and abdomen
   a. Hypochondriac pain (hepatic cirrhosis, pleurisy): *sihuawai* (77.14), which can be used with *ganshu* (BL 18).
   b. Abdominal pain: *sihuazhong* (77.09), *sihuafu* (77.10).
   c. Chest stuffiness and distention: a) *chize* (LU 5); b) *sihuazhong* (77.09).
   d. Umbilicus pain: a) *fuchao'ershisan* (VT.05) (altogether 23 points, see descriptions of the points mentioned above); b) *sihuawai* (77.14).

13) Diseases of the loin and back
   General treatment: First prick *weizhong* (BL 40) and then treat the diseases according to different conditions.
   a. Spine pain: a) *weizhong* (BL 40); b) *renzhong* (DU 26).
   b. Loin pain: *weizhong* (BL 40).
   c. Sprain and stiffness: *weizhong* (BL 40).
   d. Lumbago due to angiosclerosis: *dingzhu* (DT.10), *weizhong* (BL 40).
   e. Back pain: *chengshan* (BL 57).

14) Diseases of the heart
   General treatment: a) cubital fossa; b) *sihuazhong* (77.09); c) *wuling* (DT.04).
   a. Cardiomegaly: *wuling* (DT.04) (upper energizer portion).
   b. Angiosclerosis of the heart: *sihuazhong* (77.09), *sihuafu* (77.10).
   c. Cardioplegia: *sihuazhong* (77.09), *sihuafu* (77.10), the twelve *Jing*-Well points.

d. Palpitation: *dan* (11.13).
e. Heart failure: *houxin* (DT.11).
f. Cardialgia: *huobao* (55.01), *chize* (LU 5).
g. Accelerated heartbeat: *sihuazhong* (77.09), *sihuafu* (77.10).

15) Diseases of the liver and gall bladder
a. Jaundice: *yinbai* (LR 9), *pishu* (BL 20), *weishu* (BL 21).
b. Hepatic cirrhosis: *sihuawai* (77.14), *ganshu* (BL 18).
c. Liver diseases: *huobao* (55.01).

16) Lung diseases
a. Bronchitis (with yellow sputum): *sihuawai* (77.14).
b. Asthma: a) *wuling* (DT.04) at the back; b) *taiyang*; c) *chize* (LU 5); d) *sihuawai* (77.14); e) pricking the blue vein from *houxi* (SI 3) to *wangu* (GB 12).
c. Acute pneumonia: a) *dabai* (22.04); b) *feishu* (BL 13), *fengmen* (BL 12).
d. Miscellaneous diseases of the Lung Channel: *sihuawai* (77.14), or together with *feishu* (BL 13) with better effect.

17) Diseases of the spleen and stomach
a. Epiagstric pain: *sihuazhong* (77.09), *sihuafu* (77.10).
b. Gastritis: a) *sihuazhong* (77.09), *sihuafu* (77.10); b) from *neiting* (ST 44) to *jiexi* (S41).
c. Acute gastralgia: a) *sihuazhong* (77.09), *sihuafu* (77.10); b) *quze* (PC 3), *weizhong* (BL 40); c) *wuling* (DT.04) [middle energizer portion, around *weishu* (BL 21)].
d. Gastric hemorrhage: a) *weimaoqi* (VT.04); b) *sihuazhong* (77.09), *sihuafu* (77.10).
e. Gastric ulcer: *sihuazhong* (77.09), *sihuafu* (77.10).
f. Duodenal ulcer: a) pricking the blue vein from *neiting* (ST 44) to *jiexi* (S41); b) external malleolus.
g. Acute enterogastritis (with vomiting and diarrhea): a) *sihuazhong* (77.09), *sihuafu* (77.10), *sihuawai* (77.14); b) *quze* (PC 3), *weizhong* (BL 40).

18) Kidney diseases
a. Nephritis: a) pricking *shuishu* to let out yellow discharge; b) *fuchao'ershisan* (VT.05); c) around the kidney.

19) Intestinal diseases
General treatment: *sihuazhong* (77.09), *sihuawai* (77.14).
a. Duodenum: a) pricking the blue vein from *neiting* (ST 44) to *jiexi* (S41); b) around the external malleolus.
b. Cecitis: *sihuazhong* (77.09), *sihuafu* (77.10), *sihuawai* (77.14).
c. Hernia: around the inner malleolus.
d. Acute enterogastritis: *sihuazhong* (77.09), *sihuafu* (77.10), *sihuawai* (77.14).

e. Acute enteritis: a) *sihuazhong* (77.09), *sihuafu* (77.10); b) *sanjiang* (DT.15).
f. Acute abdominal pain: *quze* (PC 3), *weizhong* (BL 40).

20) Gynecopathy
a. Swelling and pain of the breast: *sihuazhong* (77.09), *sihuafu* (77.10).
b. Amenorrhea: *sanjiang* (DT.15).
c. Hysteritis: *sanjiang* (DT.15).
d. Retention of placenta: *huobao* (55.01).
e. Leucorrhea: a) *sanjiang* (DT.15); b) *shiqizhui* (EX-B8), *baliao* (BL31, 32, 33, 34).

21) Diseases of the blood vessel
a. Apoplexy: the twelve *Jing*-Well points.
b. Hypertention: a) *sihuawai* (77.14); b) *wuling* (DT.04); c) *weizhong* (BL 40).
c. Paralysis of the hand and foot or hemiplegia caused by hypertension: a) *wuling* (DT.04); b) *chize* (LU 5), *weizhong* (BL 40).
d. Phlebangioma: pricking the tumor.

22) Children's diseases
a. Infantile malnutrition (with much food intake and emaciation): a) *sifeng* (EX-UE10); b) *ganshu* (BL 18), *geshu* (BL 17), *weishu* (BL 21), *shenzhu* (DU12).
b. Smallpox: a) *chize* (LU 5), *weizhong* (BL 40); b) the ear back.
c. Convulsion: a) *shixuan* (EX-UE11); b) *qishing* (DT.03); c) *yintang* (EX-HN3).
d. Asthma: *dabai* (22.04).
e. Night cry: *dan* (11.13).
f. High fever and vomiting: *zongshu* (1010.07), or together with *qishing* (DT.03).
g. Congenital deformity of the tongue: *shaoze* (SI 1), *shaochong* (HT 9), *yinbai* (LR 9).
h. Mumps: *shaoshang* (LU 11), *guanchong* (SJ 1).

23) Miscellaneous diseases
a. Dry cholera: a) *zongshu* (1010.07); b) *wuling* (DT.04).
b. Cholera: a) *weizhong* (BL 40); b) *chize* (LU 5), *quze* (PC 3).
c. Xiexui: a) *weizhong* (BL 40); b) *shaoshang* (LU 11).
d. Hemorrhoid: *weizhong* (BL 40).
e. Sunstroke: the twelve *Jing*-Well points.
f. Epilepsy: a) onset: the twelve *Jing*-Well points; b) remission: *wuling* (DT.04).
g. Skin diseases: postauricular vein.

h. Hordeolum: a) *pishu* (BL 20), *weishu* (BL 21); b) postauricular vein; c) *quchi* (LI 11).
i. Scarlet fever: *shi'erhou* (VT.02).
j. Various kinds of cholera: a) *jinwu* (VT.03); b) *wuling* (DT.04).
k. Wool-like furuncle: a) *weimaoqi* (VT.04); b) *houxin* (DT.11).
l. Deep-rooted boils: *houxin* (DT.11).
m. General fatigue: *beimian* (44.07).
n. Vomiting (with discomfort of the five *zang*-organs): a) *qishing* (DT.03) [*zongshu* (1010.07)]; b) *wuling* (DT.04).
o. Herpes zoster: a) around the local area; b) the ear back; c) *zhiwu* (11.26).

4. Case Reports

1) Mr. Wang was a 36 year old office worker who had sciatica on the left side and was unable to walk. The painful area was on the Gall Bladder Channel. He was treated by pricking the raised blue vein between *fenglong* (ST 40) and *yanglingquan* (GB 34) to let out some blood and he was cured after only one treatment.

2) Mr. Yang was a 20 years old student who had conjunctivitis and congested eyes for three days. He was treated by pricking the thin purple vein on the posterior aspect of the auricle to let out little blood; he recovered the second day.

3) Mrs. Xie was a 33 year old woman with rheumatalgia of the knees for many years; she had sharp pains when she went to see us. We first pricked *sanjin* (DT.07) to let out little blood and her pain was greatly relieved. We then applied acupuncture at *neiguan* (PC 6) bilaterally and asked her to move the legs. She was thus cured of the disease after only one treatment without recurrence for ten years.

4) Mr. Tu was a 40 year old army man who had sprained his waist for two days with great pain. He was treated by pricking the raised blue vein at *weizhong* (BL 40) to let out little blood, followed by needling at *shugu* (BL 65), and he recovered after one treatment.

5) Mrs. Wang was a 40 year old woman with migraines for nearly 20 years. The pain came with vomiting and sharp pain. She was treated by pricking the temporal area to let out blood, and her headache was instantly relieved. She didn't come for a second visit, but telephoned us that she had already recovered.

6) Mr. Yang was a 36 year old man who was unable to open his mouth because of overindulgence in eating beetle nuts. He had white spots in the mouth and would have sharp pain if he ate pungent food. He was diagnosed with buccal carcinoma at a major hospital. He invited me to

come to Taiwan to treat him. I pricked *taiyang* (EX-HN5) and *chize* (LU 5), and the patient could immediately open his mouth. After that, bloodletting was performed once a week for three months. The white spots turned red, he was able to open his mouth freely and could eat foods of all flavors. He has been cured for four years now and everything is OK.

7) Mr. Han was 35 years old and had asthma for three years with attacks in the winter. He was treated by pricking *feishu* (BL 13), *gaohuang* (BL 43), *dazhui* (DU 14) and *chize* (LU 5) and needling *shuijin* (1010.20) and *yuji* (LU 10); his symptoms were immediately relieved. The same treatment was repeated three times, once a week, and he did not have any more attacks.

5. My Experience

1) Bloodletting is commonly referred to as "pricking."

2) In treating chronic rheumatalgia, bloodletting therapy can prevent recurrence, which often occurs in patients treated only with acupuncture.

3) According to the *Nei Jing* (Yellow Emperor's Inner Classic), the principle of bloodletting therapy is that blood should be released in order to treat chronic diseases. In my opinion, in chronic diseases always present with hyperactivity of the pathogenic factors and blood stasis, which caused obstruction of the blood vessel. While acupuncture relieves the diseases, recurrences are likely to occur due to an incomplete resolution of the condition. Therefore, bloodletting is necessary, just as the ancient people said, "To treat wind one must treat blood, and free flow of blood leads to subsidence of wind."

4) While contralateral needling method is effective in filiform needle treatment, ipsilateral bloodletting will achieve better effect.

5) Bloodletting therapy is more effective if distal points are chosen. This conforms to the old saying of "pricking distal points: the foot is pricked to treat diseases of the head." Similarly, diseases of the lower part of the body is treated by pricking the upper part of the body, e.g. to treat diseases of the lower limbs, the back is pricked.

6) For bloodletting techniques, one can refer to "Application of Three-edged Needle" in the first volume of *Zhen Jiu Jing Wei* (The Strategy of Acupuncture).[1]

(Dissertation of Strait Chinese Medicine Journal, October, 1990)

[1] Or in the chapter thirteen of *Zhen Jiu Bao Dein* (Acupuncture Treasure Text)

Appendix 2

A Collection of Application of Tung's Extraordinary Points

by Young, Wei Chieh

Treatment of Stiff Neck and Chronic Lumbago with *Chongzi* (22.01)

Stiff neck is a common disease and a number of points can be used to treat this disease effectively, such as *xuanzhong* (GB 39), *luozhen* (Extra 28), *houxi* (SI 3) and *tianzhu* (BL 10). I have used *houxi* (SI 3) and *shugu* (BL 65) to treat the disease. It is stated in *Ling Shu Za Bing Pian* (Spiritual Pivot – Miscellaneous Diseases) that "in treating stiff neck, use points from the Hand-*Taiyang* Channel for those unable to turn to the left and right, and use points from the Foot-*Taiyang* Channel for those unable to turn forward and backward." Therefore, in the former case, *houxi* (SI 3) from the Small Intestine Channel of Hand-*Taiyang* is used; in the latter case, *shugu* (BL 65) from the Bladder Channel of Foot-*Taiyang* is use, both with speedy effect. Both points can be used if both conditions are present.

In addition, *zhengjin* (77.01) can also be used to treat stiff neck, which I have often used with great effect. [For more information about the application of *zhengjin* (77.01) and *zhengzong* (77.02), please refer to my book *Tung Shi Qi Xue Jian Zuo* (Lectures on Tung's Acupuncture: Points Study)].

However, according to other medical books [*Yu Long Ge Fu* (Song and Ode of the Jade Dragon), *Tong Xuan Zhi Yao Fu* (Ode of the Essentials of Understanding), *Wo Yan Ling Xiao Ying Xue Ge* (Song of Effective Points of Wo Yan Ling), etc.], *chengjiang* (REN 24) is the best point for stiff neck. Therefore, this point can always used for any kind of stiff neck.

Stiff neck sometimes also affects the shoulders and upper arms, and points other than the Hand and Foot-*taiyang* can also be used. *Chongzi* (22.01) is a good point, which I have used together with *chengjiang* (REN 24) for stiff neck in the past ten years. In most cases, the disease is cured after only one treatment.

(Strait Chinese Medicine, 1990-1)

Treatment of Polyuria and Frozen Shoulder with *Shenguan* (77.18)

Shenguan (77.18) is an important point on the leg, 1.5 inches directly below *yinlingquan* (SP 9). This is the first choice of Master Tung in treating kidney deficiency and diseases caused by kidney deficiency.

I have often used this point to treat frozen shoulder with good effect. According to statistics based on over 100 cases, its effect is even better than the method of puncturing *tiaokou* (ST 38) towards *chengshan* (BL 57) or the method of using local points. For chronic and severe cases, this point can be used together with *chize* (LU 5). For those with difficulty raising the arms and turning the arms backward, *zuwujin* (77.25) (healthy side) can be added with prompt effect. For chronic cases with congealed shoulders, bloodletting at the cubital fossa should be given.

I have used this point to cure over ten cases of night polyuria, especially senile patients with kidney deficiency, with marked effect. The effect is even more satisfactory for young people. The point is also effective for day polyuria. No points from the fourteen regular Channels are comparable to this point.

In addition, this point can also be used to treat numbness and pain of the ten fingers very effectively. It is also an important point for eye diseases such as spotted vision and strabismus, often used in combination with *fuliu* (KI 7). It is also a common point for hemiplegia. The point is always punctured bilaterally.

In short, this point is quite effective with a wide range of application. Besides what is mentioned above, all the diseases caused by kidney deficiency can be treated with this point.

(Strait Chinese Medicine, 1990-1)

Treatment of Chapped Palm (Hand Skin Diseases and Common Cold with Watery Nasal Discharge) with *Mu* (11.17)

Mu (11.17) is a very important point on the palm, at the middle of the line between the midline of the first knuckle of the index finger and the junction between the black and white flesh at the medial aspect of the index finger. It is in fact two points lying at the upper and lower one third between the two finger creases.

Originally, Master Tung used this point to treat hyperactivity of liver fire and spleen *qi* dryness, thus the name "*Mu*" (Chinese meaning: wood). I often use this point to treat dry eyes, dacryorrhea and palmar polydypsia, and find that it is a better point than points from the fourteen regular channels.

I have also used the point to treat hardening of the hand skin and hand skin diseases, especially chapped palm with especially good effect. The diseases are usually cured after three or four, or even one or two, sessions of treatment.

Mu (11.17) is also effective for watery or thick nasal discharge, especially when it is caused by common cold.

To treat the hand skin diseases, use the point on the diseased side; to treat nasal discharge, use the point on the healthy side.

This point can clear away liver fire, and the effect is even better if it is used in combination with *Long Dan Xie Gan Tang* (Decoction of Radix Gentianae for Purging Liver Fire).

(Strait Chinese Medicine, 1990-1)

Treatment of Infertility with *Fuke* (11.24)

There have been more and more cases of infertility in recent years, which, according to Chinese medicine, can be divided into different types: kidney deficiency, blood deficiency (or *qi* and blood deficiency), liver depression, blood stasis and phlegm dampness. Both Chinese drugs and acupuncture can treat this disease effectively. Doctors normally treat the disease according to the main disease and the accompanying symptoms, such as obstruction of the oviduct, or retroversion of left flexion of the uterus.

I have treated infertility for many years using acupuncture with good effect. I especially want to recommend *fuke* (11.24), used as a main point in combination with *huanchao* (11.06). In the past ten years I have successfully treated nearly one hundred female fertility patients; the effect is better than points from the fourteen regular channels. Treatment can be given every other day, with the two points used alternately. According to my experience, the younger the patient and the earlier the treatment, the better the effect. I have read over one hundred articles and papers about the treatment of infertility, and 80% of the patients in the case reports are under 35 years old. It is strange that 80% of the patients that I have treated are over 35 years old.

(Strait Chinese Medicine, 1990-1)

Wuhu (11.27) – An Important Point for Pain of Fingers and Toes

Acupuncturists commonly treat pains of the fingers and toes with *sifeng* (Extra 25) in the transverse creases between the fingers and *bafeng* (Extra 40) in the transverse creases between the toes respectively. Although multiple points are used, the effect is not satisfactory. I have used wuhu1, one of the five points in *wuhu* (11.27), to treat finger pain and wuhu3, also one of the five points in *wuhu* (11.27), to treat toe pain with speedy effect.

Wuhu (11.27) was discovered by Master Tung, the indication of the point was said to be "only general bone swelling," according to *Tung Shi Zhen Jiu Zheng Jing Qi Xue Xue* (Tung's Acupuncturology on Regular Channels and Extraordinary Points). In the clinical practice, I have made several discoveries. Besides pain of the fingers and toes, this point can also be used to treat pain of the dorsal part of the foot and the heel, and peritendinitis. I have treated several hundred patients, from players of national teams to those who were treated with other methods in vain, and the results have always been satisfactory.

Wuhu (11.27) is at the junction between the dorsal and palmar flesh on the first interphalangeal joint of the thumb; it is on the Lung Channel of Hand-*taiyin*. There are altogether five points from the tip of the first metacarpus to the interphalangeal transverse crease, each about one sixth of the whole length apart. Starting from the finger tip, the five points are wuhu1, wuhu2, wuhu3, wuhu4, and wuhu5.

*Wuhu*1 is often used to treat finger and palm pain and peritendinitis; wuhu3 is used for toe pain; wuhu2 is used to enhance the effect of wuhu1 and wuhu3; wuhu4 is used to treat pain of the dorsal part of the foot and wuhu5 is used for heel pain.

A case report: Mr. Chen, a player of the national basketball team, had had injury of the first and second toes of the left foot and could not move about freely. I punctured wuhu3 and asked him to move the injured toes, and he felt much better 2 or 3 minutes later. The needle was retained for 30 minutes and he didn't feel any pain. The disease was cured in just one treatment.

(Strait Chinese Medicine, 1990-3)

Linggu (22.05) and *Dabai* (22.04) —
Important Points for Warming *Yang* and Reinforcing *Qi*

Linggu (22.05) and *dabai* (22.04) are main points for the palm, which are often used by Master Tung and are among the more common points I tend to use. *Linggu* (22.05) is between the dorsal part of the thumb and the furcula of the index finger, at the junction of the first and second metacarpal bones. *Dabai* (22.04) is just *sanjian* (LI 3) of the Large Intestine Channel and is seldom used alone, but is inserted together with *linggu* (22.05) as *Dao Ma* needle technique to achieve the best results. It is used alone only in bloodletting for children's asthma, high fever and acute pneumonia.

According to *Tung Shi Zhen Jiu Zheng Jing Qi Xue Xue* (Tung's Acupuncturology on Regular Channels and Extraordinary Points), the indications of *linggu* (22.05) include "sciatica due to pulmonary incompetence, lumbago, foot pain, facial paralysis, hemiplegia, skeleton distention, irregular menstruation, amenorrhea, difficult labor, backache, tinnitus, deafness, migraine, dysmenorrhea, intestinal pain and dizziness."

Pulmonary incompetence refers to "*qi* deficiency." These two points have extremely strong effect of reinforcing *qi* and can be used to treat any conditions due to *qi* deficiency, the effect of which is by no means inferior to *zusanli* (ST 36), *qihai* (REN 6) and *tanzhong* (REN 17). The points are also very effective in warming *yang*. I have often used the bilateral *linggu* (22.05) alone to treat spinal pain, dysuria and polyuria, and *shenguan* (77.18) can also be used with better effect. The points arc also cffcctivc for elbow pain (⊥), groin pain (∠), heal pain (∠) and dizziness (╨). (Remarks: ⊥ means the diseased side or the same side; ∠ means healthy side or opposite side; ╨ means both sides. I created these signs twenty years ago and have found them to be very convenient).

Linggu (22.05) and *dabai* (22.04) can be used to treat hemiplegia. According to my experience of over twenty years in treating over one hundred cases, the therapeutic effect is better than the points of the fourteen regular Channels, such as *quchi* (LI 11), *yanglingquan* (GB 34), *jianyu* (LI 15), *huantiao* (GB 30), *xuanzhong* (GB 39), etc. In using these two points, the healthy side is often punctured, and they are especially effective for pains of the leg along the *yangming* and *taiying* Channels.

Deep insertion of both points are necessary, and the farther away the diseased area, the more deeply the needle should be inserted. When both points are used, *linggu* (22.05) is punctured first and then *dabai* (22.04).

Dabai (22.04) coincides with *sanjian* (LI 3) of the Large Intestine Channel. *Linggu* (22.05) is anterior to the furcula posterior to *hegu* (LI 4). Holographically, the former controls the upper energizer and the latter, the lower energizer. Also, since deep insertion is used, the effect of the points covers the three energizers (*sanjiao*), thus their strong effect.

(Strait Chinese Medicine, 1990-3)

Xiaojie (A.05) — An Important Point for Ankle Pain

Ankle sprain and pain is a common disease and acupuncture is effective for it. Generally, treatment is given by puncturing *xuanzhong* (GB 39) and *kunlun* (BL 60) for external malleolus and *xuanzhong* (GB 39) and *taixi* (KI 3) for internal malleolus. Alternatively, local points can be chosen. In recent years, people also use the extraordinary point *huai* (ankle).

In the past twenty years, I have used *xiaojie* (A.05) to treat ankle sprain and pain with extremely good effect, much better than the methods mentioned above, based on statistics of over 300 cases.

Xiaojie (A.05) is on the junction of black and white flesh by the metacarpal bone of the basic joint of the thumb (on the Lung Channel of Hand-*Taiyin*). The insertion of the needle is made when the patient's hand forms a fist, and the needle should be inserted toward *chongxian* (22.02), about 1.5 inches deep. The healthy side is punctured. After the needling sensation is felt, the doctor should rotate the needle while asking the patient to move and ankle, and the pain is instantly relieved. The needle is normally retained for 30 minutes, or 45 minutes or longer for chronic and severe diseases. Local redness and swelling can be treated by pricking *weizhong* (BL 40) on the affected side to eliminate swelling.

A case report: Mr. Wen, a player of the national tennis team, came to visit me in October, 1985. He had had left ankle sprain for three days and had received massage treatment twice with no satisfactory effect. I punctured *xiaojie* (A.05) on the right side and rotate the needle every ten minutes. After fifteen minutes the pain was greatly relieved, and the needle was retained for 30 minutes. He didn't feel any pain after that but came again the next afternoon asking for consolidation treatment. He then went to attend a match for two hours without feeling any discomfort.

(Strait Chinese Medicine, 1990-3)

***Remarks**: This point was discovered by Dr. Wei Chieh Young based on Master Tung's correspondence needling method.

Appendix 3

Index of Questions and Answers in the Book

Appendix 4

Index of Tung's Extraordinary Points

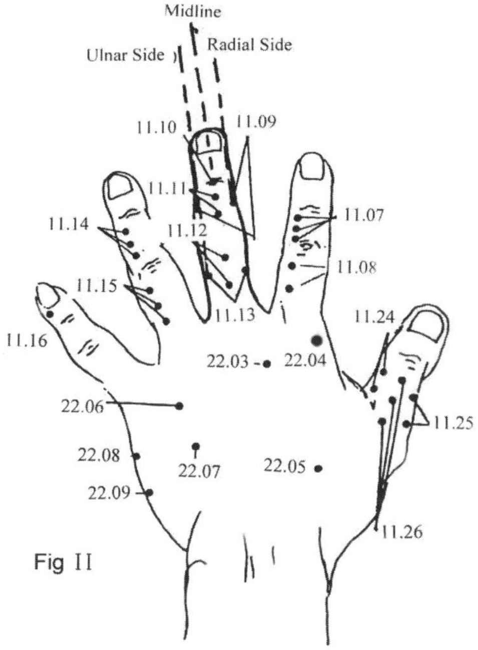

Fig II

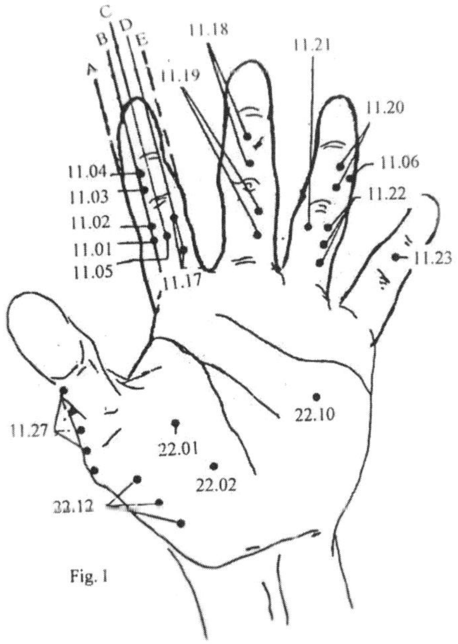

Fig. 1

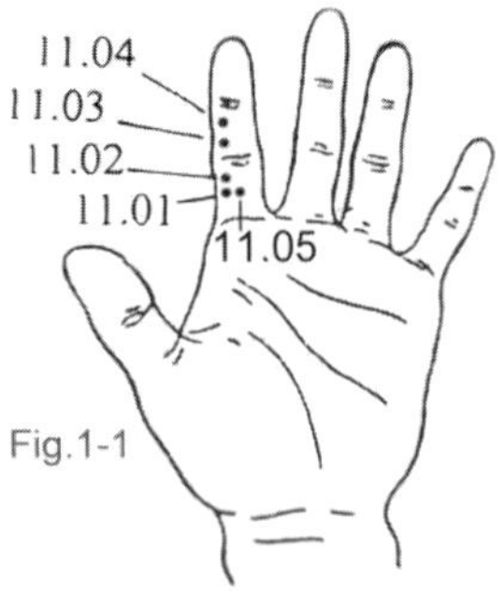

Fig.1-1

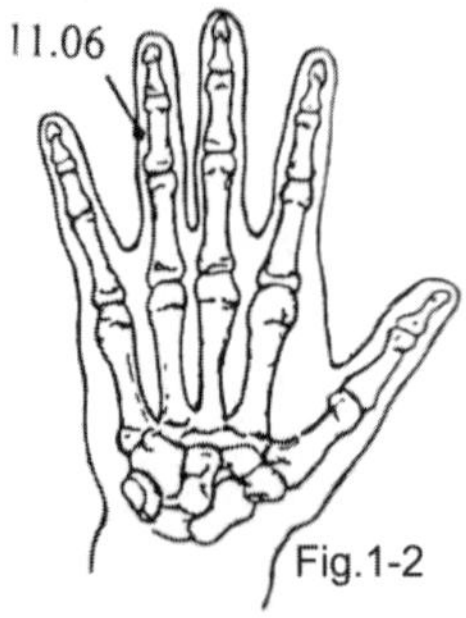

Fig.1-2

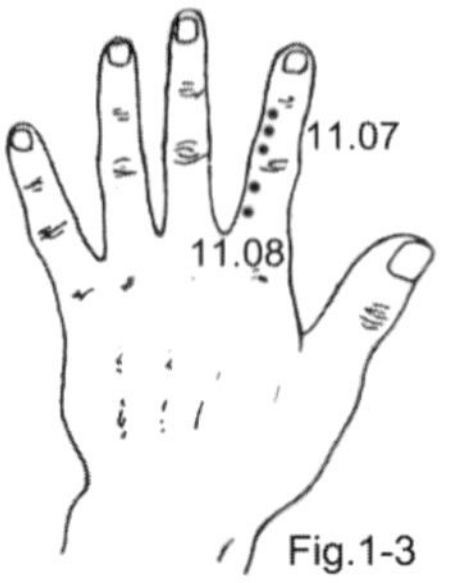

Fig.1-3

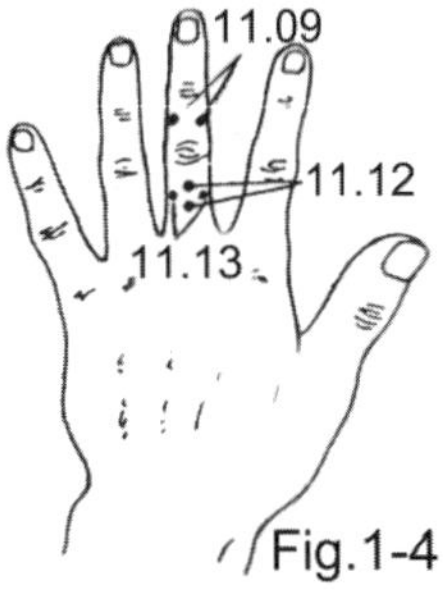

Fig.1-4

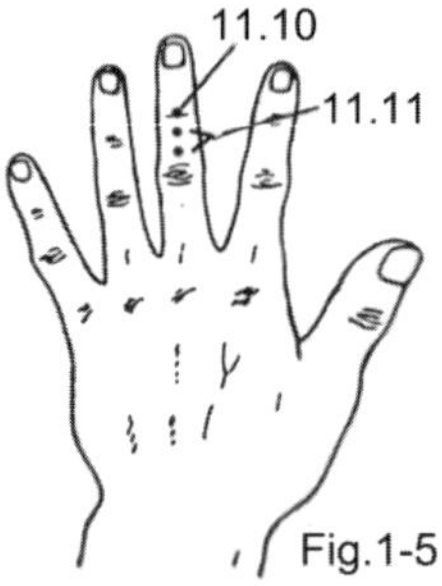

Fig.1-5

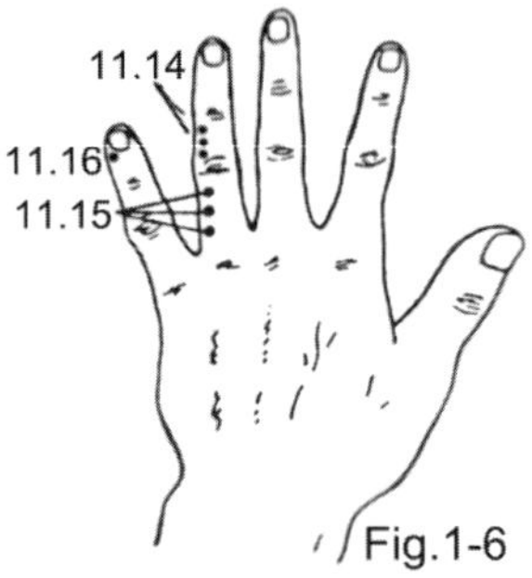

Fig.1-6

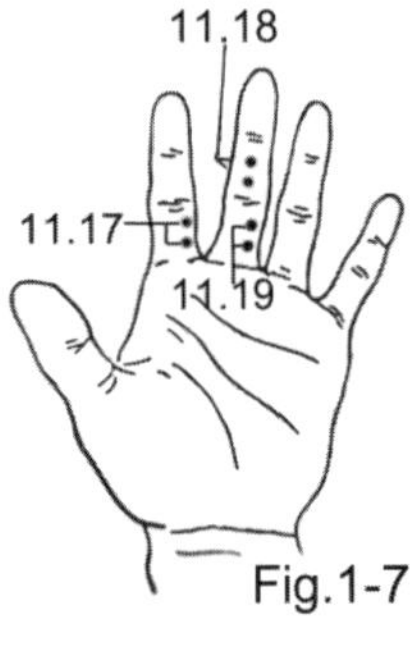

Fig.1-7

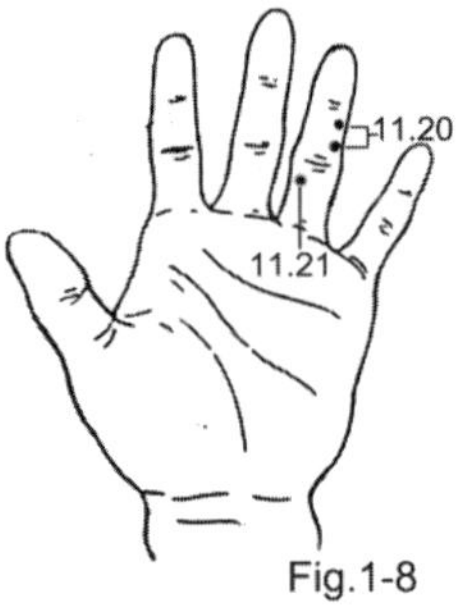

Fig.1-8

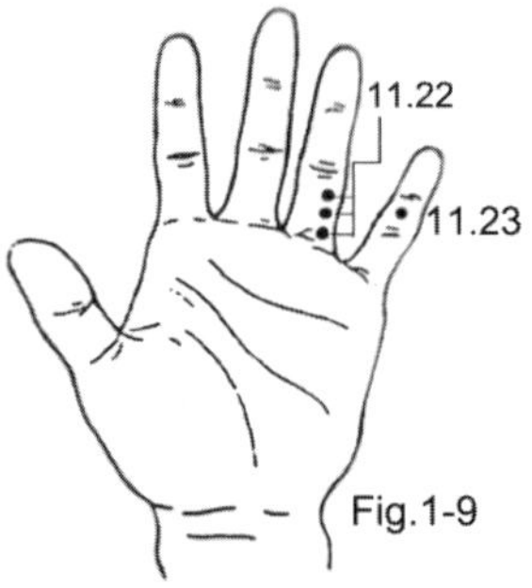

Fig.1-9

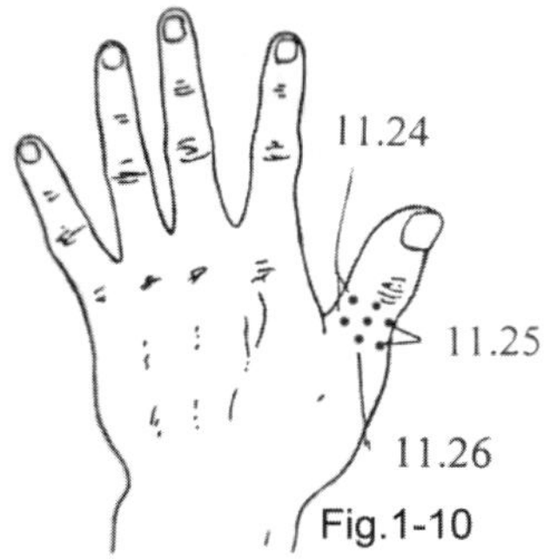

Fig.1-10

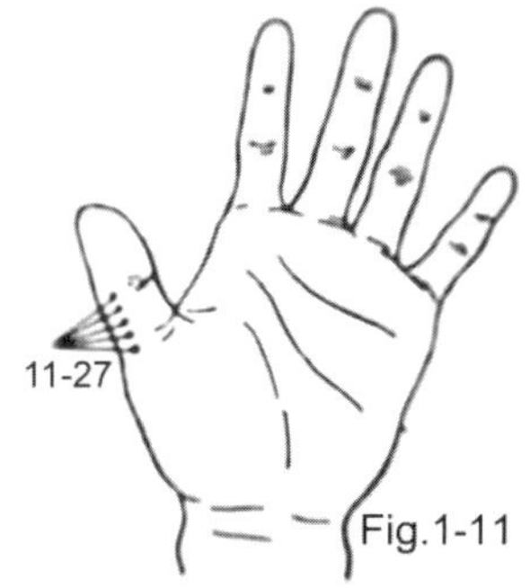

Fig.1-11

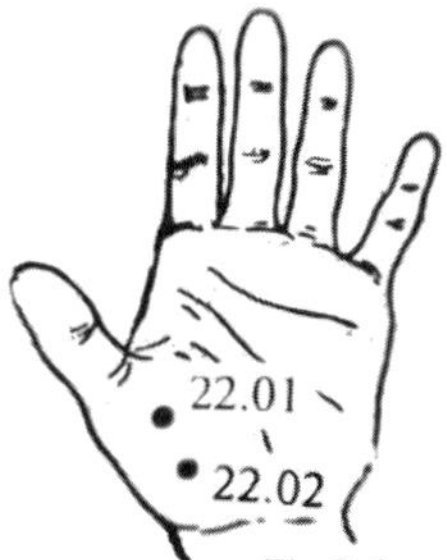

Fig.2-1

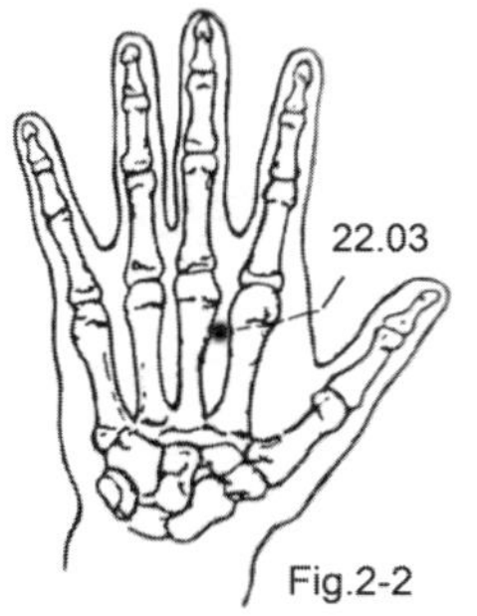

Fig.2-2

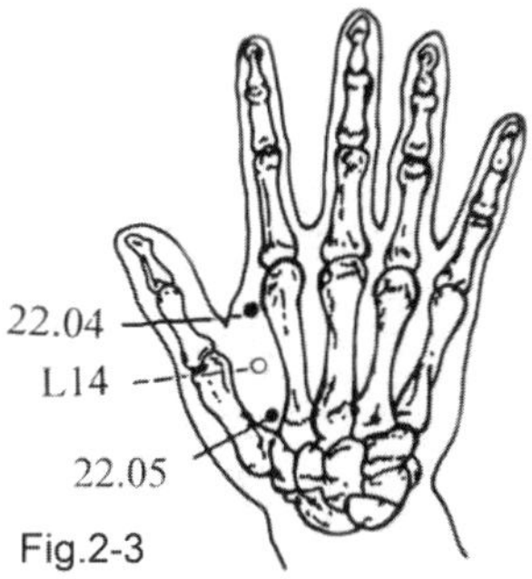

Fig.2-3

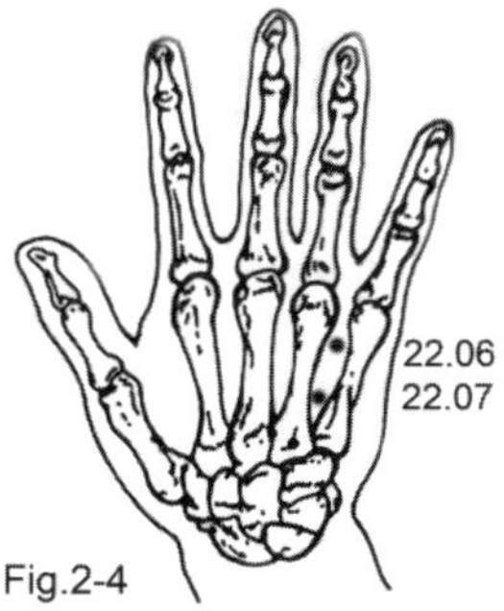

Fig.2-4

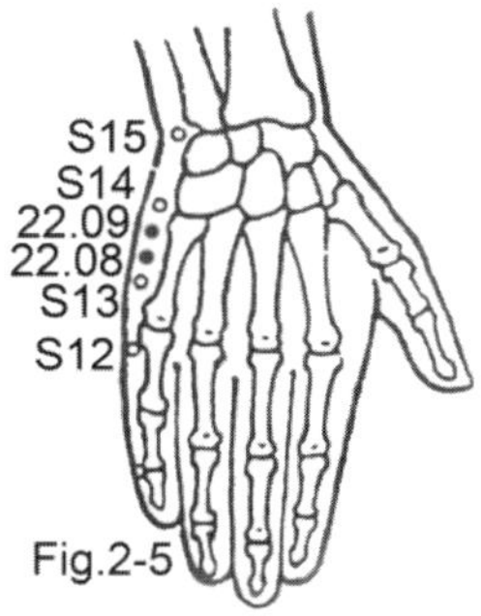

Fig.2-5

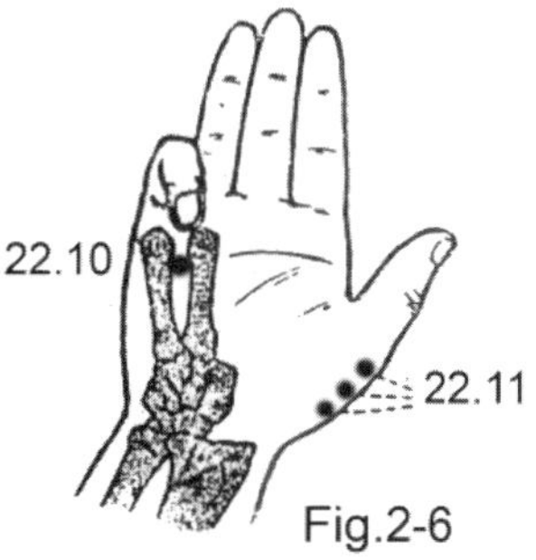

Fig.2-6

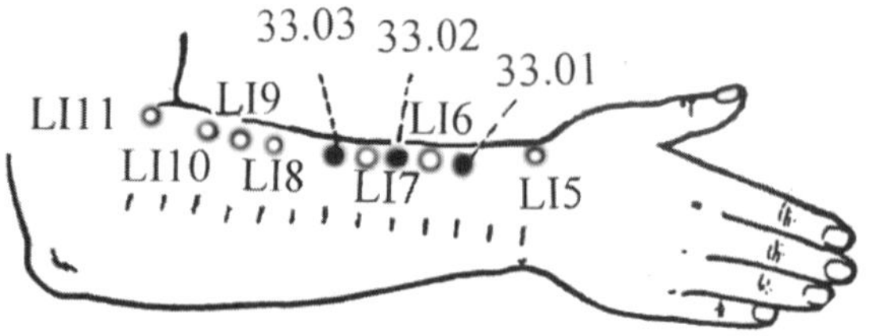

Fig.3-1

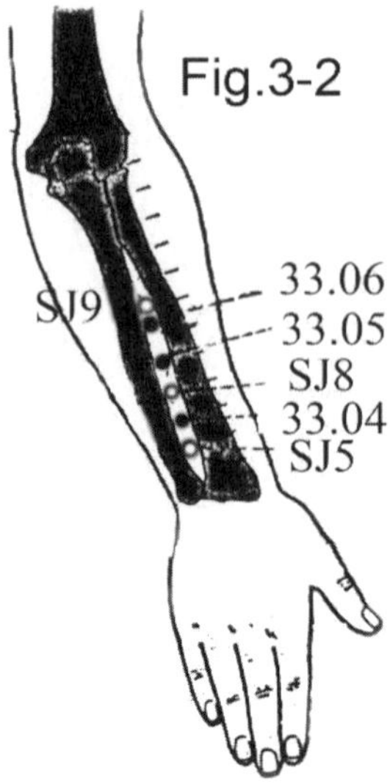

Fig.3-2

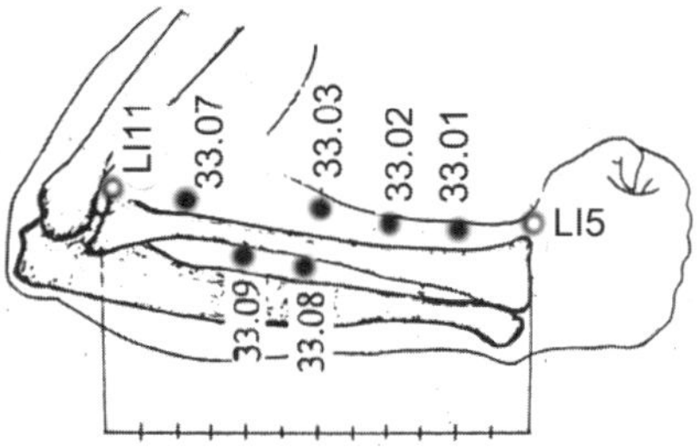

Fig.3-3

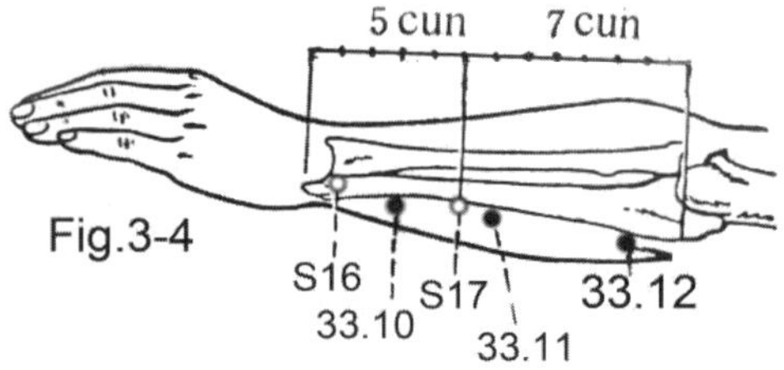

Fig.3-4

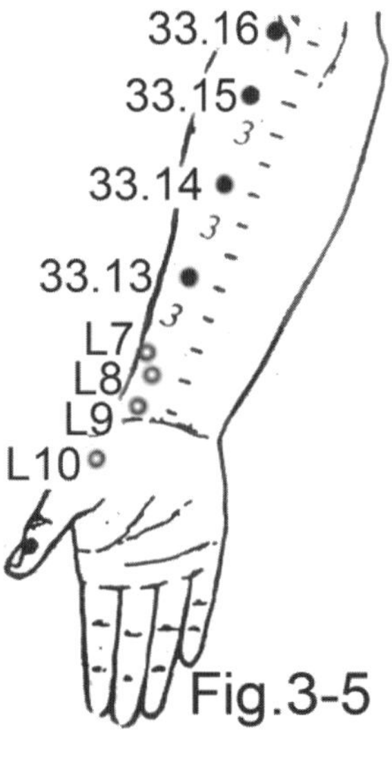

Fig.3-5

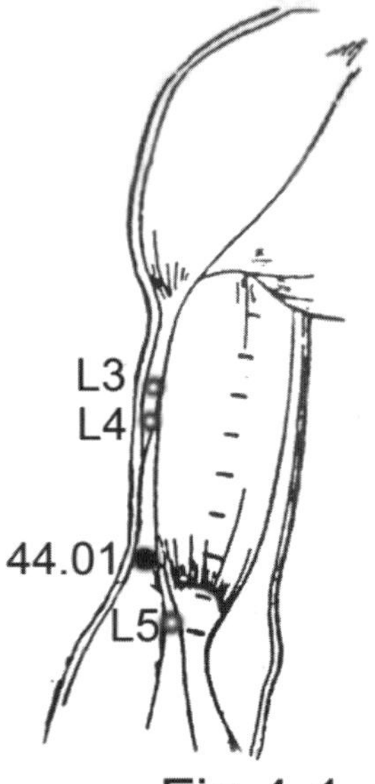

Fig.4-1

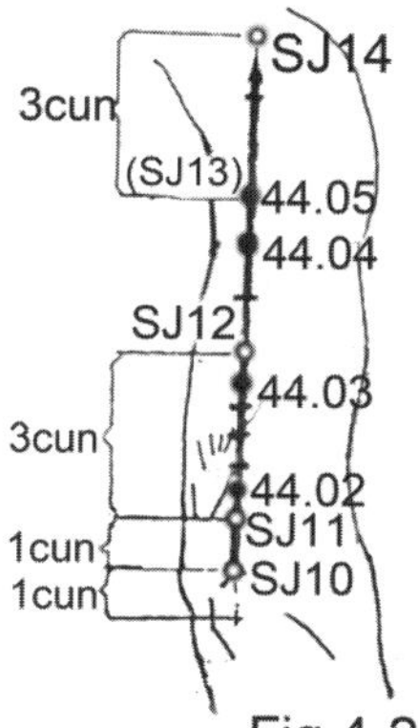

Fig.4-2

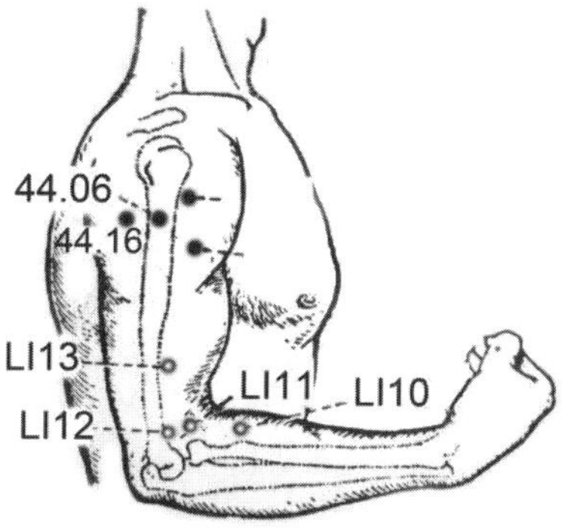

Fig.4-3

FiG.4-4

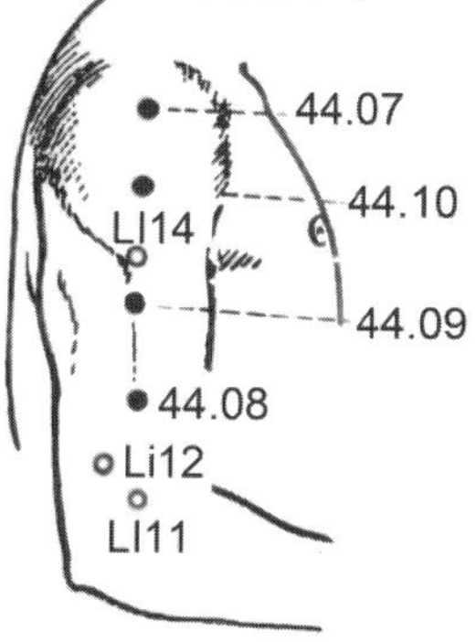

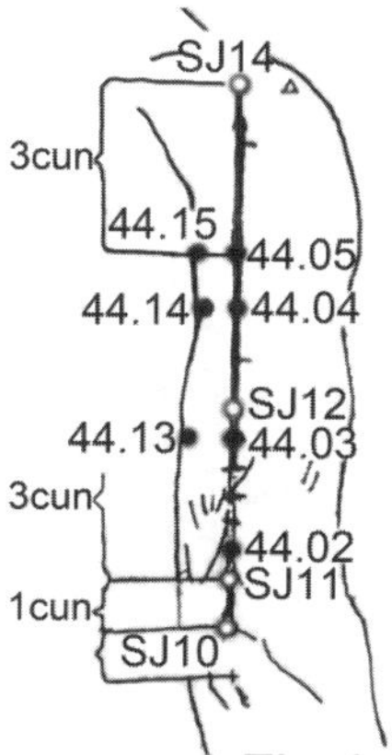

Fig.4-5

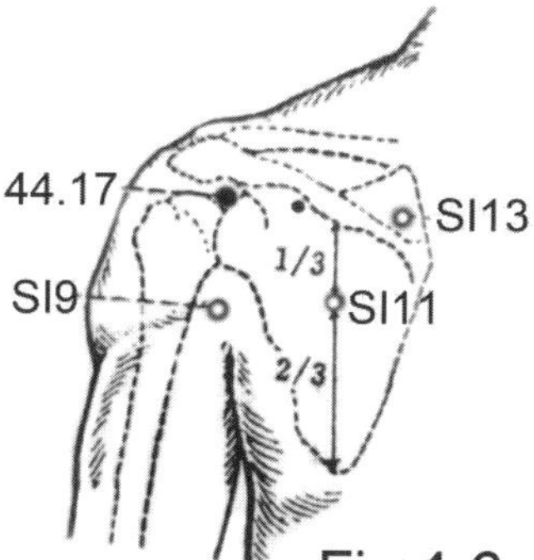

Fig.4-6

Fig.5-1

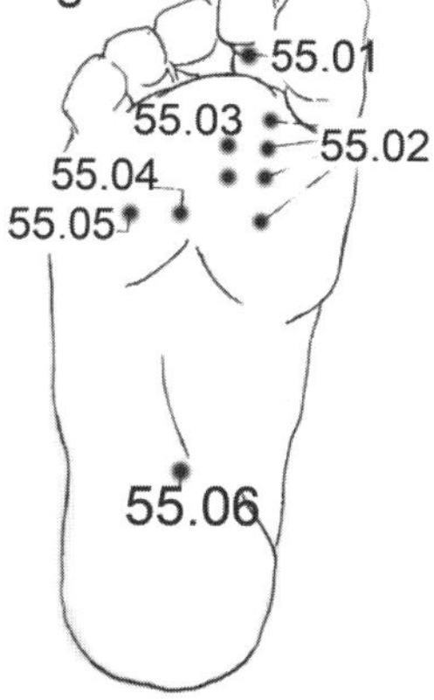

Fig.5-2

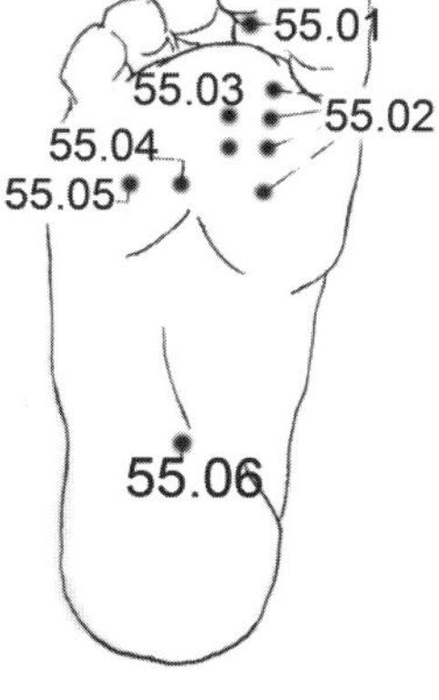

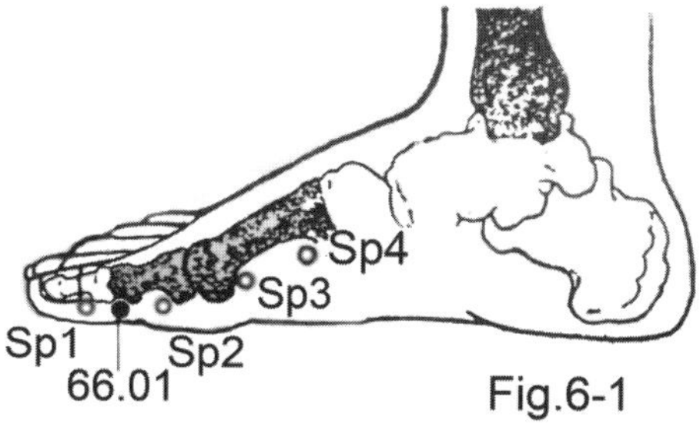

Fig.6-1

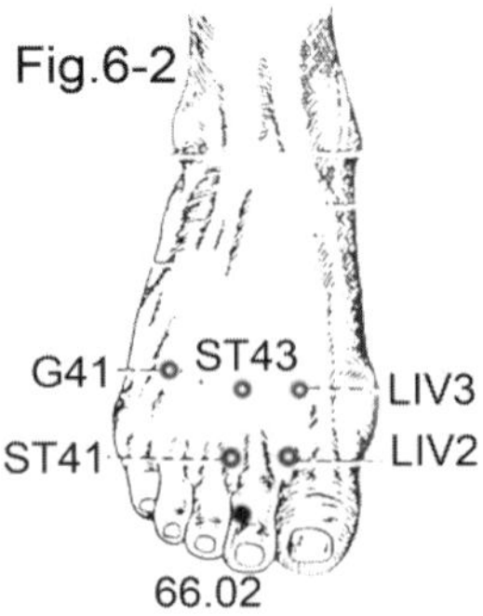

Fig.6-2

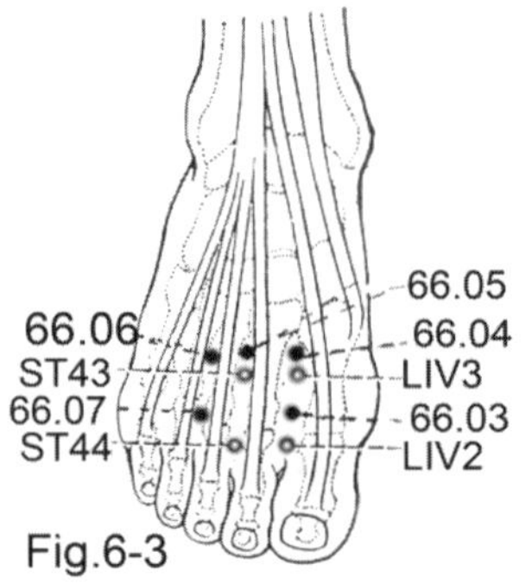

Fig.6-3

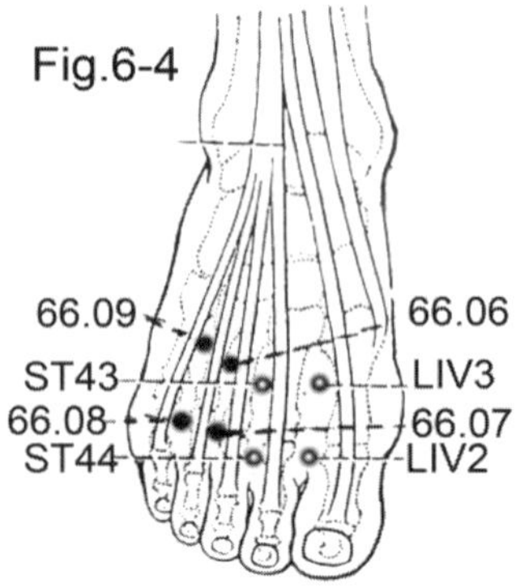

Fig.6-4

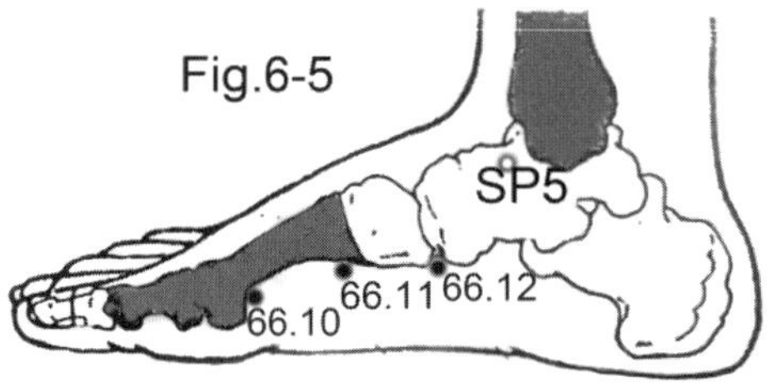

Fig.6-5

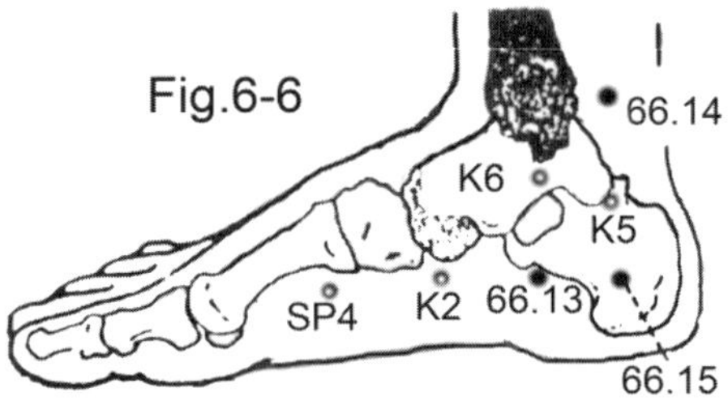

Fig.6-6

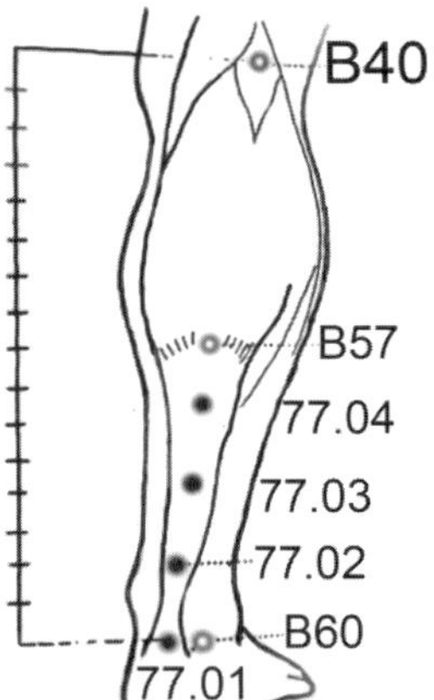

Fig.7-1

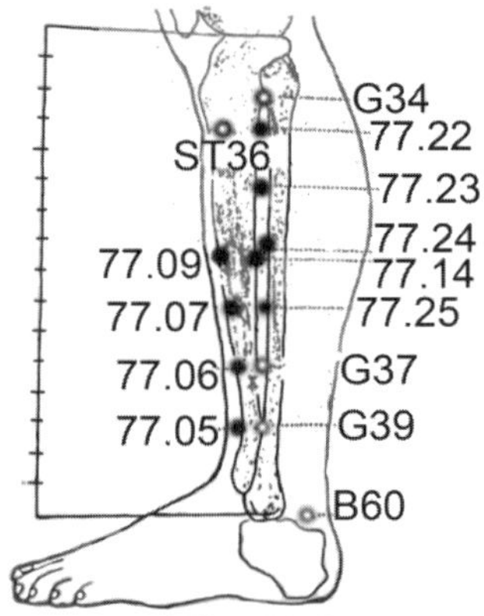

Fig.7-2

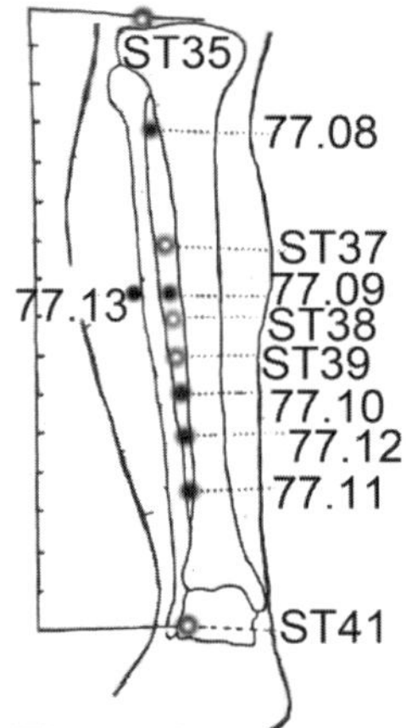

Fig.7-3

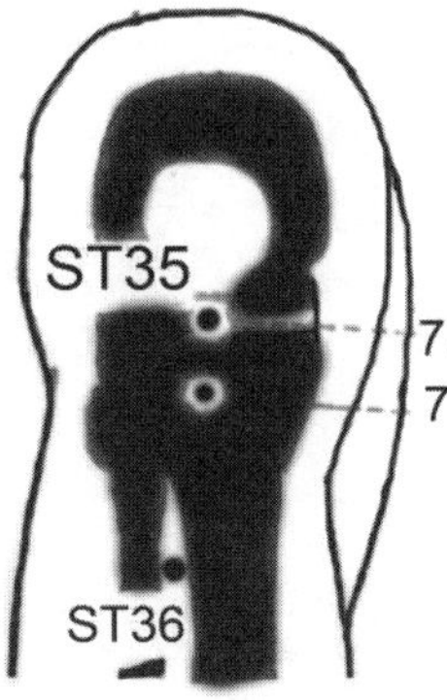

Fig.7-4

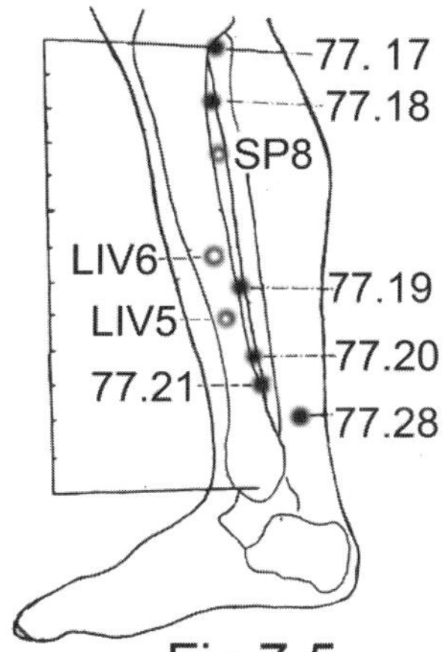

Fig.7-5

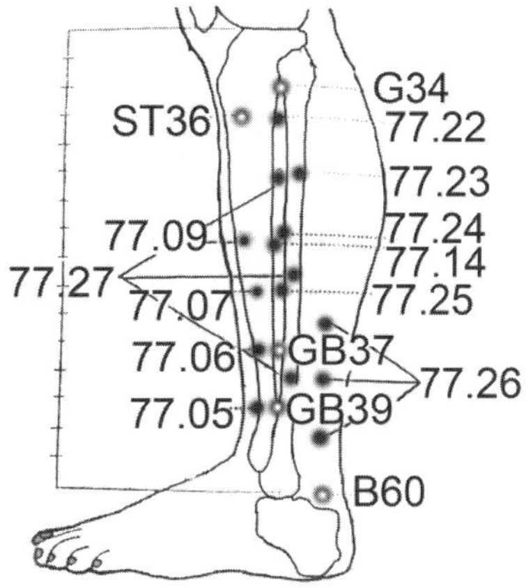

Fig.7-6

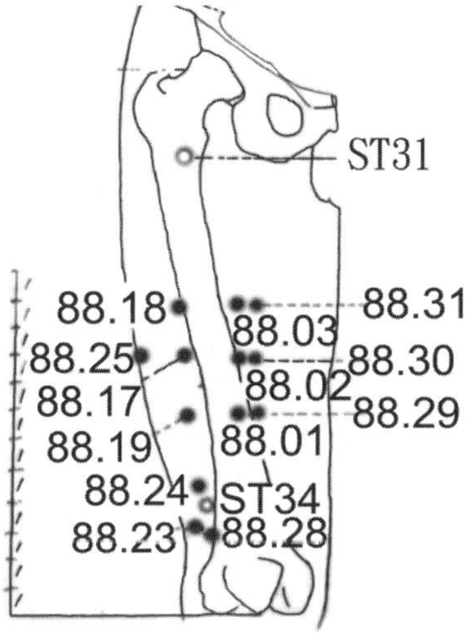

Fig.8-1

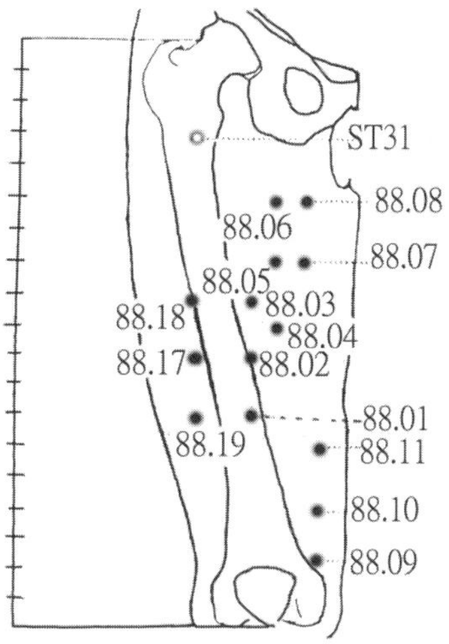

Fig.8-2

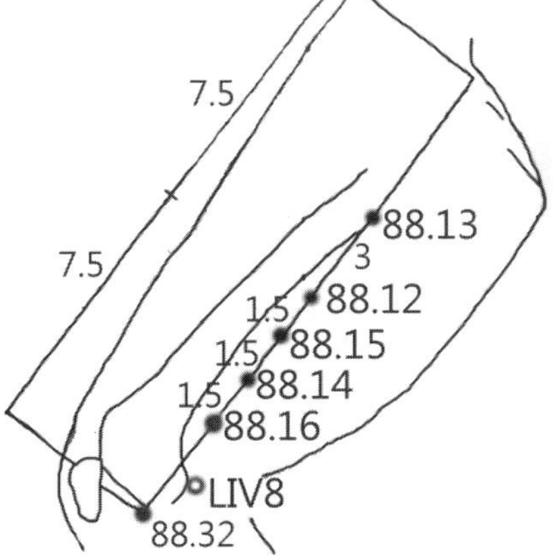

Fig.8-3

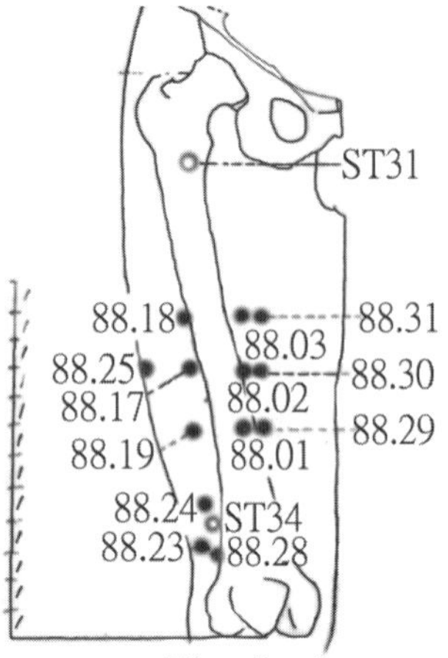

Fig.8-4

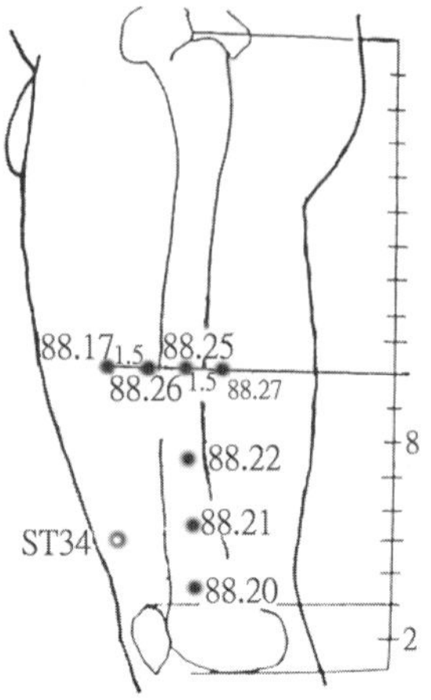

Fig.8-5

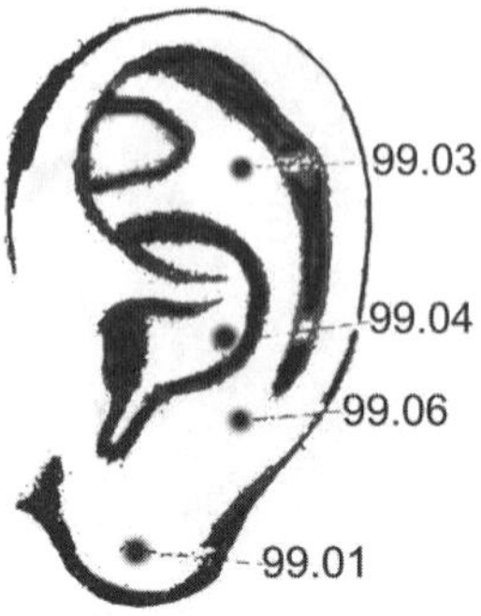

Fig.9-1

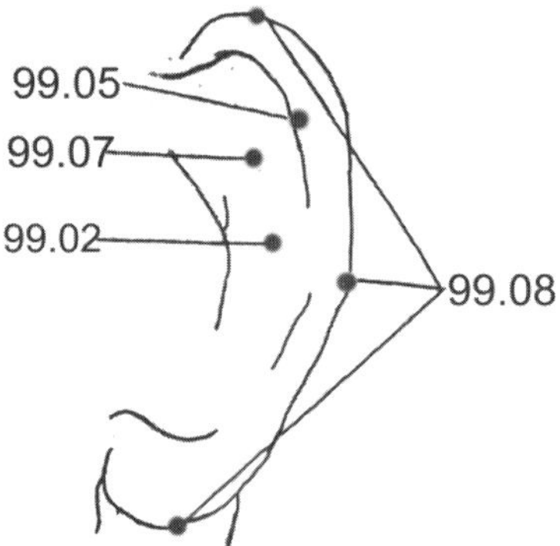

Fig.9-2

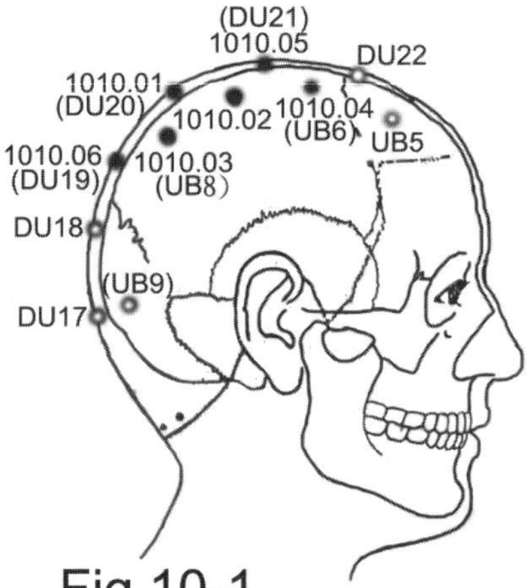

Fig.10-1

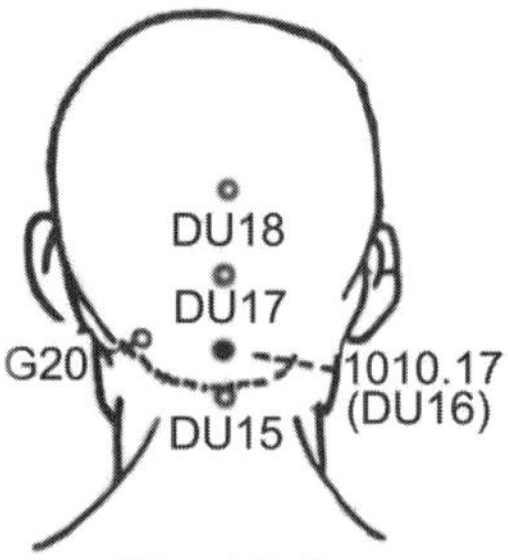

Fig.10-2

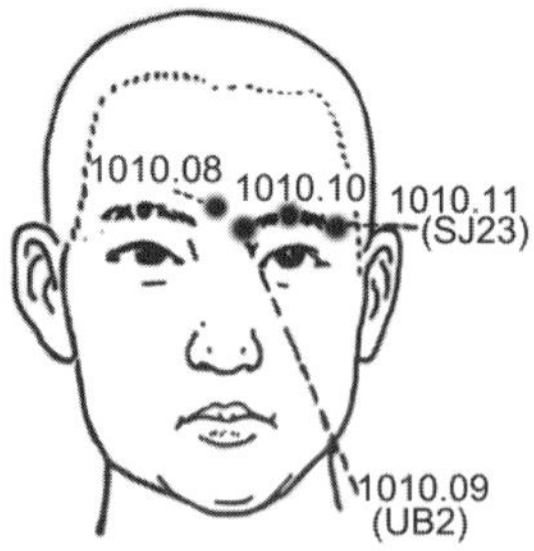

Fig.10-3

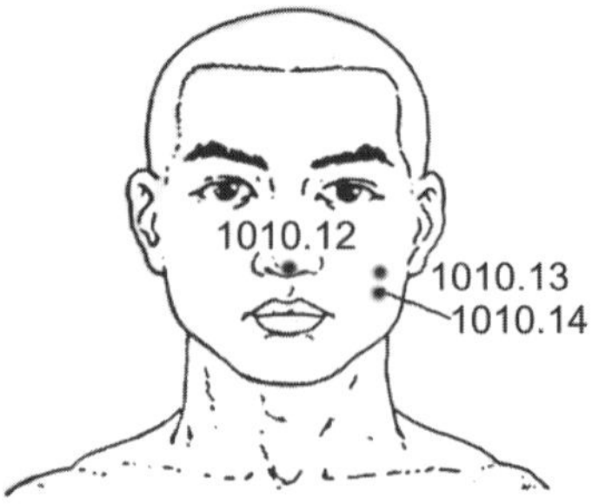

Fig.10-4

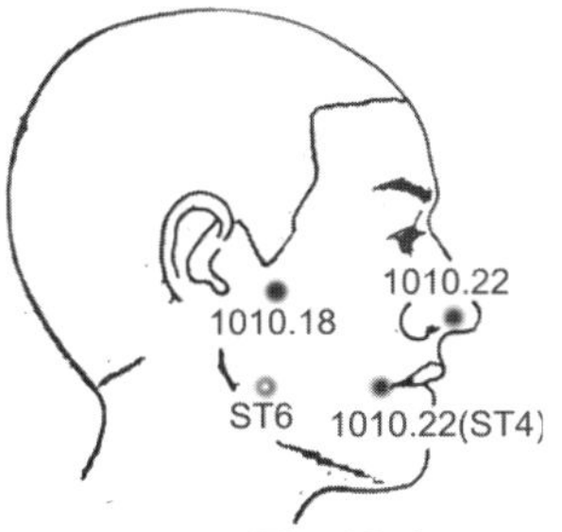

Fig.10-6

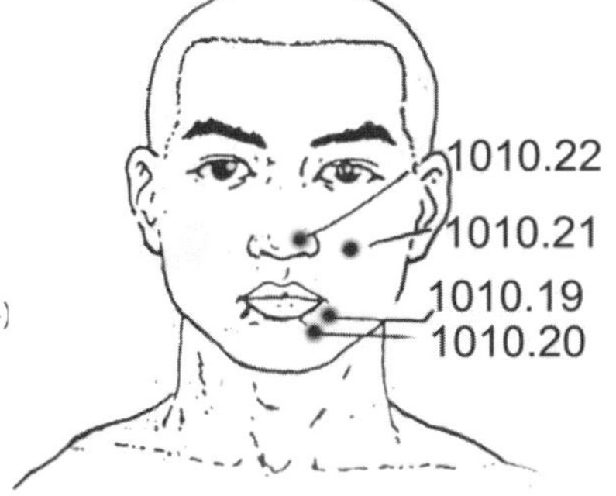

Fig.10-7

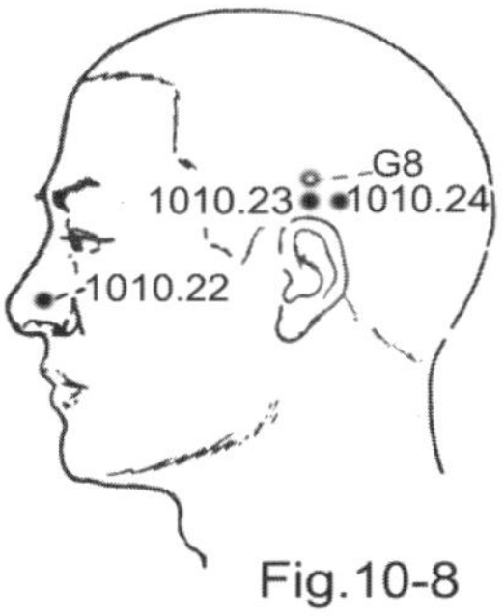

Fig.10-8

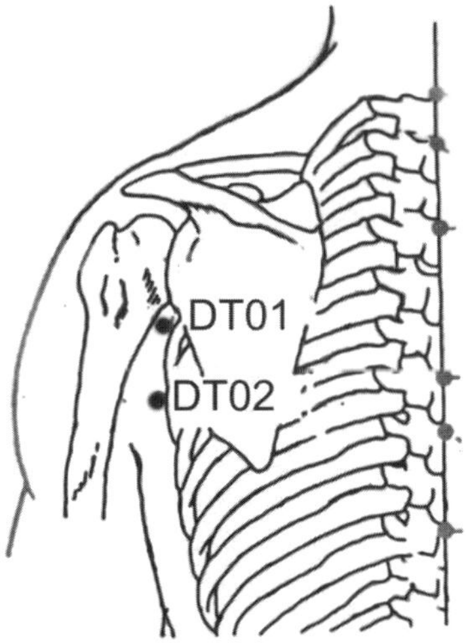

Fig.11-1

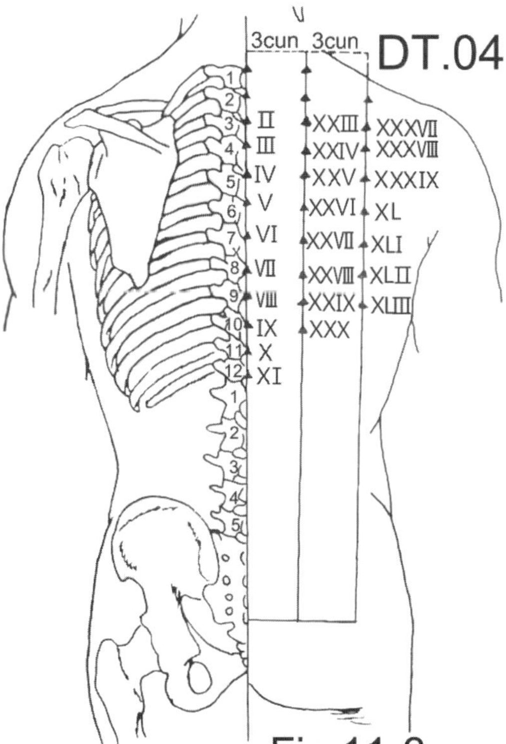

Fig.11-3

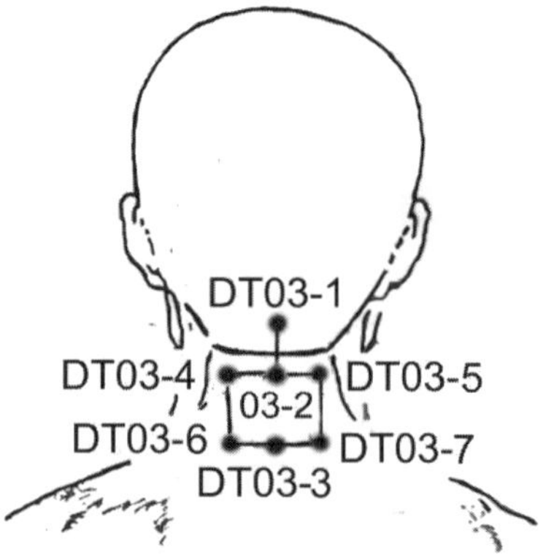

Fig.11-2

Fig.11-4

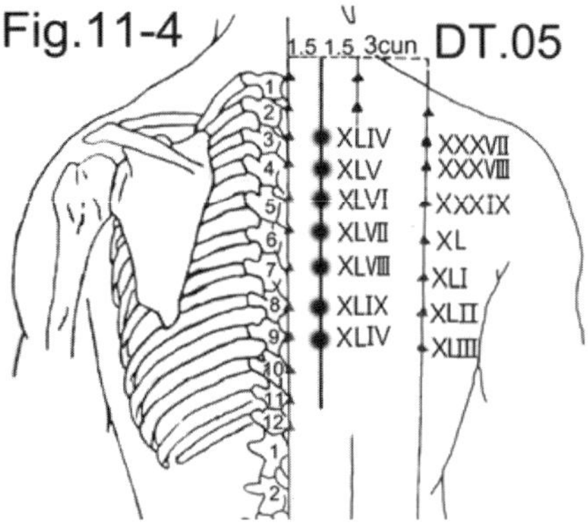

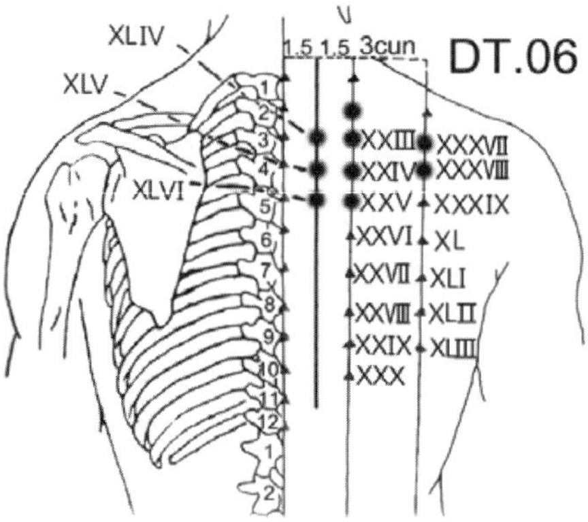

Fig.11-5

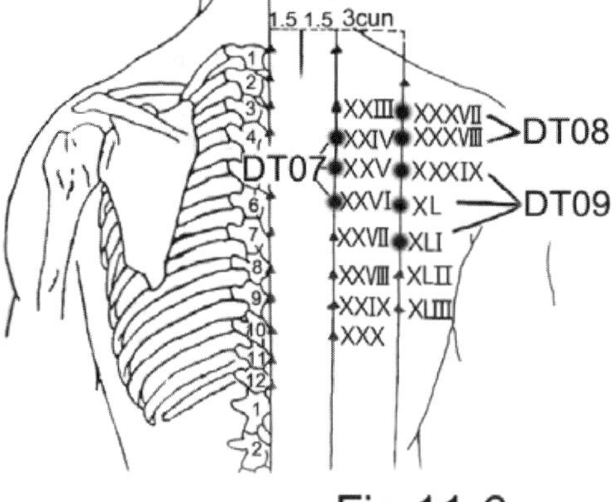

Fig.11-6

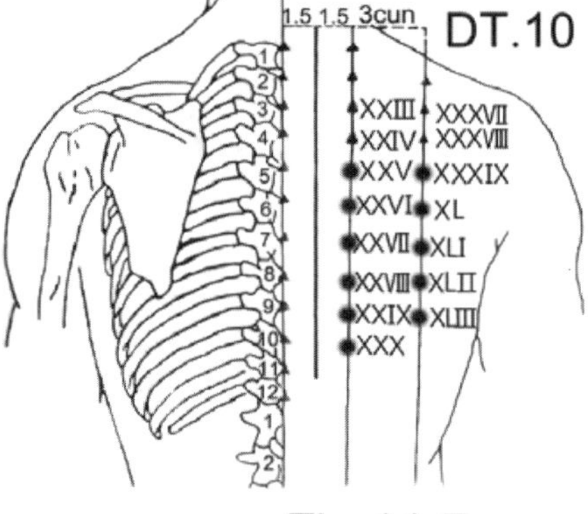

Fig.11-7

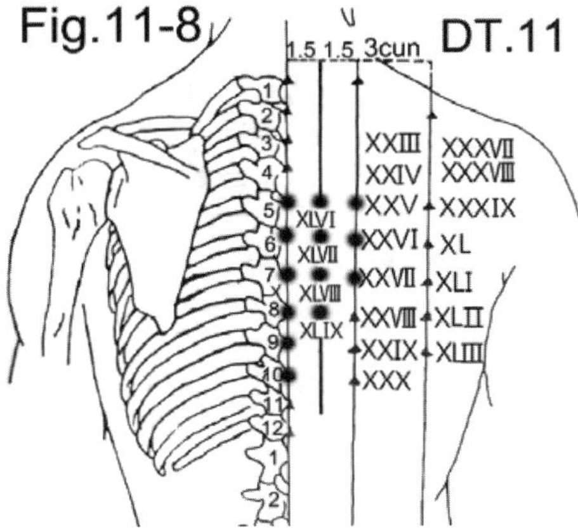

Fig.11-8

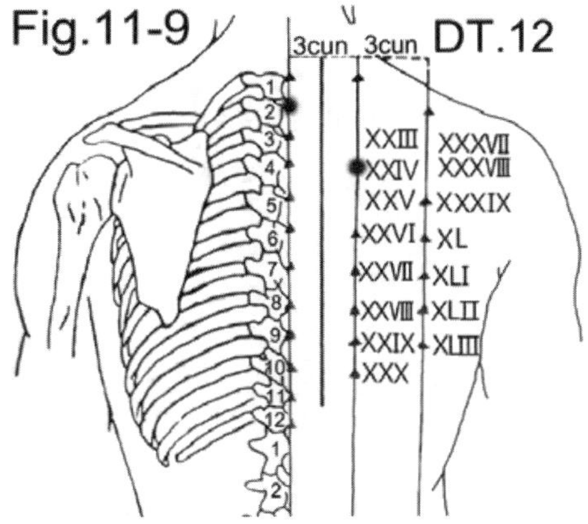

Fig.11-9

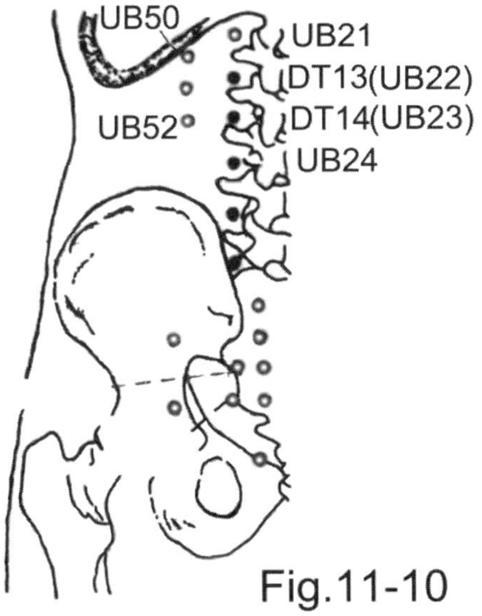

Fig.11-10

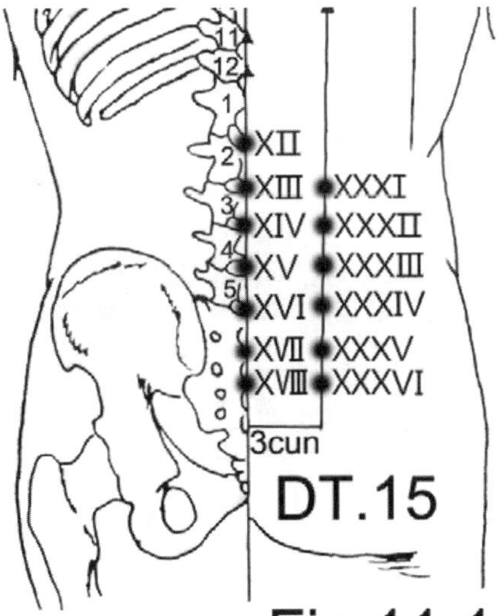

Fig.11-11

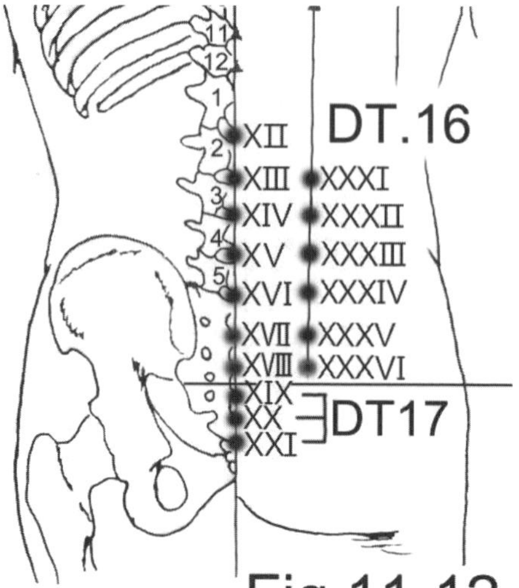

Fig.11-12

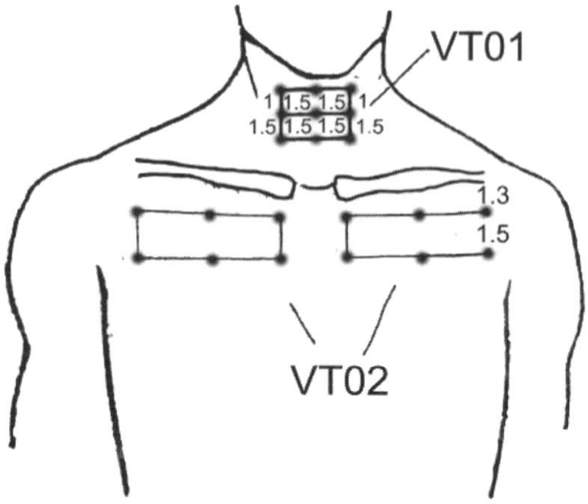

Fig.12-1

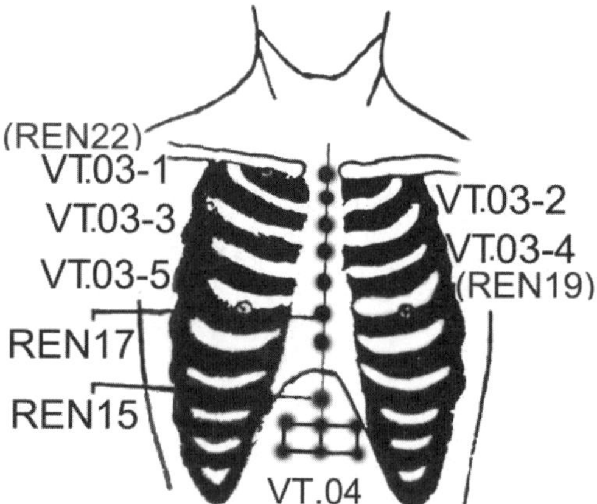

Fig.12-2

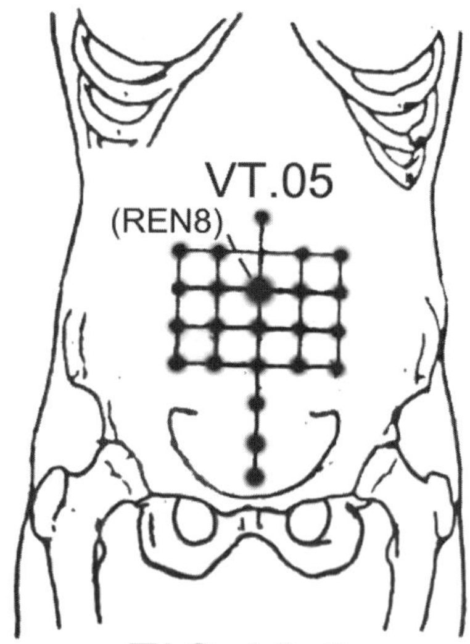

FIG.12-3

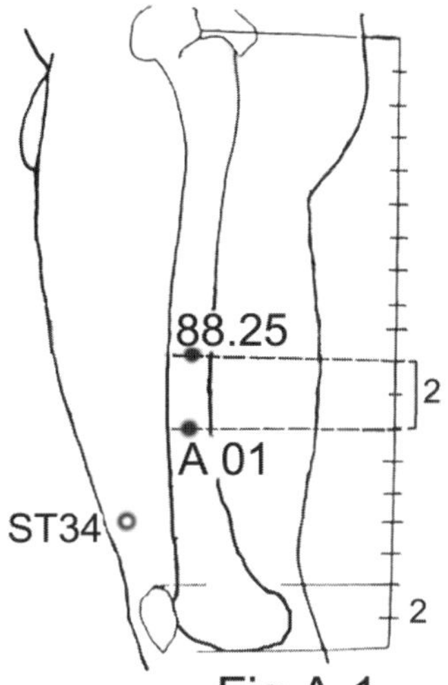

Fig.A-1

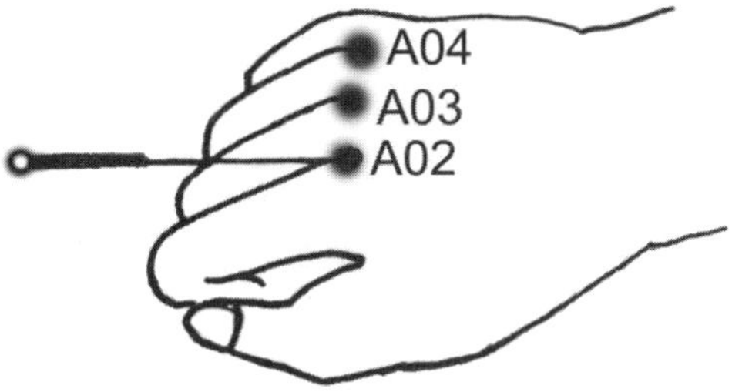

Fig.A-2

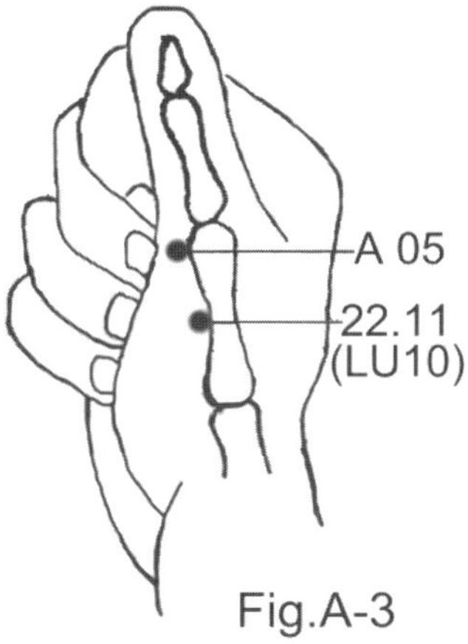

Fig.A-3

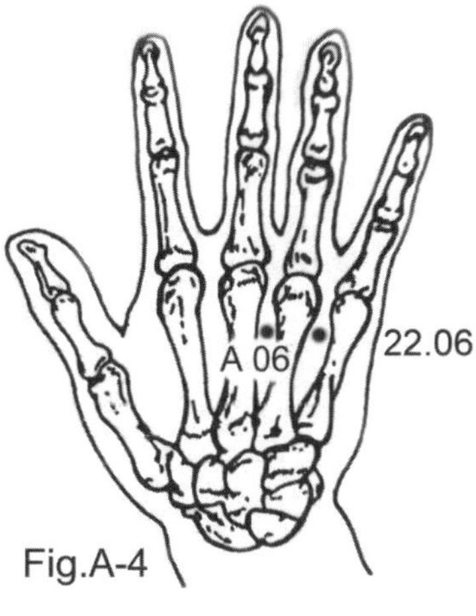

Fig.A-4

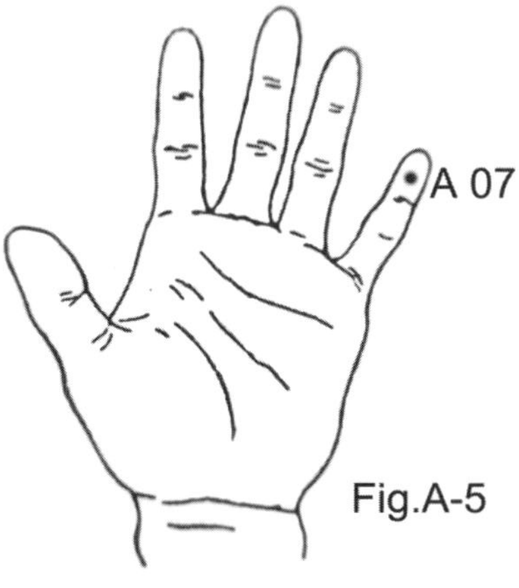

Fig.A-5

Appendix 5

Guiding Needling Technique

(*Qian Yin* Needling Technique)

By Dr. Wei Chieh Young

Guiding Needle Technique was created by me in 1972. It was published in my book *Zhen Jiu Jing Wei* (The Longitude and Latitude of Acupuncture and Moxibustion) which has been printed 20 editions. Now I have revised it to introduce it to the practitioner for clinical practice.

I developed the Guiding Needling Technique, based upon my study of the Active *Qi* Technique (*Dong Qi* Needling Technique). The Guiding Needling Technique is highly effective in treating syndromes involving pain, numbness, and itching. The technique both disperses and balances. Using this technique, I select distal points on the opposite side and the same side to create an effective therapeutic loop or circuitry. Typically, the points in the loop are designed to pass from one side to the other through the site of the pain. When the channel thereby becomes unblocked, the pain vanishes. I have found the Guiding Needling Technique to be much more effective than the Active *Qi* Technique.

The specific method for performing the Guiding Needling Techniques follows.

1. Select a distal point on the healthy side as a therapeutic point.

2. Select a distal point on the diseased side as a guiding point.

3. Manipulate these two points at the same time to create a therapeutic circuit.

4. Ask the patient to move or massage the site of the pain. With slight manipulation of the needles, the pain should immediately remit. For many patients, the pain goes away immediately, with the insertion of needles and there is no need to manipulate them. This phenomenon occurs because these two points form a therapeutic circuit and mutually guide the energy between each other.

5. Once the patient's pain is resolved, we need to consider the underlying pathology in deciding whether to take out or retain the needles. If we retain the needles, it is important to manipulate the needles at regular intervals to continue to circulate the energy.

The application of this needling technique is simple and highly effective. For example, with left elbow pain, we can needle *Fengshi* (GB 31) on the right side and *Hegu* (LI 4) on the left side to immediately stop the elbow pain. In this case, *Hegu* (LI 4) is the guiding point. In the example of right-sided shoulder pain, we can needle *Fenglong* (ST 40) on the left side to treat the pain and *Zhongzhu* (SJ 3) as a guiding point on the right side to immediately resolve the shoulder pain. Similarly, left knee pain can be treated with Neiguan (PC 6) on the right side as a treatment point and *Taichong* (LR 3)on the left side as a guiding point.

In general, one should use the *Ying*-Spring or *Shu*-Stream point on the diseased side to guide and disperse, which is called *Ying*-Shu treating the external channel, especially for pain syndromes. In the majority of cases, we use the *Shu*-Stream point because it treats heaviness of the body and joint pain. For example, if someone has shoulder pain on the *Yangming* channel, we would choose a distal point on the opposite side to treat the pain. On the diseased side, we would use *Sanjian* (LI 3), the *Shu*-Stream point, as the guiding point. In another example, if someone has lateral shoulder pain on the *Shaoyang* channel, we would use *Zhongzhu* (SJ 3) on the same side as the guiding point; and if someone has posterior shoulder pain on the *Taiyang* channel, we would use *Houxi* (SI 3) on the same side as the guiding point.

In summary, we choose the *Shu*-Stream point on the diseased side as the guiding point and a distal point on the healthy side as the treatment point. The *Neijing* stated that we should treat illness on the upper body with lower body points. Please note that distal points are used to disperse. If the problem is on the left side, we select points on the right side to balance as points on the opposite side are for balancing. When a patient has bilateral pain, for example pain in both knees, we can needle *Neiguan* (PC 6) on both sides first, followed by *Taichong* (LR 3). We manipulate the *Neiguan* (PC 6) on the left side and ask the patient to move her left knee. Then we manipulate *Neiguan* (PC 6) on the right side and ask the patient to move her right knee. This sequence of points affects both sides mutually.

Sometimes it is not necessary to needle a distal point on an extremity as a guiding point. For example, if a patient suffers from facial disease, we can use *Yingxiang* (LI 20) as a guiding point because it is an exit point of the Large Intestine and the beginning point of the Stomach Primary Meridians. The Large Intestine and Stomach Primary Meridians circulate through the whole face. Therefore, in cases such as acne or rhinitis, *Yingxiang* (LI 20) can be used as a guiding and treatment point very effectively.

The application of Guiding Needling Technique uses one needle on the upper part of the body and one on the lower part to formulate a circuit. Because of this resulting circulation in both the upper and lower parts of the body, the effect of treatment is much strongly. Using one point on the healthy side and another on the diseased side can create a loop that crosses from side. In this manner, both the guiding and treatment points have treatment effects, doubling the effectiveness of the treatment.

Guiding Needling Technique can also be combined with the Couple Needling Technique (*Dao Ma* Needling Technique) with excellent results. For example, for left-sided sciatica pain, one can needle *Linggu* (22.05) and *Dabai* (22.04) on the right side, followed by the left *Kunlun* (UB 62). Here we use *Linggu* and *Dabai* with the Couple Needling Technique with *Kunlun* (UB 62) to create a therapeutic loop.

Conclusion

Here I have discussed three needling techniques, but there are many more. These are only the ones I personally use most often. They are very effective. One major advantage is that they can be used when we may not be able to distinguish between excess and deficiency syndromes. They are especially useful for acupuncturist not familiar with tonification and sedation techniques.